# Sickle Cell Anemia: From Basic Science to Clinical Practice

# Sickle Cell Anemia: From Basic Science to Clinical Practice

Edited by Elena Ledger

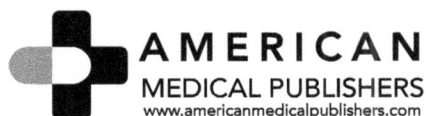

AMERICAN
MEDICAL PUBLISHERS
www.americanmedicalpublishers.com

American Medical Publishers,
41 Flatbush Avenue,
1st Floor, New York,
NY 11217, USA

Visit us on the World Wide Web at:
www.americanmedicalpublishers.com

ISBN: 978-1-63927-185-6

**Cataloging-in-Publication Data**

Sickle cell anemia : from basic science to clinical practice / edited by Elena Ledger.
    p. cm.
Includes bibliographical references and index.
ISBN 978-1-63927-185-6
1. Sickle cell anemia. 2. Sickle cell anemia--Treatment. 3. Hemolytic anemia.
4. Blood hyperviscosity syndrome. I. Ledger, Elena.
RC641.7.S5 S53 2022
616.152 7--dc23

# Table of Contents

# Preface

A sickle cell disease is a group of blood disorders that a person inherits from parents. They usually occur when the person inherits two abnormal copies of the hemoglobin gene. Sickle cell anemia is the most common type of sickle cell disease. It causes an abnormality in hemoglobin, the oxygen-carrying protein found in red blood cells. The problems due to sickle cell anemia begin to appear around 5 to 6 months of age. It leads to problems such as sickle cell crisis, swelling in hands and feet, stroke and bacterial infections. The care of people suffering from sickle cell anemia includes infection prevention with vaccination and antibiotics, folic acid supplementation and pain medication. A bone marrow transplant is also used in certain cases. This book consists of contributions made by international experts. It contains some path-breaking studies in sickle cell anemia. It will serve as a valuable source of reference for graduate and post graduate students.

This book is the end result of constructive efforts and intensive research done by experts in this field. The aim of this book is to enlighten the readers with recent information in this area of research. The information provided in this profound book would serve as a valuable reference to students and researchers in this field.

At the end, I would like to thank all the authors for devoting their precious time and providing their valuable contribution to this book. I would also like to express my gratitude to my fellow colleagues who encouraged me throughout the process.

**Editor**

# Foetal Haemoglobin, Erythrocytes Containing Foetal Haemoglobin, and Hematological Features in Congolese Patients with Sickle Cell Anaemia

L. Tshilolo,[1,2] V. Summa,[3] C. Gregorj,[3] C. Kinsiama,[1] J. A. Bazeboso,[1] G. Avvisati,[3] and D. Labie[4]

[1] Unité de Dépistage de la Drépanocytose, Centre Hospitalier Monkole, BP 817, Kinshasa XI, Democratic Republic of Congo
[2] Centre de Formation et d'Appui Sanitaire (CEFA), 10, Avenue Kemi, Mont Ngafula, Kinshasa, Democratic Republic of Congo
[3] Servizio di Ematologia, Università Campus Bio-Medico di Roma, 21, Via Alvaro del Portillo, 00128 Roma, Italy
[4] INSERM, Institut Cochin, 4, rue du Faubourg Saint-Jacques, 75014 Paris, France

Correspondence should be addressed to L. Tshilolo, leon.tshilolo@gb-solution.cd

Academic Editor: Betty S. Pace

High HbF levels and F cells are correlated with reduced morbidity and mortality in sickle cell disease (SCD). This paper was designed to determine the HbF and F cells levels in Congolese sickle cell anemia (SCA) patients in order to determine their impact on the expression of SCD. *Population and Method.* HbF levels were measured in 89 SCA patients (mean age 11.4 yrs) using a standard HPLC method. F cell quantitation was done in a second group of SCA patients ($n = 42$, mean age 8.9 yrs) and compared with a control group ($n = 47$, mean age 5 yrs). F cells were quantified by a cytofluorometric system (MoAb-HbF—FITC; cut off at 0.5%). *Results.* The mean value of HbF was 7.2% ± 5.0 with heterogeneous distribution, most patients (76%) having HbF < 8%. Mean values of F-cells in SCA patients and control group were 5.4% ± 7.6 (median: 2.19% ; range 0,0–30,3%) and 0.5% ± 1.6 (median 0.0, range 0–5.18), respectively. SCA patients with F cells >4.5% developed less painful crisis and had higher percentage of reticulocytes. *Conclusion.* Congolese SCA patients displayed low levels of HbF and F-cells that contribute to the severity of SCD.

## 1. Introduction

Fetal hemoglobin (HbF, a2.2) is a major contributor to the phenotypic heterogeneity of sickle cell anemia (SCA). A major ameliorating factor is an inherent ability to produce fetal hemoglobin; elevated levels are correlated with reduced morbidity and mortality in patients with SCA [1–3].

In normal adults, HbF levels are distributed in a nonuniform way in the red cells with a range varying from 0.1 to 7% of total hemoglobin (Hb). In red cells producing higher HbF (termed F cells), HbF is elevated (around 25% of cellular Hb) and genetically determined [2, 4, 5].

Genetic variation at three principal loci—the HBB cluster on chromosome 11p, HBS1L-MYB region on chromosome 6q and BCL11A on chromosome 2p—have been shown to influence HbF levels and disease severity in ß thalassemia and SCA. Taking into account these loci, there is

still substantial residual variance in HbF levels, suggesting the importance of other quantitative trait loci (QTL) modulating HBG expression [4, 6].

Total Hb and HbF levels vary in SCA patients according to the βS haplotypes: values are greater in patients bearing the Arabo-Indian and Senegalese haplotypes and less in those with the Bantu or Central African haplotype [2, 4, 6–8].

Sickle cell disease (SCD) has a high prevalence in Sub-Saharan Africa where majority of the affected patients live. B$^S$ gene prevalence in the Democratic Republic of Congo (DRC) is around 25% and about 1.7% of newborns are affected (50,000 births per year) [9].

Expression of SCA in Congolese patients displayed a severe form with high mortality and complications [10].

To our knowledge, there are no specific data on HbF and F cells reported in SCA patients living in DRC. We therefore present here the preliminary analysis of HbF and F cells in two series of SCA patients and correlations with other hematological parameters and clinical data.

## 2. Population and Methods

All patients were SS homozygotes regularly followed up in comprehensive sickle cell programs in DRC.

A first study quantified HbF in steady state SCA patients followed up in Lubumbashi ($n = 48$) and Kinshasa ($n = 41$), a total of 89 patients (34 M, 48 F; mean age 11.4 yrs $\pm$ 5.4). No patient was on hydroxyurea treatment.

The second study involved 42 SCA patients (23F, 24 M; mean age 8.8 yrs $\pm$ 5.1) and a control group of 47 non-SCA patients (26 F, 21 M; mean age 5 yrs $\pm$ 5.1) recruited in Kinshasa. In this study, we assessed F Cells numbers and compared the results to hematologic parameters and clinical data.

Diagnosis of SCA was established using standard hemoglobin electrophoresis techniques (acetate electrophoresis or Isoelectric focusing-IEF) coupled to Itano solubility test. The percentage of HbF was determined by high performance liquid chromatography (HPLC).

HbF expression was evaluated using a previously described flow cytometric procedure [11, 12] with slight modifications. In brief, twenty microliters of whole blood were fixed with 1 mL ice-cold 0.05% glutaraldehyde in PBS pH 7.4 vortexed for 15 seconds (s), then incubated at room temperature (RT) for 10 min. The cells were washed twice with PBS, permeabilized by vortexing for 15 s with 0.5 mL ice-cold 0.1% Triton X-100 (Sigma, Milan) in 0.1% bovine serum albumin in PBS (BSA-PBS), and incubated at RT for 5 min. The cells were then washed once with 0.1% BSA-PBS and suspended in 0.5 mL 0.1% BSA-PBS.

Ten microliters of cell suspension were then mixed with $20 \mu L$ of 1-in-5 diluted MoAb-HbF-FITC (IQ products, Milan) in 0.1% BSA-PBS and $70 \mu L$ of 0.1% BSA-PBS and incubated in the dark at RT for 15 min. An irrelevant mouse antibody of the appropriate subclass was used as a negative control to determine background fluorescence. The cells were washed once with 0.1% BSA-PBS and immediately measured by flow cytometry (as described below).

The flow cytometer analysis reported the percentage of F+ cells in total counted red blood cells of each sample. The positive cut off point was set at 0.5% above negative population of isotype control staining cells.

HbF expression was, also, analyzed using the Kolmogorov-Smirnov statistic test ($D$-value), which allows the objective and accurate identification of small differences in fluorescence intensity [13]. Samples with $D < 0.15$ were considered negative, whereas those with a $D \geq 0.15$ were considered positive.

Modified technique for evaluating HbF expression: considering the complexity of the previous procedure for identifying the F+ cells, we applied a second flow cytometric technique to perform F+ cells evaluation. This method (routinely utilized for characterizing other cellular parameters, as for example MDR in patients affected by acute leukemias) enabled us to test the samples more conveniently, using fewer and simpler steps, and a precise identification of the red blood cells population in the flow cytometric dot plot, useful for a specific analysis. In addition, this technique led to increased capacity to analyze more samples together than the previous one.

Twenty microliters of whole blood were fixed (Fix and Perm permeabilization kit; Caltag Laboratories) with $100 \mu L$ of Medium A at room temperature (RT), in the dark, for 15 min; then cells were washed once with PBS, and then after incubated with $100 \mu L$ of Medium B and $4 \mu L$ of MoAb-HbF-FITC at RT, in the dark for 30 min. Finally, cells were washed once with PBS, and immediately measured by flow cytometry. The flow cytometric analysis was performed considering the same parameters used for the previously described technique [11, 12].

*Flow cytometric analysis* was conducted using a FACScan flow cytometer (Becton Dickinson), operated at 488 nm which detects green (MoAb-HbF-FITC) fluorescence. Data acquisition and analysis were performed with the CellQuest software (Becton Dickinson). We measured 50,000 events. The red blood cell area was gated by forward scatter signals (FSC) versus side scatter signals (SSC). The latter was measured using the logarithmic scales (log SSC).

Comparison of hematological parameters (Blood cell counts and HbF levels) were made with other reports of African SCA patients [14–17].

These studies were approved by the Local Ethnic Committees of the participating institutions, Campus Biomedico di Roma, and The CEFA/Centre Hopsitalier Monkole, in accordance with the Declaration of Helsinki.

*Statistical analyses* were conducted with a software program SPSS system (Version 12, Chicago). Results were expressed as the mean value and median value: standard deviation(SD). Comparisons of means were analysed by Students $t$-test, correlations by Pearsons test, and comparison between categorical variables by Chi square test or Fishers exact test (where appropriated).

HbF expression ($D$-value) and F+ cells were represented as dichotomized variable (positive versus negative). Data were analyzed using the two-sided Student's $t$-test to correlate results obtained by mean of the two different parameters of analysis and the two flow cytometric techniques, while Mann-Whitney $U$-test was used to measure the differences observed between positive and control groups.

Values were considered statistically significant when $P < 0.05$.

## 3. Results

*3.1. Patients Population.* In the first study of 89 SCA patients, the mean HbF% was 7.2% $\pm$ 5.0 (median 5.9; range 1–27.5%). It was 7% and 7.4% in the Lubumbashi and Kinshasa group, respectively ($P > 0.05$). Values of HbF were higher in females (7.4%, mean age 10.4 yrs) than in males (6.9%, mean age 9.2 yrs), but the difference was not statistically significant (Mann Whitney test chi square = 0.018, degree of freedom = 1, $P = NS$). Higher values were observed in children aged less than 3 yrs but no statistical differences were observed between the different age groups.

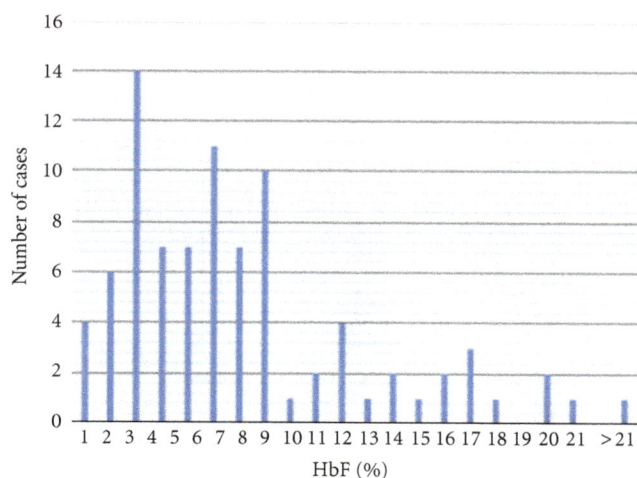

FIGURE 1: Population distribution of the HbF rate. Patient distribution related to HbF rate displayed a heterogeneous pattern with a predominant group (74%) with HbF% <8. Globally, only 20/89 (or 22.5%) of patients displayed values higher than 10% of HbF.

Distribution of HbF rate displayed a heterogeneous pattern with a predominant group (66/89 or 74%) with HbF < 8% and two other groups with 9–13% and 14–17%. Globally, levels of HbF were less than 10% in 69/89 of cases (77.5%) and varied considerably; the distribution pattern was not normal even after log transformation of values (not shown), (Figure 1).

In the second study, enumeration of erythrocytes containing HbF (F cells) using the first, standard flow cytometric technique resulted in mean %. SD of F+ cells in 42 SCD samples of 5.44% ± 7.6 (median: 2.19%; range 0.00–30.3%). The mean $D$-value. SD was 0.21 ± 0.007 (median: 0.33; range 0.07–0.57). In the 47 controls, the mean %± SD of F+ cells was 0.50% ± 1.06 (median: 0; range 0–5.18%), and the mean $D$-value ± SD was 0.024 ± 0.034 (median: 0; range 0–0.15) (Figure 2).

Correlation among F+ cells % and $D$-value for the entire population was highly significant with a $r = 0.67$ ($P < 0.0001$). The comparison among SCD patients and controls as for the % of F+ Cell and $D$-value was also highly significant ($P < 0.001$ for both F+ cells % and $D$-value).

The evaluation of the samples with the Fix & Perm flow cytometric technique showed a mean %. SD of F+ cells of 8.67%. 13.48 (median: 4.63; range 0–57.75%), while the mean $D$-value. SD was 0.19. 0.17 (median: 0.15; range 0–0.7).

Comparison of the two flow cytometric techniques showed strong correlation for F+ cells values ($r = 0.63$; $P = 0.0005$) and for $D$-value parameters ($r = 0.53$; $P < 0.005$). 40/42 of SCA patients (95%) had values above the cut-off value of 0.5% while in the control group, only 12/47 subjects (25.5%) had values above the cut off.

Population distribution of % F cells were heterogeneous and displayed a nonnormal distribution even after log-transformation of values (Figure 3). Patients aged <12 yrs displayed higher values than older patients: mean values of

3.7 were observed in group 1 and 4.7 in group 2 versus 1.9 in group 3 (Table 1).

*3.2. Comparison of %F Cells with Hematological Parameters and Clinical Issue.* We found no significant correlations between the results obtained by cytometry system with the glutaraldehyde method with clinical and biological data; but with the Fix & Perm method, the number of vaso-occlusive crisis was significantly reduced in patients with F cells rate >4.5% ($P < 0.05$) while the reticulocytes number was significantly elevated ($P < 0.005$).

We did not observe significant differences between haematological parameters (Hb, MCV, MCH, and MCHC) in different age groups, although children aged >18 yr displayed higher value of RDW (Table 1).

Comparisons of hematological parameters in our patients with those described in other African SCA patients are depicted in Table 2.

## 4. Discussion

Hematological characteristics and clinical severity in SCA are variable and are influenced by environmental and genetic factors, including the presence of $\alpha$-thalassemia, variation in Hb F level, and the haplotype background that is linked to the $\beta$ globin gene [14]. The Bantu or CAR haplotype is considered as a major risk factor associated with clinically severe form of SCD and organ damage [7, 18, 19]. Most of the SCA patients living in central Africa and in DRC carry the CAR haplotype [20].

The protective role of HbF in the sickling of red cells and the clinical severity of SCD is evident. The HbF level has emerged as an important prognostic factor both for sickle cell pain and mortality; and a %HbF > 10% has been suggested as a threshold level for reduced clinical severity [5, 6, 19, 21, 22].

Different studies on HbF levels in SCA patients bearing CAR haplotypes reported levels values varying from 2 to 10.8%, but generally less than 10% [14, 18, 19, 23, 24]. To date, no values of HbF levels have been reported in Congolese SCA patients living in DRC. The mean value of 7.2% HbF observed in our study confirmed that patients bearing the CAR haplotype had levels of HbF less than 10%, the minimal level that permits a protective role on the sickling of red cells [2, 19]. We found no significant differences in Hb levels in our patients related to sex or age although recent studies confirmed that adult females have higher HbF and F Cells values than males because of the presence of an X-linked QTL (Quantitative Trait locus) [4, 6]. Mouele [16] reported similar data in the neigboring Congo Brazzaville.

Nagel et al. [19] suggested that the HbF level in SCA patients aged more than 5 yrs was dependent of the C-T mutation at position −158 G$\gamma$ in the promoter of the G$\gamma$ globin gene (known as the Xmn I-G$\gamma$ site) [23]. They also found mean levels of HbF at 6.4% and 12.4% in the groups with a rate of G$\gamma$ < 38% and G$\gamma$ > 38%, respectively. The presence or absence of alpha deletion did not modify these observations. Patients with CAR haplotype had a low G$\gamma$ globin gene expression in comparison to the other

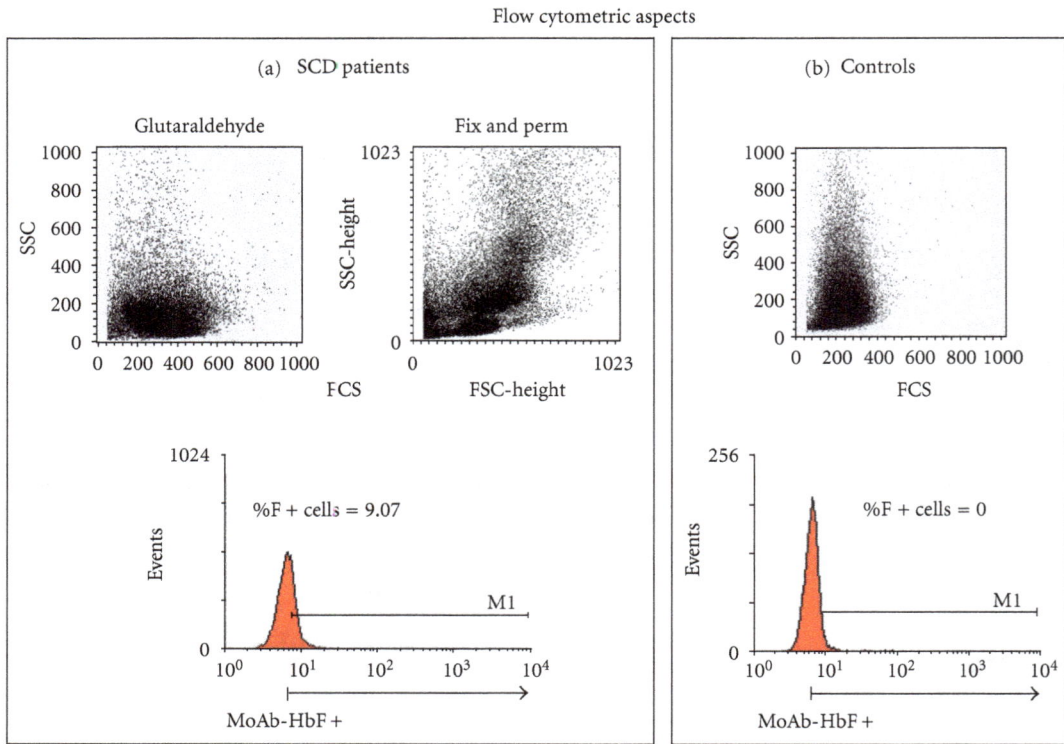

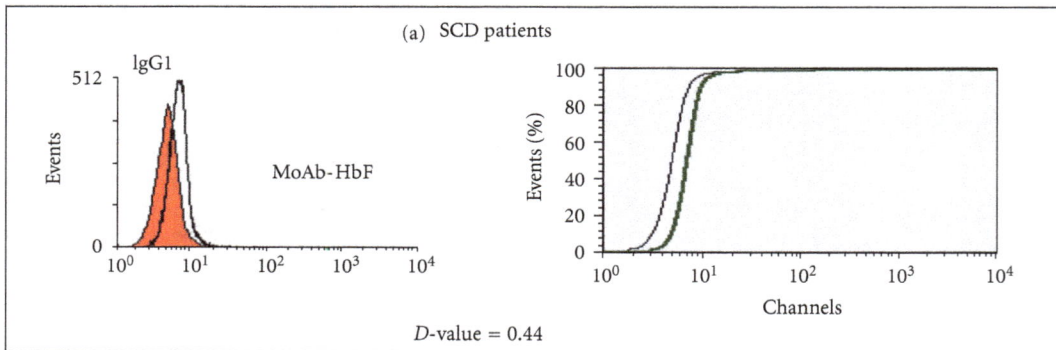

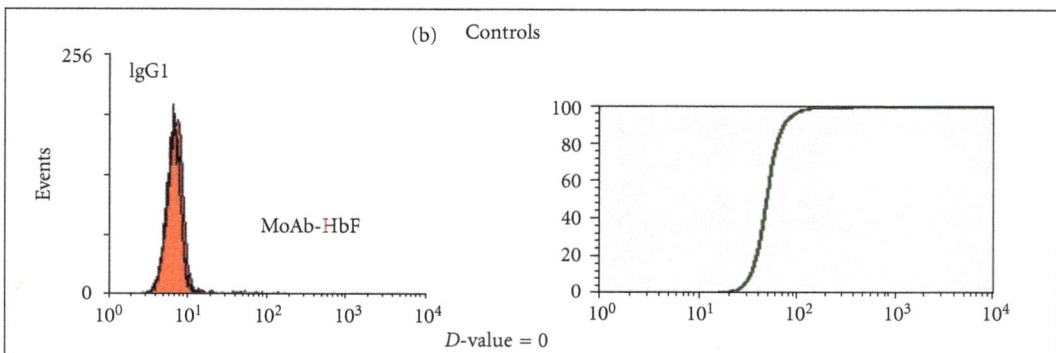

FIGURE 2: Illustration of flow cytometric and KS aspects of F cells values in a SCA patient and a control. HbF expression was, also, analyzed using the Kolmogorov-Smirnov (KS) statistic test ($D$-value), which allows the objective and accurate identification of small differences in fluorescence intensity. Samples were considered positive when $D \geq 0.15$.

TABLE 1: Hematological parameters related to F cells rate in different age groups.

| Group (n) | age (yrs) | WBC (G/L) | RBC (T/L) | Hb (g/dL) | Pcv (%) | MCV (fl) | MCH (pg) | MCHC (g/dL) | Pts (G/L) | RDW-cv (%) | PDW (%) | MPV | F Cell (D-value) | F cell % |
|---|---|---|---|---|---|---|---|---|---|---|---|---|---|---|
| 1 (12) | 2–5 (12) | 18.38 | 2.49 | 6.4 | 21.8 | 89,9 | 26.3 | 29.2 | 514.8 | 24.5 | 13.1 | 10.1 | 0.3 | 3,7 |
| 2 (21) | 6–12 (21) | 18.74 | 2.39 | 6.4 | 21.1 | 90,6 | 27.3 | 30.2 | 434.5 | 24.2 | 12.6 | 10.1 | 0.3 | 4,7 |
| 3 (7) | 13–18 (7) | 15.92 | 2.12 | 5.8 | 18.6 | 87,9 | 27.1 | 31.0 | 367.0 | 25.9 | 14.5 | 11.4 | 0.2 | 1,9 |
| 4 (1) | >18 (1) | 14.80 | 1.68 | 4.5 | 16.7 | 99,4 | 26.8 | 26.9 | 375.0 | 32.0 | 14.1 | 10.5 | — | — |

Subjects were divided in 4 age groups (1, 2, 3, and 4) and compared each to others. Parameters that displayed significant differences concerned the F cells rate and the RDW. Significant differences were observed in the F cells rate between the group 1 and 2 versus group 3 ($P < 0.05$); RDW was significantly higher in a child aged >18 yrs than in the other groups.

TABLE 2: Comparison of hematological parameters in SCA patients from different African studies.

| Countries | Nb | Mean age | Hb (g/dL) | PCV (%) | RBC (T/L) | MCV (fl) | MCH (pg) | MCHC (g/dL) | HbF(%) | References |
|---|---|---|---|---|---|---|---|---|---|---|
| Tanzania | 12 | 10.7 | 6.42 | 24.7 | 2.27 | 108.8 | 28.8 | 26 | 8.6 | [14] |
| Kenya | 25 | 10.9 | 7.85 | 26 | 2.54 | 102.4 | 30.9 | 30.2 | 7.5 | [14] |
| Angola | 4 | 9.3 | 7.30 | 20.7 | 2.70 | 88.3 | 30.5 | 35.3 | 2 | [14] |
| Nigeria | 249 | 9.7 | 7.53 | 28 | 2.76 | 103 | 26.8 | 26.8 | 9.2 | [14] |
| Nigeria | 94 | | 7.4 | 26 | 3.6 | | | | 7.2 | [17] |
| Nigeria | 200 | 23.6 | 7.5 | 23.0 | — | 79.3 | 28.3 | 32.5 | 2.1 | [15] |
| R Congo | 116 | 9.4 | 6.6 | | | | | | 8.8 | [16] |
| DR Congo | 115 | 8.7 | 7.0 | 23.2 | 2.47 | 95.3 | 28.3 | 30.3 | 7.4 | Personal communication |
| DR Congo | 42 | 8.9 | 6.2 | 20.7 | 2.3 | 89.6 | 26.8 | 29.7 | 7.2 | Our data |

Most of the African SCA patients have Hb less than 8 g/L and Hb F less than 10%. Large variations of HbF rate were observed in the same country like Nigeria probably because of the heterogeneous population who were tested. In DR Congo, values were almost s similar.

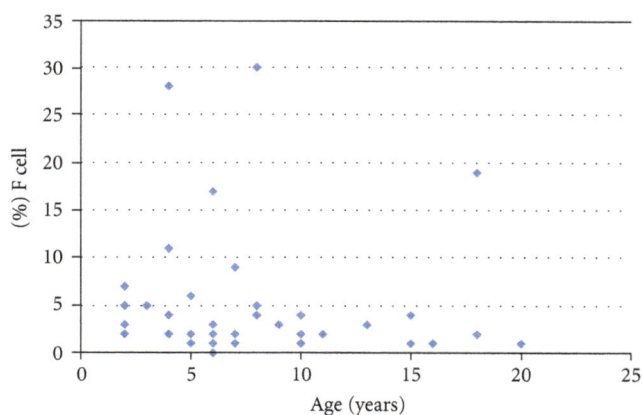

FIGURE 3: % F cells distribution in 42 SCA patients related to age. The mean value was at $5.44 \pm 7.6$ with a non gaussian pattern even after log-transformation of values (not shown).

African haplotypes (Senegalese and Benin types) [19]. This polymorphism has been associated with erythropoietic stress and expanded erythroid mass secondary to ineffective erythropoiesis or hemolytic process and preferential survival of the red cell precursor that contain HbF, as observed in $\beta$-thalassemia and sickle cell anemia [4, 6, 24].

Genetic variation at three principal loci—HBB cluster on chromosome 11p, HBS1L-MYB region on chromosome 6q, and BCL11A on chromosome 2p—have been shown to influence HbF levels and disease severity in $\beta$ thalassemia

and SCA [4]. A recent study revealed that all three principal HbF loci have a significant impact in Tanzanian patients with SCA; the strongest association being seen at the BCL11A locus on chromosome 2 [25].

We think that values observed in our study were probably due to the heterogeneity of G$\gamma$ globin gene expression in patient bearing the Bantu haplotype [19]. Comparison of the HbF values reported in other African SCA patients, displayed low values of $2,17 \pm 1.81\%$, and $4.7 \pm 2.9\%$ in Nigerian patients described by Omoti [15] and Falusi and Olatunji [26], respectively. Mouele [16] reported values of $8.8 \pm 5.8\%$ in SCA patients in the neighboring Republic of Congo.

Differences observed in those African SCA patients may be due to the various age proportion of populations, the coinheritance trait of thalassemia gene, or other genetic components controlling the number of F cells and the clinical status of the patients [21, 24]. As HbF has been shown to be stable in SCA patients at 4–6 years [6, 19], comparison of HbF values should be determined in children aged >4 yrs and in steady state.

Levels of HbF and F cells vary considerably among different populations; this variability does not originate from a single genetic locus and HbF persistence is considered as a quantitative trait (QT) depending on multiple genes being expressed together with a small environmental component [4].

In normal adults, F cells % varied from 0.5 to 7% while in SCA patients, values have a much broader range [21]. We have no local reference values in Congolese SCA patients, but 40/42 (95%) of patients and 12/47 (25.5%) of controls displayed values higher than the cut-off point (0.5%). Higher values displayed by some SCA patients and controls (Figure 2) would be due to the concomitant hereditary persistence of fetal hemoglobin (HPFH) as described in other studies [21]. The wide ranging distribution of % HbF and F cells observed in our population can be due to the small sample size in this study, and also due to genetic factors (α-thalassemia and the QTL traits) and to environmental factors (malaria, infections). This later condition coupled with a chronic inflammatory status that has been reported in majority of SCA patients living in DRC [27] would contribute to the hyperhemolytic status. Hemolysis can play a role in the "erythropoietic stress" due to malaria and other infectious complications as expressed by the high reticulocytes number in Congolese SCA patients [28]. Further studies are required to evaluate this hypothesis.

Elsewhere, a significant correlation has been reported between the F cells rate and the %HbF and also with some erythrocyte indices like MCV and Hb [5, 21]. In our study, we found no significant correlations between F cells and other hematological parameters, except the reticulocyte percentage.

Although comparison of hematological parameters in SCA patients from different African countries showed variability, globally, it appears that SCA African patients had low values of Hb (<8 g/L) and %HbF (<10). These data can explain the severity of phenotype of SCD in patients bearing African $\beta^s$ haplotypes.

In spite of the wide individual variations of the %HbF and F cells rate, these two parameters would be used as a tool to monitor response to agents such as hydroxyurea, a drug that reduces the severity of SCD [4, 6, 21].

## 5. Conclusion

In spite of some limitations of this study, we have provided new data highlighting low HbF levels and clinical severity of SCA in Congolese patients which can be used to compare African patients located in different geographical area and genetic background. Moreover, comparison of both flow cytometric techniques for F+ cell quantitation resulted in a significant statistical correlations. To confirm its reliability, the less complex and quicker Fix & Perm technique should be further utilized for measuring the amount of F+ cells in SCA. Furthermore, Genome wide studies in different sub-Saharan SCA patients would contribute to the understanding of the complex role of HbF and F cells in the phenotype and the complex physiopathology of sickle cell disease.

## Conflict of Interests

The authors have no conflicts of interest.

## Acknowledgments

The authors are grateful to Paul Telfer (Royal London Hospital, Queen Mary University of London, London UK) for the revision of the article, to Mr. Lukusa David for his statistical assistance, and to the technicians of Laboratory at Centre Hospitalier Monkole for their help.

## References

[1] J. Elion and D. Labie, "Bases physiopathologiques moléculaires et cellulaires du traitement de la drépanocytose," *Hématologie*, vol. 2, no. 6, pp. 499–510, 1996.

[2] D. Labie and J. Elion, "Généthique et physiopathologie de la drépanocytose," in *La Drépanocytose*, R. Girot, P. Begué, and F. Galactéros, Eds., pp. 1–11, John Libbey Eurotext, Paris, France, 2003.

[3] O. S. Platt, D. J. Brambilla, W. F. Rosse et al., "Mortality in sickle cell disease—life expectancy and risk factors for early death," *The New England Journal of Medicine*, vol. 330, no. 23, pp. 1639–1644, 1994.

[4] S. L. Thein and S. Menzel, "Discovering the genetics underlying foetal haemoglobin production in adults," *British Journal of Haematology*, vol. 145, no. 4, pp. 455–467, 2009.

[5] M. Maier-Redelsperger, J. Bardakdjlan-Michau, M. G. Neonato, and R. Girot, "Diagnostic biologique des syndromes drépanocytaires," in *La Drépanocytose*, R. Girot, P. Begué, and F. Galacteros, Eds., pp. 13–29, Ed John Libbey Eurotext, Paris, France, 2003.

[6] I. Akinsheye, A. Alsultan, N. Solovieff et al., "Fetal hemoglobin in sickle cell anemia," *Blood*, vol. 118, no. 1, pp. 19–27, 2011.

[7] D. Powars, L. S. Chan, and W. A. Schroeder, "The variable expression of sickle cell disease is genetically determined," *Seminars in Hematology*, vol. 27, no. 4, pp. 360–376, 1990.

[8] J. Elion and D. Labie, "Drépanocytose et adhérence cellulaire," *Hématologie*, vol. 3, no. 4, pp. 201–211, 1998.

[9] L. Tshilolo, L. M. Aissi, D. Lukusa et al., "Neonatal screening for sickle cell anaemia in the Democratic Republic of the Congo: experience from a pioneer project on 31 204 newborns," *Journal of Clinical Pathology*, vol. 62, no. 1, pp. 35–38, 2009.

[10] L. Tshilolo, "Les complications de la drépanocytose chez l'enfant Africain," *Développement et Santé*, vol. 182, pp. 13–19, 2006.

[11] Y. Mundee, N. C. Bigelow, B. H. Davis, and J. P. Porter, "Simplified flow cytometric method for fetal hemoglobin containing red blood cells," *Cytometry*, vol. 42, pp. 389–393, 2000.

[12] Y. Mundee, N. C. Bigelow, B. H. Davis, and J. B. Porter, "Flow cytometric method for simultaneous assay of foetal haemoglobin containing red cells, reticulocytes and foetal haemoglobin containing reticulocytes," *Clinical and Laboratory Haematology*, vol. 23, no. 3, pp. 149–154, 2001.

[13] A. Tafuri, C. Gregorj, M. T. Petrucci et al., "MDR1 protein expression is an independent predictor of complete remission in newly diagnosed adult acute lymphoblastic leukemia," *Blood*, vol. 100, no. 3, pp. 974–981, 2002.

[14] C. Oner, A. J. Dimovski, N. F. Olivieri et al., "$\beta^s$ haplotypes in various world populations," *Human Genetics*, vol. 89, no. 1, pp. 99–104, 1992.

[15] C. E. Omoti, "Haematological values in sickle cell anaemia in steady state and during vaso-occlusive crisis in Benin City, Nigeria," *Annals of African Medicine*, vol. 4, no. 2, pp. 62–67, 2005.

[16] R. Mouele, "Haemoglobin F (HbF) levels in sickle-cell anaemia patients homozygous for the Bantu haplotype," *European Journal of Haematology*, vol. 63, no. 2, pp. 136–137, 1999.

[17] N. Nduka, S. M. Owhochuku, and P. Odike, "Current observations on sickle cell genotype in Nigeria," *East African Medical Journal*, vol. 70, no. 10, pp. 646–649, 1993.

[18] M. S. Figueiredo, J. Kerbauy, M. S. Gonçalves et al., "Effect of $\alpha$-thalassemia and $\beta$-globin gene cluster haplotypes on the hematological and clinical features of sickle-cell anemia in Brazil," *American Journal of Hematology*, vol. 53, no. 2, pp. 72–76, 1996.

[19] R. L. Nagel, S. K. Rao, and O. Dunda-Belkhodja, "The hematologic characteristics of sickle cell anemia bearing the Bantu haplotype: the relationship between (G)$\gamma$ and HbF level," *Blood*, vol. 69, no. 4, pp. 1026–1030, 1987.

[20] M. J. Stuart and R. L. Nagel, "Sickle-cell disease," *The Lancet*, vol. 364, no. 9442, pp. 1343–1360, 2004.

[21] S. J. Marcus, T. R. Kinney, W. H. Schultz, E. E. O'Branski, and R. E. Ware, "Quantitative analysis of erythrocytes containing fetal hemoglobin (F cells) in children with sickle cell disease," *American Journal of Hematology*, vol. 54, no. 1, pp. 40–46, 1997.

[22] M. H. Steinberg, Z. H. Lu, F. B. Barton, M. L. Terrin, S. Charache, and G. J. Dover, "Fetal hemoglobin in sickle cell anemia: determinants of response to hydroxyurea," *Blood*, vol. 89, no. 3, pp. 1078–1088, 1997.

[23] D. Labie, J. Pagnier, and C. Lapoumeroulie, "Common haplotype dependency of high (G)$\gamma$-globin gene expression and high Hb F levels in $\beta$-thalasssemia and sickle cell anemia patients," *Proceedings of the National Academy of Sciences of the United States of America*, vol. 82, no. 7, pp. 2111–2114, 1985.

[24] U. Testa, "Fetal hemoglobin chemical inducers for treatment of hemoglobinopathies," *Annals of Hematology*, vol. 88, no. 6, pp. 505–528, 2009.

[25] J. Makani, S. Menzel, S. Nkya et al., "Genetics of fetal hemoglobin in Tanzanian and British patients with sickle cell anemia," *Blood*, vol. 117, no. 4, pp. 1390–1392, 2011.

[26] A. G. Falusi and P. O. Olatunji, "Effects of alpha thalassaemia and haemoglobin F (HbF) level on the clinical severity of sickle-cell anaemia," *European Journal of Haematology*, vol. 52, no. 1, pp. 13–15, 1994.

[27] G. Baune, N. Borel Giraud, and L. Tshilolo, "Etude du profil protéique de 45 enfants drépanocytaires homozygotes congolais," *Annales de Biologie Clinique*, vol. 67, no. 2, pp. 1–6, 2009.

[28] L. Tshilolo, S. Wembonyama, V. Suma, and G. Avvisati, "L'hémogramme chez l'enfant drépanocytaire congolais au cours des phases stationnaires," *Médecine Tropicale*, vol. 70, no. 5-6, pp. 459–463, 2010.

# Traditional Herbal Management of Sickle Cell Anemia: Lessons from Nigeria

**Sunday J. Ameh,[1] Florence D. Tarfa,[1] and Benjamin U. Ebeshi[2]**

[1] *Department of Medicinal Chemistry and Quality Control, National Institute for Pharmaceutical Research and Development (NIPRD), PMB 21, Garki, Idu Industrial Area, Abuja, Nigeria*
[2] *Department of Pharmaceutics & Medicinal Chemistry, Niger Delta University, Wilberforce Island, Amassoma, Nigeria*

Correspondence should be addressed to Sunday J. Ameh, sjitodo@yahoo.com

Academic Editor: Aurelio Maggio

*Background.* Patients in West Africa where sickle cell anemia (SCA) is endemic have for ages been treated with natural products, especially herbs, as, is still the case in rural communities. *Objective.* In this paper we look closely at some of these herbs to see if there are any lessons to be learnt or clues to be found for optimizing the treatments based on them, as had been done in the case of NIPRISAN, which was developed from herbs in Nigeria based on Yoruba Medicine. *Methods.* Select publications on SCA, its molecular biology and pathology, and actual and experimental cases of herbal treatment were perused in search of molecular clues that can be linked to chemical constituents of the herbs involved. *Results.* The study revealed that during the last 2-3 decades, much progress was made in several aspects of SCA pharmacology, especially the approval of hydroxyurea. As for SCA herbalism, this paper revealed that antisickling herbs abound in West Africa and that the most promising may yet be found. Three new antisickling herbs (*Entandrophragma utile, Chenopodium ambrosioides,* and *Petiveria alliacea*) were reported in May 2011. At NIPRD, where NIPRISAN was developed, three other recipes are currently awaiting development. *Conclusion.* The study raised the hope that the search in the Tropics for more effective herbal recipes for managing sickle cell anaemia will be more fruitful with time and effort.

## 1. Introduction

*1.1. Health and Disease as Conceived among Communities in Nigeria.* Health and disease concepts in African Traditional Medicine are far more advanced than many biomedical scientists would imagine. For instance, long before Ronald Ross revealed mosquito as the vector of malaria and Charles Laveran plasmodium as the parasite [1], communities in tropical African had associated mosquitoes with high fever. Among the Idoma of Benue State, Nigeria, it was known since antiquity that "idapo" (malarial fever) is caused by "imu" (mosquito) and that "ofe-egbe" (dysentery) is caused by bad water or eki-iju (egg of green house flies: a variety of *Musca domestica* associated with poor sanitation). On the other hand, disorders underlain by more remote causes are attributed to evil spirits and practices frowned upon or forbidden by tradition. Such practices include marriage between close relatives. In Idomaland, marriage even between second

cousins is expressly forbidden—it is considered an abomination and a cause of abnormalities or incurable disorders. We are not aware of any specific name for sickle cell disorder in Idoma, but we know that the condition is common and is classed among diseases believed to be caused by evil spirits or misconduct. Ibrahim Muazzam, NIPRD's ethnobotanist and an associate of Etkin [2], informed us that among the Hausa-Fulani of northern Nigeria, where sickle cell anemia is called "sankara-miji," the disorder is perceived to be "paranormal" and incurable. Among the Yoruba and Igbo of southern Nigeria, "Abiku" [3] and "ogbanje" [4] or "iyi-uwa" [5] are umbrella terms that include sickle cell anemia and are believed to be "paranormal". The foregoing suggests to us that traditional communities in Nigeria are not only aware of the syndrome called "sickle cell anemia" but also well aware of its chronicity, endemicity, and "paranormality." The general manifestations of SCA and strategies for management including herbal treatment are indicated in Figure 1.

Nonherbal pharmacologic interventions:

The goal of pharmacologic intervention is to manage and control symptoms, and to limit the number of crises.

Treatment for anemia:
(1) Folic acid
(2) Other dietary supplements (DS)

Treatment for painful crisis:
(1) Analgesics
(2) Plenty of fluids

Other treatments for crises:
(1) Hydroxyurea: a drug that may help reduce the number of pain episodes like chest pain and breathlessness
(2) Anti-infectives such as penicillin

Treatments for complication:
(1) Drug rehabilitation
(2) Wound care with antiseptics

Manifestations of SCA:

Anemia

Pain

Delayed growth

Fevers

Leg/skin ulcers

Jaundice

Excessive thirst

Frequent urination

Priapism in males

Poor eyesight

No. of stokes

Possible herbal intervention:

The goal of traditional/herbal intervention is to manage and control symptoms, and to limit the number of crises

Treatment for anemia:
(1) Vegetal food/fruits rich in DS
(2) Food with assorted herbs/spices

Treatment for painful crisis:
(1) Analgesic herbs
(2) Plenty of fluids such as "kunu"

Other treatments for crises:
(1) Niprisan: a drug that may help reduce the number of pain episodes (Wambebe et al., 2001)
(2) Disease-specific anti-infective herbs

Treatments for complication:
(1) Symptomatic phytotherapy
(2) Wound care with antiseptic herbs

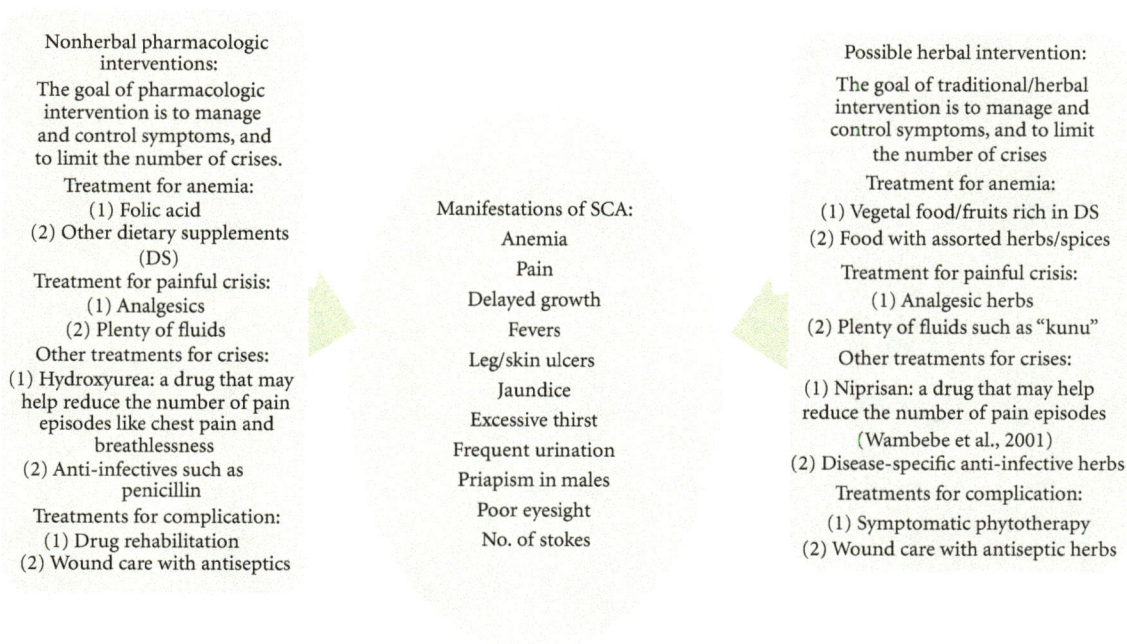

FIGURE 1: Manifestations of SCA and strategies for management including herbal treatment. The two major pathologies of SCA are hemolytic anemia and vasoocclusion with pain especially in the limbs. Acute chest syndrome, which can result from infections, is the leading cause of death. Neurologic complications such as stroke and hemorrhage can occur. Aplastic crisis is most often the result of infection with Parvovirus B19, which results from temporary cessation of RBC production. Genitourinary-hematuria, renal failure, and priapism may occur. Cholelithiasis due to severe hemolysis can develop into acute cholecystitis due to the formation of pigmented gallstones [6–13].

*1.2. Traditional Herbal Approaches to Sickle Cell Anemia in Nigeria.* As described elsewhere [14, 16, 17], among the Efik and Ibibio, Hausa, Igbo, Idoma, and Yoruba: clove (*Eugenia caryophyllata* or "kanunfari" in Hausa; *Piper guineense* ("eche" in Idoma or "akwa-ose" in Igbo); grains of paradise (*Aframomum melegueta* or "otuta" in Idoma); *Sorghum bicolor* (the leaf stalk yields an extract that looks like blood); *Pterocarpus osun* (common in the Yoruba state of Osun) are used in various health conditions, including sickle cell anemia. As stated earlier [14] *E. caryophyllata, P. guineense, P. osun*, and *S. bicolor* are the herbal components of the Yoruba recipe upon which the antisickling drug Niprisan is based. Prior to the era of Niprisan these herbs were either extracted with "ogoro" (ethanolic distillate of palm wine) or with an aqueous solution trona (sodium sesquicarbonate—a mineral used in Nigeria as tenderizer). Niprisan has passed phases IIA and IIB, and is widely used in Nigeria, and is known or popular in India and the USA. In 2010, Swift [18] of COSMID Corporation, USA, stated the following:

A dried extract of four plants has been used to treat patients with SCD in Nigeria for many years (NIPRISAN). It has been through multiple clinical trials in Nigeria and has been formally approved for use in that country since 2006 for the treatment of SCD. The US FDA has determined there is sufficient safety and efficacy data for NIPRISAN to start a Phase III clinical trial. The US FDA Botanical Review Team (BRT) suggested a simpler formulation of

NIPRISAN, development of a chemical fingerprint for the formulation using LC/MS and elucidation of some of the anti-sickling compounds in the formulation would improve standardization and increase the probability of obtaining FDA marketing approval.

To the best of our knowledge phase III trial of Niprisan is yet to be reported. We did however suggest in 2011 that phytocannabinoids and vanilloids in *E. caryophyllata* and *P. guineense* may account for some of the useful effects of Niprisan in sickle cell crisis [14]. Some of these compounds, including shikimic acid derivatives (vanilloids) and cannabinoids are indicated in Figure 2 and Table 3, respectively.

*1.3. An Overview of Vanilloids and Cannabinoids—Agents in Pain Control.* The probable roles of vanilloids and cannabinoids receptors in the control of pain, the key issue in sickle cell crisis, are described in a latter section of this paper. In the present we briefly mention these groups of phytochemicals and their synthetic analogues as components of *E. caryophyllata* and *P. guineense,* and that they may account for some of the useful effects of Niprisan in sickle cell crisis [14].

*1.3.1. Vanilloids.* The vanilloids, namely: vanillin, eugenol, zingerone, capsaicin, and piperine (isomer of capsaicin), are molecules with distinctive flavours, yet are quite similar in their molecular structures. All contain a benzene ring. Subtle changes in the sizes or positions of groups of atoms attached

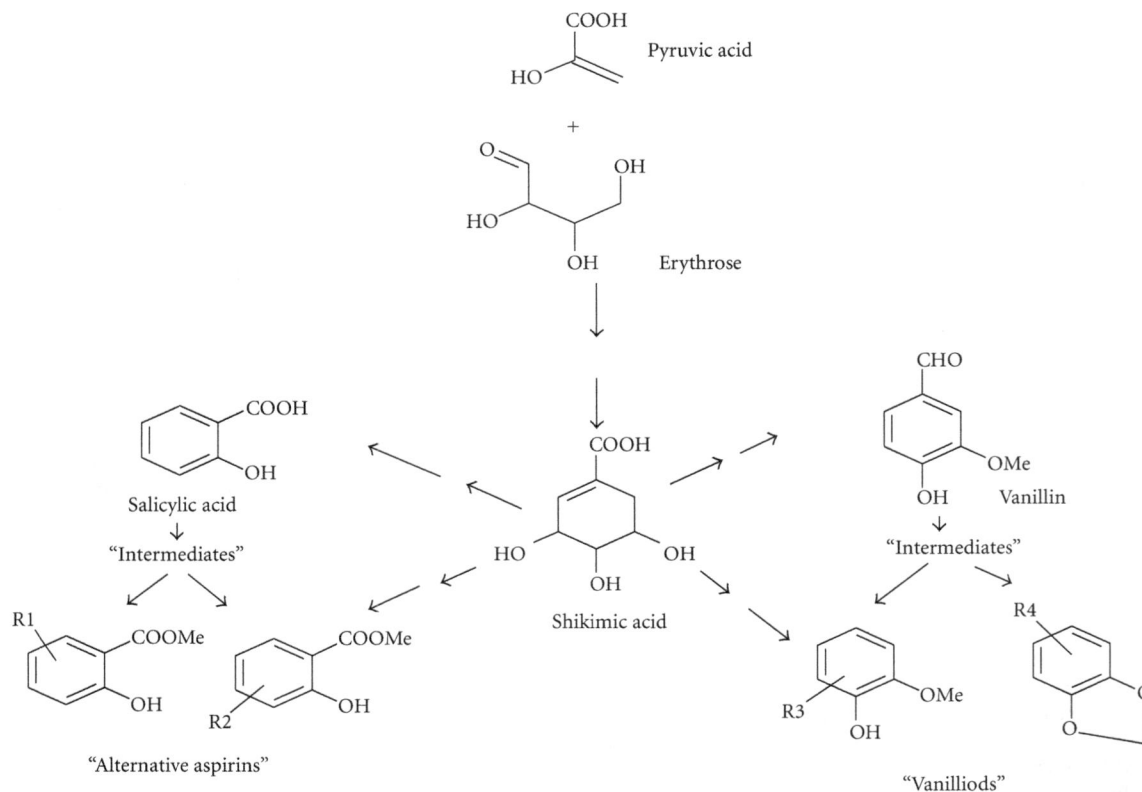

FIGURE 2: Biosynthesis and relationship of shikimic acid to "alternative aspirins" and "vanilloids". The shikimic acid pathway is a key biosynthetic pathway for several phytochemicals known for their medicinal attributes. The Figure illustrates the biosynthesis of shikimic acid from pyruvic acid and erythrose and the relationship between the acid and its byproducts and intermediates, some of which possess aspirin-like effects, like analgesia and desickling of sickled RBCs. Such byproducts/intermediates include salicyclic acid derivatives, vanillin, piperine, capsaicin, and cubebin. Piperine, capsaicin, and cubebin as byproducts of shikimic acid are the likely antisickling agents Niprisan [14]. It is of note that Ouattara [15] had attributed the antisickling properties *Fagara zanthoxyloides* to divanilloylquinic acids.

to the ring dramatically change their organoleptic and other physicochemical characteristics. Eugenol, capsaicin, and piperine are present in *E. caryophyllata* and *P. guineense*. Eugenol has a short hydrocarbon chain attached to the ring, which makes it much less water soluble than vanillin. Although it is practically insoluble in water, it freely mixes with fats and oils. Its fat solubility allows it to penetrate tissues and bind more tightly to lipid rich membrane bound vanilloid receptors. The tail gives eugenol a stronger odour than vanillin. Eugenol has a numbing analgesic effect; because it has some antiseptic effects it is used in the formulation of some brands of toothpaste. It is supposed that the hydrocarbon tail in combination with the polar OH group on the ring allows eugenol to interact with vanilloid receptors in order to produce analgesia and other physiochemical effects. Capsaicin and piperine are of a lower molecular weight than eugenol, and their side chains contain a polar amide group, which makes them less volatile and almost odourless but very "hot"—a persistent burning sensation even at concentrations lower than 10 ppm. The intense flavour results from the molecules' long hydrocarbon tails. The chain allows them to bind very strongly with their membranous lipoprotein receptors. The fatty tail also allows the molecules to slip through

lipid-rich cell membranes, making the burning sensation more pervasive and persistent. Both the burning and analgesic effects of capsaicin or piperine owe to the way the molecules interact their lipoprotein receptors. Paradoxically, the ability of these compounds to cause pain (i.e., the burning sensation) makes them useful in alleviating pain. Exposure to them lowers sensitivity to pain, and it is applied as a counterirritant in the treatment of arthritis and other chronically painful conditions. People who use lots of pepper (as the Idoma and Yoruba do) build up a tolerance to it. According to Fred Senese [19]—"a small jolt of capsaicin excites the nervous system into producing endorphins, which promote a pleasant sense of well-being. The endorphin lift makes spicy foods mildly addictive (and for some, an obsession)."

*1.3.2. Cannabinoids.* Cannabinoids are a group of terpeno-phenolic compounds present in *Cannabis sativa*' and occur naturally in the nervous and immune systems of animals. The broader definition of cannabinoids refers to a group of substances that are structurally related to tetrahydrocanna-binol (THC) or that bind to cannabinoid receptors. The chemical definition encompasses a variety of distinct chemical classes: the classical cannabinoids structurally related to THC; the nonclassical cannabinoids—the aminoalkylindoles, eicosanoids—related to the endocannabinoids 1, quinolines, and arylsulphonamides; additional compounds that do not fall into these standard classes but bind to cannabinoid receptors ($CB_1$ and $CB_2$). An example of such is $\beta$-Caryophyllene, which binds selectively to $CB_2$. Currently, there are three general types of cannabinoids: the "phytocannabinoids" that occur uniquely in the cannabis plant or the caryophyllenes that occur in clove; the "endogenous cannabinoids" that are produced in the in humans and other animals; the "synthetic cannabinoids" that are similar compounds produced by in the laboratory by chemical manipulations [20].

*1.4. Aim of the Paper.* Eleven years into the 21st century, the only cure for SCA is bone marrow transplant that requires a rigorously compatible family member as donor. There is at best only an 85% disease-free survival rate, with a 7% transplant-related mortality rate and a 9% graft failure rate [21]. The procedure is expensive and precarious, and suitable donors are hard to come by. Moreover, patients needing the treatment the most are the least likely to benefit from it due to higher risks. These barriers mean that pharmacologic approaches (and that include herbal palliation) will remain the primary strategy for managing SCA. This paper is necessitated by the mistaken notion that herbal remedies are coming too late in the day to feature significantly in SCA management. We are inclined to reason otherwise and to hold the view that a thorough familiarity with SCA and the ever increasing volume of data on phytochemicals may provide valuable leads, lessons, and clues. In this regard, we here wish to draw attention to the following pertinent comment [22]:

> Doctors in Nigeria use fagara (*F. zanthoxyloides*) to reduce the painful crisis of the genetic disease, sickle cell anemia. This herb has a variety of unusual properties that reduce platelet and blood cell sticking. After reading the reports from Nigeria many years ago, I decided to try fagara's relative prickly ash bark for the same indication. I made a simple tincture of 50% prickly ash bark and 50% ginkgo leaf, and gave it to a young African-American girl in the first grade who constantly missed school and needed to be hospitalized 3-4 times per year due to the painful sickle cell crisis. I gave her about 25 drops three times a day. She immediately stopped having serious problems, her thinking was no longer fuzzy, the frequency of her attacks went down to about one per year, and the severity of the attacks decreased appreciably. This success has continued through the years, as long as she takes her medicine. I saw her last year, and she has blossomed into a beautiful junior high school student, the sickle cell disease now only a bit-player in the background of her life. Another of my patients had lived with the disease his entire life, with almost constant pain, and bimonthly crisis.

I gave him 35 drops three times per day, and he immediately improved in the same way as the young girl. This improvement in both frequency of attacks and level of pain has persisted in three of my long-term patients over many years. The wholesale cost of this medicine is less than $20 per month at full dosage. My biggest fear is that this knowledge will be co-opted by a pharmaceutical company, and made available to the many suffering children only at an exorbitant cost.

Elsewhere, we had reasoned on the need for support for clinical trials of promising traditional remedies, and for national drug regulatory agencies in developing countries to show more interest in herbal clinical trials [17]. We attempt in this paper to show how this line of thought should follow from what we have learnt of herbal management of SCA in Nigeria.

## 2. An Overview of SCA

*2.1. Epidemiology of SCA and Some Historical Landmarks.* Epidemiology of SCA commenced in the USA in 1910 with the discovery of the disorder in a patient hospitalized in 1904, suffering from anemia [41]. The study progressed through the era involving Pauling and others [42] and Ingram [43, 44]; and is today a success because the necessary preventive measures for SCA are now well known [45]. Also fairly documented is the use in Africa of herbal palliatives for SCA [24, 25, 46]. In this paper we take a closer look at some of these herbs and hypothesize on the likely biochemical bases for their use and how such insight may facilitate their optimization. Ages before European colonization of West Africa, the people had identified a chronic condition variously called "Abiku," "Ogbanje," "Sankara-jimi" in Nigeria. Thus, several therapies—herbal and otherwise—waxed and waned, but most of the herbals survived. Shortly after SCA was defined in the US, studies at Ibadan University confirmed the syndrome in Nigeria. During the 1970s studies at Ibadan and Ife described the first series of herbal remedies for SCA. In the 1990s biomedical scientists from Ibadan, Ife, and Zaria developed Niprisan which was launched in 2006. In 2001, before the franchise to produce Niprisan was licensed to a US drug firm, NIPRD had 3 other promising recipes. It should be mentioned that the disease was first named "sickle-cell anemia" in 1922 [47]. But some elements of the disorder had been recognized in an 1846 paper in Southern Journal of Medical Pharmacology which described the absence of a spleen in the autopsy of a runaway slave [48, 49].

*2.2. Prevalence, Manifestations, and Management Strategies*

*2.2.1. Global Prevalence of SCA.* Aside from Africa and countries bordering the Mediterranean (e.g., Italy, Greece, Spain, and Turkey) that have high incidences of SCA, significant prevalence has been reported especially in Saudi Arabia, Yemen, India, Pakistan, Bangladesh, and China [6, 23, 26, 50, 51]. The occurrence of SCA in the Americas and in Northwest Europe owes of course to the Triangular Slave

TABLE 1: Significant cases of SCDs including thalassemias by continent/region.

| Continent/region | Major disorder | Remark/reference |
|---|---|---|
| Africa | (1) SCA (HbSS)<br>(2) HbSC<br>(3) $\alpha$-Thalassemia<br>HbC has lysine rather glutamine in 6th position as in $\beta$-globin of HbA | One in 12 Blacks worldwide carries the SCA trait. About 1 in 400 has SCA. About 75% of global SCAs are in Africa. About 150,000 SCA cases are born yearly in Nigeria. The carrier frequency ranges between 10% and 40% across equatorial Africa, decreasing to 1-2% in north Africa and <1% in South Africa [6]. |
| Islands and countries in Mediterranean area and the Middle East | (1) HbS$\beta^0$ or $\beta$<br>(2) $\alpha$-Thalassemia<br>(3) $\beta$-Thalassemia<br>(4) HbC$\beta^0$ or $\beta^+$<br>(5) SCA | These islands and countries including Turkey have significant cases of SCDs and thalassemias. Saudi Arabia has a yearly rate of ~3,000 newborns. Qatif City has the highest rate [7, 8]. |
| America—USA | (1) SCA<br>(2) $\beta$-Thalassemia<br>(3) HbC$\beta^0$ or $\beta^+$<br>(4) Other SCDs | About 72,000 persons in the US have SCA, mostly African-Americans at the rate of 1 in 500 newborns as against 1 in 1, 200 for Hispanic-American births [23, 24]. In 2004, 83,149 cases of hospitalization were attributed to SCD in the US at a cost of ~\$488 million [9]. |
| Asia | (1) SCA<br>(2) $\alpha$-thalassemia<br>(3) $\beta$-thalassemia<br>(4) HbC$\beta^0$ or $\beta^+$<br>(5) HbE$\beta^0$ or $\beta^+$<br>HbC has lysine rather glutamine in 26th position as in $\beta$-globin of HbA | SCA is significantly prevalent in Bangladesh, China, and other Asian countries. In India the prevalence ranges from 9.4 to 22.2%. Hemoglobin E/thalassemia is common in Cambodia, Thailand, and India. The Maldives has the highest incidence of thalassemias in the world with a carrier rate of 18%. The corresponding figures for Bangladesh, China, India, Malaysia, and Pakistan range 3–8% of the populations [7, 10]. |
| Europe | (1) $\beta$-thalassemia<br>(2) $\alpha$-thalassemia<br>(3) HbC$\beta^0$ or $\beta^+$<br>(4) HbE$\beta^0$ or $\beta^+$<br>(5) SCA | Aside from well-known cases in Italy, Greece, Portugal and Spain, significant prevalence of SCDs and the thalassemias occur in others. In UK more than 200 babies are born annually with SCD. The highest prevalence of 1 in 2,415 is in France due to immigration from more endemic zones [10]. |
| New SCDs/1000 in select areas:<br>Nigeria: ≥19<br>Ghana: 10–18.9<br>S. Arabia: 5–9.9<br>Europe: ≤0.1 | Types of SCD seen:<br>(1) $\beta$-thalassemia<br>(2) $\alpha$-thalassemia<br>(3) HbC$\beta^0$ or $\beta^+$<br>(4) HbE$\beta^0$ or $\beta^+$<br>(5) SCA | New SCDs/1,000 in selected areas [7, 12, 25, 26]:<br>Mexico: 0.1–0.19<br>Central America: 1–18.9<br>South America: 0.1-4.0<br>Southeast Asia: 0.2–18.9<br>Oceania: ≤0.1 |

$\alpha$-Thalassemia results froms decreased production of $\alpha$-globin leading to an excess of $\beta$-globin in affected adults or an excess of $\gamma$-globin in affected newborns. The excess $\beta$-globin form unstable tetramers called Hemoglobin H (or HbH) consisting of 4 $\beta$-globin chains that exhibit abnormal oxygen dissociation curves. $\beta$-Thalassemias are either of the $\beta^0$ type (thalassemia major) or of the $\beta^+$ type (thalassemia intermedia). In the $\beta^0$ type-thalassemias there is no production of $\beta$-globin; hence it is the severer form of $\beta$-thalassemia. In the $\beta^+$ type thalassemia some $\beta$-globin is produced, making it in the milder form. In either case, however, there is a relative excess of $\alpha$ chains, but these do not form tetramers; instead, they bind to RBC membranes, producing membrane damage, and at high concentrations they form toxic aggregates that lead to anemia. As indicated in the table thalassemias can coexist with SCDs.

Trade [23]. Table 1 shows the general picture of sickle cell disorders (SCDs) worldwide.

*2.2.2. Manifestations of SCA and Strategies for Management.* Key manifestations of SCA are indicted in Figure 2 with comments on symptoms treated with pharmacologic agents and nonpharmacologic strategies. Pharmacologic agencies, of course, include herbal preparations such as Niprisan or Ciklavit.

## 3. Herbal Materials Used in Managing SCA

*3.1. Examples of Plants Used in Managing SCA.* A summary of the gross effects and the proposed general actions of some of the herbs used in SCA treatment is presented in Table 2.

## 4. Biochemical Bases for Herbal Management of SCA

*4.1. Structure of Hemoglobin in Relation to Antisickling Agents.* Hemoglobins exist in two quaternary states—the deoxygenated conformation called Tense or T-state and the oxygenated conformation called Relaxed or R-state. Sickling occurs only in T-state haemoglobin S (HbS) due to its polymerizing tendency. Thus, a key approach to the crisis of sickling lies in finding a means of inhibiting this tendency of T-state HbS or of causing it to revert to the R state. Safo and coworkers [52] had shown that both HbA and HbS possess allosteric sites with which suitable chemical ligands can interact to shift the equilibrium in favor of the R state and have identified several such entities, called allosteric

TABLE 2: Herbal materials used in managing SCA and its probable modes of action.

| Herb/reference | Probable general effect/mode of action/phytochemical constituents |
| --- | --- |
| *Fagara zanthoxyloides* (root) [27, 28] | Three isomeric divanilloylquinic acids (burkinabin A, burkinabin B, and burkinabin C) were identified as the likely antisickling agents. But some workers have proposed coumarins, vanillic acid, parahydroxybenzoic acid, and paraflurobenzoic acid. |
| *Carica papaya*—(unripe fruit or leaf) [29–31] | Antisickling effects of 87% inhibitory and 74% reversal activities were obtained from the 5-day fermentation of unripe fruit of *C. papaya* at 2.5 mg per mL of water. Methanol extract had 64% inhibitory and 55% reversal activities while the chloroform extract was inactive. Phenylalanine, tyrosine, and glycine were thought to be responsible. |
| Garlic (bulb) [32] | The basis is unknown, but allicin in garlic, is a potent stimulus of TRPV1 as mentioned in Section 4 (Biochemical Bases for Herbal Management of SCA). Moreover, garlic is used in many infective conditions especially respiratory infections in SCA. |
| *Hymenocardia acidai* (leaf) [33] | Mpiana et al. [33] related the anti-SCA activities of *H. acida* to anthocyanins. |
| *Cajanus cajan* (seed) [34, 35] | Phenylalanine is thought to be the most active principle in *Cajanus cajan* seed—a component of Ciklavit antisickling phytomedicine, developed in Nigeria by two professors, Ekeke and Shode [34]. |
| *Khaya senegalensis* (stem bark/leaf) [36] | Fall et al. [36] attributed the anti-SCA effects of *K. senegalensis* to limonoids. |
| The herbs Niprisan: (1) *S. bicolor* (2) *P. osun* (3) *Clove* (4) *P. guineense* [37–40] | The bases for the actions of *Sorghum bicolor* and *Pterocarpus osun* are unknown, but they are rich in brightly coloured red/orange flavonoids. They probable act as hematonics especially if they contain folic acid or its analogues. Given their blood red colour, the "Doctrine of Signatures" as mentioned elsewhere [16, 17] may have influenced their inclusion by Yoruba sages of old. It had been supposed that the principles in Niprisan that mitigate, palliate, or reduce the frequency of SCA crisis [18] probably reside mainly in clove and *P. guineense* [14]. |

Clove is *Eugenia caryophyllata*, which, like *P. guineese*, contains principles that impact SCA crisis. Notably, the isomeric divanilloylquinic acids of *Fagara zanthoxyloides* contain the vanillyl group as do the vanilloids of clove and *P. guineense*. A discussion of these principles is presented in Section 4.

regulators. These regulators in the case of HbS act as antisickling agents—which can be defined as entities that can inhibit or reverse the sequence of pathological processes leading to sickling. Compounds known to possess this type of effect include (i) "alternative aspirins" such as acetyl-3,5-dibromosalicylic acid [53], (ii) furfural derivatives [52], and (iii) a variety of compounds called capsaicinoids or vanilloids that possess a vanilyl functional group, or its approximation as in vanillin or related compounds [54]. These vanilloids include some substituted benzaldehydes [55] and several shikimic acid byproducts. The structures of some of these antisickling entities including the "alternative aspirins" and "vanilloids" are shown Figure 2.

### 4.2. Physical Pain and Biochemical Bases for Its Amelioration.
Physical pain is an unpleasant sensation associated with actual or potential tissue damage and is essential to an organism's defense and coordination. But, since pain tends to persist beyond its immediate purpose, organisms are equipped with endogenous systems for controlling pain. Such systems are orchestrated by a complex interplay of ion channels and receptors [56].

### 4.2.1. Ion Channels.
Ion channels are pore-forming proteins that act to establish and control voltage gradient across the plasma membrane of cells by allowing the flow of ions across their electrochemical gradient [56]. A special group called transient receptor potential (or TRP) channels has 28 members that differ in the way they are activated. Some are constitutively open, while others are gated by voltage, ligands, pH, redox state, osmolarity, heat, or mechanical stretch [15].

### 4.2.2. Vanilloid or Capsaicin Receptor (TRPV1) as an Ion Channel.
The so-called transient receptor potential vanilloid (TRPV) group of channels has 6 subfamilies, designated-TRPV1 to TRPV6 [15, 57–59]. Caterina et al. [60] indicate that TRPVs are so sensitive to temperature that they are regarded as molecular thermometers. TRPV1 is activated at 43°C and by acidic pH, allicin in garlic, vanilloids (e.g., piperine and capsaicin) and by endocannabinoids (e.g., anandamide and N-arachidonoyl-dopamine). To illustrate how the vanilloids act, it has been shown that capsaicin selectively binds to TRPV1 on the membrane of pain or heat sensing neurons [60]. As a heat activated calcium channel, TRPV1 normally opens at 37–45°C. However, when capsaicin binds to TRPV1, it causes the channel to open below 37°C (body temperature), which is why capsaicin is linked to the sensation of heat. Prolonged activation of these neurons by capsaicin leads to a depletion of presynaptic substance P—a neurotransmitter for pain and heat. Neurons lacking TRPV1 are unaffected by capsaicin [59, 60].

### 4.2.3. Cannabinoid Receptors in Pain Control.
The cannabinoid receptors are a class of cell membrane proteins that are activated by lipids called cannabinoids [61]. Some cannabinoids are endogenous, while others (e.g., the psychoactive constituents of *Cannabis sativa*) are exogenous. At least

TABLE 3: Some bioactive agents of *P. guineense and E. caryophyllata*—components of Niprisan.

| Constituent | Chemistry and pharmacology |
| --- | --- |
| <br>Caryophyllene | $\beta$-Caryophyllene is a warm constituent of *P. guineense*, found also in *C. sativa* and clove. It occurs as a mixture with $\alpha$-caryophyllene. It has been found to bind selectively to cannabinoid receptor type 2. This is a key finding given the role of this receptor in pain control. |
| $CH{:}CHCH{:}CHCHNC_5H_{10}CO$<br><br>Piperine-a vanilloid | Piperine and chavicine are geometric isomers responsible for the pungency of *P. guineense*, constitute ~5–8%, and are used as ethnomedicines. |
| $CH_2NHCO(CH_2)_4CHCHCH_2Me_2$<br><br>Capsaicin-a vanilloid | Capsaicin is (8-methyl-*N*-vanillyl-6-nonenamide) a pungent constituent that produces a burning-sensation in all tissues. Capsaicin and related compounds are called capsaicinoids or vanilloids. |
| <br>Cubebin | Cubebin is tetrahydrodiperonyl-2-furanol. The furanyl and piperonyl (or vanilyl) groups draw attention to the palliate roles of furan and vanilloids in SCD crisis. "Cubebine" is French designation for diethylether extract of *P. cubeba*. |

two receptor subtypes—$CB_1$ (expressed mainly in the CNS, lungs, liver, and kidneys) and $CB_2$ (expressed in the immune system, hematopoietic cells, and peripheral nerve terminals where they function in pain control)—are known. All these tissues are involved in SCA crisis.

*4.2.4. $\beta$-Caryophyllene: a Component of P. Guineense and Clove Is a Cannabinoid.* $\beta$-Caryophyllene, a constituent of *Cannabis sativa* and of *E. caryophyllata* and *P. guineense*: components of Niprisan, has been found to bind selectively to $CB_2$, and to exert significant cannabimimetic effects in mice [62]. This implies that caryophyllene can relief pain in humans and be of benefit to SCD patients. Hence it is possible that Indian hemp, which is richer in caryophyllene than Niprisan, may someday be developed for SCA medication.

## 5. Conclusion

This paper revealed that antisickling herbs are common in West Africa and that more are still being discovered. At NIPRD, where some aspects of Niprisan are still being researched, there are currently three other recipes earmarked for development. We figure that with time more effective antisickling herbs will be found and developed if proper strategies are instituted.

## Acknowledgments

Niprisan is produced by the Drug Manufacturing Unit of NIPRD as a nonprofit social service authorized by the Nigerian Health Minister after the expiration in 2011 of the license earlier granted Zeechem International Limited. Ciklavit is a product of Neimeth International Pharmaceuticals Plc. It was presented by the Nigerian Health Minister, Professor Eyitayo Lambo, at the 56th session of the World Health Organization regional committee meeting held in Addis Ababa, Ethiopia, in 2006 [63]. The reference to the two products is purely academic, with no conflict of interests whatsoever or any anticipation of financial gain.

## References

[1] F. E. G. Cox, "History of the discovery of the malaria parasites and their vectors," *Parasites & Vectors*, vol. 3, article 5, 2010.

[2] N. Etkin, *Edible Medicines: An Ethnopharmacology of Food*, University of Arizona Press, 2006.

[3] G. Jones, *Dictionary of Mythology Folklore and Symbols*, The Scarecrow Press, New York, NY, USA, 1962.

[4] E. Nzewi, "Malevolent ogbanje: recurrent reincarnation or sickle cell disease?" *Social Science & Medicine*, vol. 52, no. 9, pp. 1403–1416, 2001.

[5] C. Achebe, *Things Fall Apart*, William Heinemann limited, London, UK, 1958.

[6] "Sickle-cell anaemia—Report by the Secretariat," 2006, http://apps.who.int/gb/ebwha/pdf_files/WHA59/A59_9-en.pdf.

[7] W. Jastaniah, "Epidemiology of sickle cell disease in Saudi Arabia," *Annals of Saudi Medicine*, vol. 31, no. 3, pp. 289–293, 2011.

[8] C. Steiner and J. Miller, "Sickle cell disease patients in U.S. hospitals, 2004 Healthcare Cost and Utilization Project (HCUP)," Statistical Brief No. 21, December 2006. Rockville, Md: Agency for Health-care Research and Quality, http://www.hcup-us .ahrq.gov/reports/statbriefs/sb21.pdf.

[9] N. Awasthy, K. C. Aggarwal, P. C. Goyal, M. S. Prasad, S. Saluja, and M. Sharma, "Sickle cell disease: experience of a tertiary care center in a nonendemic area," *Annals of Tropical Medicine and Public Health*, vol. 1, no. 1, pp. 1–4, 2008.

[10] J. Bardakdjian-Michau, M. Bahuau, D. Hurtrel et al., "Neonatal screening for sickle cell disease in France," *Journal of Clinical Pathology*, vol. 62, no. 1, pp. 31–33, 2009.

[11] "*Genes and Human Disease. Genomic Resource Centre*", *Health Topic*, WHO, Geneva, Switzerland, 2011.

[12] F. B. Piel, A. P. Patil, R. E. Howes et al., "Global distribution of the sickle cell gene and geographical confirmation of the malaria hypothesis," *Nature Communications*, vol. 1, no. 8, article 104, 2010.

[13] A. C. Allison, "The distribution of the sickle-cell trait in East Africa and elsewhere, and its apparent relationship to the incidence of subtertian malaria," *Transactions of the Royal Society of Tropical Medicine and Hygiene*, vol. 48, no. 4, pp. 312–318, 1954.

[14] S. J. Ameh, O. O. Obodozie, U. S. Inyang, M. S. Abubakar, and M. Garba, "Climbing black pepper (Piper guineense) seeds as an antisickling remedy," in *Nuts & Seeds in Health and Disease Prevention*, V. R. Preedy, R. R. Watson, and V. B. Patel, Eds., pp. 333–343, Academic Press, London, UK, 1st edition, 2011.

[15] D. C. Camerino, D. Tricarico, and J. F. Desaphy, "Ion channel pharmacology," *Neurotherapeutics*, vol. 4, no. 2, pp. 184–198, 2007.

[16] S. J. Ameh, O. O. Obodozie, P. C. Babalola, and K. S. Gamaniel, "Medical herbalism and herbal clinical research—a global perspective," *British Journal of Pharmaceutical Research*, vol. 1, no. 4, pp. 99–123, 2011.

[17] S. J. Ameh, O. O. Obodozie, B. A. Chindo, P. C. Babalola, and K. S. Gamaniel, "Herbal clinical trials—historical development and application in the 21st Century," *Pharmacologia*, vol. 3, pp. 121–131, 2012.

[18] R. Swift, "Formulation and standardization of a sickle cell disease drug for clinical trial," SBIR/ STTR of the United States of America. Agency: department of Health and Human Services, Agency Tracking Number:HL099190, Contact: 1R43HL099190-01, Principal Investigator: Robert Swift.

[19] Fred Senese, "General Chemistry Online. Fire and spices," http://antoine.frostburg.edu/chem/senese/101/features/cap-saicin.shtml.

[20] R. Planells-Cases, C. García-Martínez, M. Royo et al., "Small molecules targeting the vanilloid receptor complex as drugs for inflammatory pain," *Drugs of the Future*, vol. 28, no. 8, pp. 787–795, 2003.

[21] R. Iannone, K. Ohene-Frempong, E. J. Fuchs, J. F. Casella, and A. R. Chen, "Bone marrow transplantation for sickle cell anemia: progress and prospects," *Pediatric Blood and Cancer*, vol. 44, no. 5, pp. 436–440, 2005.

[22] "PRICKLY ASH BARK (Zanthoxylum species)," An mhtm document by Dr. Tillotson of Tillotson Institute of Natural Health, 2011.

[23] B. Modell and M. Darlison, *Global Epidemiology of Haemoglobin Disorders and Derived Service Indicators*, Bulletin of the World Health Organization, WHO, Geneva, Switzerland, 2008.

[24] C. Wambebe, H. Khamofu, J. A. Momoh et al., "Double-blind, placebo-controlled, randomised cross-over clinical trial of NIPRISAN in patients with sickle cell disorder," *Phytomedicine*, vol. 8, no. 4, pp. 252–261, 2001.

[25] O. O. Obodozie, S. J. Ameh, E. K. Afolabi et al., "Standardization of the components of Niprisan: a phytomedicine for treating sickle cell disease," *Journal of Medicinal Plants Research*, vol. 3, no. 4, pp. 284–289, 2009.

[26] P. J. Nietert, M. D. Silverstein, and M. R. Abboud, "Sickle cell anaemia: epidemiology and cost of illness," *Pharmacoeconomics*, vol. 20, no. 6, pp. 357–366, 2002.

[27] E. A. Sofowora and W. A. Isaacs, "Reversal of sickling and crenation in erythrocytes by the root extract of Fagara zanthoxyloides," *Lloydia*, vol. 34, no. 4, pp. 383–385, 1971.

[28] E. A. Sofowora, "Isolation and characterization of an antisickling agent from the root of Fagara zanthoxyloides," in *Proceedings of a Symposium Fagara and the Red Blood Cell*, A. Sofowora and A. I. Sodeye, Eds., pp. 79–87, University of Ife Press, Ile-Ife, Nigeria, 1979.

[29] K. D. Thomas and B. Ajani, "Antisickling agent in an extract of unripe pawpaw fruit (*Carica papaya*)," *Transactions of the Royal Society of Tropical Medicine and Hygiene*, vol. 81, no. 3, pp. 510–511, 1987.

[30] C. M. Ogunyemi, A. A. Elujoba, and M. A. Durosimi, "Antisickling properties of *Carica papaya* Linn," *Journal of Natural Products*, vol. 1, pp. 56–66, 2008.

[31] N. O. Imaga, G. O. Gbenle, V. I. Okochi et al., "Antisickling property of *Carica papaya* leaf extract," *African Journal of Biochemistry Research*, vol. 3, no. 4, pp. 102–106, 2009.

[32] S. T. Ohnishi, T. Ohnishi, and G. B. Ogunmola, "Sickle cell anemia: a potential nutritional approach for a molecular disease," *Nutrition*, vol. 16, no. 5, pp. 330–338, 2000.

[33] P. T. Mpiana, V. Mudogo, Y. F. Kabangu et al., "Antisickling activity and thermostability of anthocyanins extract from a congolese plant, *Hymenocardia acida* Tul. (Hymenocardiaceae)," *International Journal of Pharmacology*, vol. 5, no. 1, pp. 65–70, 2009.

[34] G. I. Ekeke and F. O. Shode, "Phenylalanine is the predominant antisickling agent in *Cajanus cajan* seed extract," *Planta Medica*, vol. 56, no. 1, pp. 41–43, 1990.

[35] A. O. Akinsulie, E. O. Temiye, A. S. Akanmu, F. E. A. Lesi, and C. O. Whyte, "Clinical evaluation of extract of *Cajanus cajan* (Ciklavit) in sickle cell anaemia," *Journal of Tropical Pediatrics*, vol. 51, no. 4, pp. 200–205, 2005.

[36] A. B. Fall, R. Vanhaelen-Fastré, M. Vanhaelen et al., "In vitro antisickling activity of a rearranged limonoid isolated from Khaya senegalensis," *Planta Medica*, vol. 65, no. 3, pp. 209–212, 1999.

[37] C. O. C. Mojisola, E. A. Anthony, and D. M. Alani, "Antisickling properties of the fermented mixture of *Carica papaya* Linn and *Sorghum bicolor* (L.) Moench," *African Journal of Pharmacy and Pharmacology*, vol. 3, no. 4, pp. 140–143, 2009.

[38] A. A. Awodogan, C. Wambebe, K. Gamaniel, J. Okogun, A. Orisadipe, and P. Akah, "Acute and short-term toxicity of NIPRISAN in rats I: biochemical Study," *Journal of Pharmaceutical Research & Development*, vol. 2, pp. 39–45, 1996.

[39] K. Gamaniel, S. Amos, P. Akah et al., "Pharmacological profile of NIPRD 94/002/1-0: a novel herbal antisickling agent," *Journal of Pharmaceutical Research & Development*, vol. 3, no. 2, pp. 89–94, 1998.

[40] O. O. Obodozie, S. J. Ameh, E. K. Afolabi et al., "A normative study of the components of niprisan—an herbal medicine for sickle cellanemia," *Journal of Dietary Supplements*, vol. 7, no. 1, pp. 21–30, 2010.

[41] J. Herrick, "Peculiar elongated and sickle-shaped red blood corpuscles in a case of severe anemia," *Archives of Internal Medicine*, vol. 6, pp. 517–521, 1910.

[42] L. Pauling, H. A. Itano, S. J. Singer, and I. C. Wells, "Sickle cell anemia, a molecular disease," *Science*, vol. 110, no. 2865, pp. 543–548, 1949.

[43] V. M. Ingram, "Gene mutations in human hæmoglobin: the chemical difference between normal and sickle cell hæmoglobin," *Nature*, vol. 180, no. 4581, pp. 326–328, 1957.

[44] V. M. Ingram, "Abnormal human haemoglobins. III the chemical difference between normal and sickle cell haemoglobins," *Biochimica et Biophysica Acta*, vol. 36, no. 2, pp. 402–411, 1959.

[45] A. Gabriel and J. Przybylski, "Sickle-cell anemia: a look at global haplotype distribution," *Nature Education*, vol. 3, no. 3, pp. 2–12, 2010.

[46] J. Okpuzor, O. Adebesin, H. Ogbunugafor, and I. Amadi, "The potential of medicinal plants in sickle cell disease control: a review," *International Journal of Biomedical and Health Sciences*, vol. 4, no. 2, pp. 47–55, 2008.

[47] V. R. Mason, "Sickle cell anemia," *Journal of the American Medical Association*, vol. 79, no. 14, pp. 1318–1320, 1922.

[48] "Sickle Cell Disease: History And Origin," The Internet Journal of Haematology 1 (2), 2011, http://www.ispub.com/ostia/index.php?xmlFilePath=journals/ijhe/vol1n2/sickle.xml.

[49] "From 1918 Autopsy, A First Glimpse of Sickle Cell - and a Warning," http://www.wired.com/wiredscience/2010/11/from-a-1918-autopsy-a-first-glimpse-of-sickle-cell-%E2%80%94%C2%A0and-a-warning.

[50] D. J. Weatherall and J. B. Clegg, "Inherited haemoglobin disorders: an increasing global health problem," *Bulletin of the World Health Organization*, vol. 79, no. 8, pp. 704–712, 2001.

[51] U. A. Ndefo, A. E. Maxwell, H. Nguyen, and T. L. Chiobi, "Pharmacological management of sickle cell disease," *P and T*, vol. 33, no. 4, pp. 238–243, 2008.

[52] M. K. Safo, O. Abdulmalik, R. Danso-Danquah et al., "Structural basis for the potent antisickling effect of a novel class of five-membered heterocyclic aldehydic compounds," *Journal of Medicinal Chemistry*, vol. 47, no. 19, pp. 4665–4676, 2004.

[53] J. A. Walder, R. H. Zaugg, R. S. Iwaoka, W. G. Watkin, and I. M. Klotz, "Alternative aspirins as antisickling agents: acetyl-3,5-dibromosalicylic acid," *Proceedings of the National Academy of Sciences of the United States of America*, vol. 74, no. 12, pp. 5499–5503, 1977.

[54] D. J. Abraham, A. S. Mehanna, F. C. Wireko, J. Whitney, R. P. Thomas, and E. P. Orringer, "Vanillin, a potential agent for the treatment of sickle cell anemia," *Blood*, vol. 77, no. 6, pp. 1334–1341, 1991.

[55] I. N. Nnamani, G. S. Joshi, R. Danso-Danquah et al., "Pyridyl derivatives of benzaldehyde as potential antisickling agents," *Chemistry and Biodiversity*, vol. 5, no. 9, pp. 1762–1769, 2008.

[56] "Ion Channels: structure and function," 2011, http://www.whatislife.com/reader/channels/channels.html.

[57] R. Vennekens, G. Owsianik, and B. Nilius, "Vanilloid transient receptor potential cation channels: an overview," *Current Pharmaceutical Design*, vol. 14, no. 1, pp. 18–31, 2008.

[58] K. Venkatachalam and C. Montell, "TRP channels," *Annual Review of Biochemistry*, vol. 76, pp. 387–417, 2007.

[59] W. Loging, L. Harland, and B. Williams-Jones, "The vanilloid receptor TRPV1: 10 years from channel cloning to antagonist proof-of-concept," *Nature Reviews Drug Discovery*, vol. 6, no. 5, pp. 357–372, 2007.

[60] M. J. Caterina, M. A. Schumacher, M. Tominaga, T. A. Rosen, J. D. Levine, and D. Julius, "The capsaicin receptor: a heat-activated ion channel in the pain pathway," *Nature*, vol. 389, no. 6653, pp. 816–824, 1997.

[61] E. S. Graham, J. C. Ashton, and M. Glass, "Cannabinoid receptors: a brief history and 'what's hot'," *Frontiers in Bioscience*, vol. 14, no. 3, pp. 944–957, 2009.

[62] J. Gertsch, M. Leonti, S. Raduner et al., "Beta-caryophyllene is a dietary cannabinoid," *Proceedings of the National Academy of Sciences of the United States of America*, vol. 105, no. 26, pp. 9099–9104, 2008.

[63] W. Eya, *Nigeria: Sickle Cell—Lambo Presents Ciklavit at WHO*, Daily Champion, Lagos, Nigeria, 4th edition, 2006.

# 3

# Serum Iron Status of Under-Five Children with Sickle Cell Anaemia in Lagos, Nigeria

**S. O. Akodu, I. N. Diaku-Akinwumi, O. A. Kehinde, and O. F. Njokanma**

*Department of Paediatrics, Lagos State University Teaching Hospital, Ikeja 100001, Nigeria*

Correspondence should be addressed to S. O. Akodu; femiakodu@hotmail.com

Academic Editor: Aurelio Maggio

*Background.* Iron status in patients with sickle cell anaemia is a matter of continuing investigation. *Objective.* This paper aims to determine the serum iron status of under-five, sickle cell anaemia patients. *Methods.* The study spanned from December 2009 to February 2010 at the Consultant Outpatient Clinics involving 97 HbSS subjects and 97 age- and sex-matched HbAA controls. Biochemical iron status was assayed in subjects and controls. *Results.* Age range of the children was seven months to five years, with a mean of 30.6 (±15.97) months. Irrespective of gender, mean serum iron values were higher in HbAA controls than their HbSS counterparts but the observed difference was not significant ($P = 0.299$ and $0.111$, resp.). The mean total iron binding capacity values of males and females were also not significantly different for sickle cell anaemia subjects and controls ($P > 0.05$). Males and females with HbAA had significantly lower serum ferritin when compared with their HbSS counterparts. Irrespective of gender, mean transferrin saturation was lower in HbSS subjects but the difference was not statistically significant ($P > 0.05$). *Conclusion.* Children with sickle cell anaemia have higher serum ferritin than controls, implying relatively higher iron content in the reticuloendothelial cells.

## 1. Introduction

Sickle cell anaemia contributes significantly to morbidity and mortality among children in sub-Saharan Africa. Much is known about the disease presentation and end organ manifestation but the iron status in children with Sickle cell anaemia is still a matter of controversy [1].

In children with sickle cell anaemia, chronic haemolysis results in increased availability of iron directly from lysed red cells and also from increased absorption of iron from the gastrointestinal tract [2]. Additionally, the high load of iron provided by multiple blood transfusions [3, 4] would suggest that iron deficiency is unlikely in sickle cell anaemia. However, in some parts of the world, the frequency of blood transfusion among patients is now less as a result of improved management in recent years [5]. Reduced frequency of transfusion implies a reduction in sources of iron and, therefore, increased vulnerability to iron deficiency anaemia. This assertion is buttressed by a study in the USA which suggested that iron deficiency was commoner than expected in untransfused children with sickle cell anaemia [6]. In

addition, frequency and need for blood transfusion are not uniform for all children with sickle cell anaemia.

Ferritin is a high-molecular-weight protein that contains approximately 20% iron [7]. It occurs normally in almost all tissues of the body but especially in hepatocytes and reticuloendothelial cells, where it serves as an iron reserve. Ferritin is also present in the serum in minute amounts, where it appears to reflect iron stores in normal individuals. Ferritin plays a significant role in the absorption, storage, and release of iron. As the storage form of iron, ferritin remains in the body tissues until it is needed for erythropoiesis. When needed, the iron molecules are released from the apoferritin shell and bind to transferrin, the circulating plasma protein that transports iron to the erythropoietic cells. Transferrin is the plasma iron transport protein, which binds iron strongly at physiological pH [8]. Transferrin is generally only 25% to 30% saturated with iron [9].

In addition to serum ferritin and transferrin, serum iron and total iron binding capacity constitute indices of iron status in human subjects. The aim of the current study was to study all four biochemical markers in an effort to assess the iron status of children with sickle cell anaemia. It is expected that the findings would add to available information and assist in patient care.

## 2. Materials and Methods

The cross-sectional study was conducted between December 2009 and February 2010 among children with sickle cell anaemia attending the Sickle Cell Disorder Clinic and other Consultant Outpatient Clinics of the Department of Paediatrics, Lagos State University Teaching Hospital, Ikeja in Southwest Nigeria. The Lagos State University Teaching Hospital is an urban tertiary health centre. It is a major referral center serving the whole of Lagos State, which is a major point of entry into Nigeria from different parts of the world and the economic nerve centre of Nigeria.

Approval for the study was obtained from the Ethics Committee of the Lagos State University Teaching Hospital. Consecutive sickle cell anaemia patients aged five years and below, who came for routine follow-up clinic and have satisfied the study criteria, were recruited. Healthy controls were children with genotype "AA", from the General Outpatient and follow-up clinics, and healthy children attending other specialist clinics (e.g., Paediatric Dermatology Clinic) and were matched for age and sex. Written informed consent was obtained from parents of participants. The study sample size consisted of 194 children, 97 each with haemoglobin genotype SS and AA.

*Inclusion Criteria*

    (a) Aged six months to five years,

    (b) confirmed Hb SS by electrophoresis,

    (c) subjects in steady state, that is, absence of any crisis in the preceding four weeks and absence of any symptom or sign attributable to acute illness [10].

*Exclusion Criteria*

    (a) Denial of consent,

    (b) children on long-term transfusion therapy,

    (c) children who had received a blood transfusion within three months prior to the study,

    (d) children with a history of prematurity or low birth weight.

The inclusion criteria for the controls were the same as for subjects except that the haemoglobin genotype was AA and they had no symptoms or signs attributable to acute illness in the preceding four weeks. Also, the exclusion criteria for the controls were the same as for subjects except that the haemoglobin genotype was AA and they had received iron supplementation within three months prior to recruitment.

Five millilitres of blood were drawn from a convenient peripheral vein into plain tubes. The vacuum tubes were labelled and placed in a cool box containing ice-packs. The samples were protected from light at all times using sheets of black plastic. They were transported to the Research Laboratory of the Department of Paediatrics, Lagos State University College of Medicine.

After centrifugation the serum was separated and stored at minus 20°C until assay. The unsaturated or latent ironbinding capacity (UIBC) was measured by spectrophotometric techniques. Transferrin saturation (expressed as percentage of total iron binding capacity) was calculated using the formula: 100 X the serum iron concentration divided by total iron binding capacity [11]. Serum iron was measured using Iron Ferrozine test kit (Biosystems, Spain) while the TIBC was measured by using Iron/Total Iron Binding Capacity reagent set (TECO Diagnostics, USA). Serum ferritin was measured by using human ferritin enzyme immunoassay test kit (Diagnostic Automation, USA).

Social class was determined from occupation and educational attainment of parents using the scheme proposed by Oyedeji [12]. The subjects were classified into one of five classes (I–V) in descending order of social privilege. Study subjects were then further stratified into upper (classes I and II), middle (class II), and lower (classes IV and V) socioeconomic groups. The data was analyzed using the Statistical Package for Social Science (SPSS) version 17.0. Level of significance was set at $P < 0.05$.

## 3. Results

A total of 194 children, 97 each with genotype SS and AA, respectively, were recruited. The demographic characteristics of the study subjects are given in Table 1. Overall, the age of the subjects ranged from seven months to sixty months with a mean of 30.61 (±15.97) months: 32.05 ± 16.12 months and 29.18 ± 15.77 months for SS subjects and AA controls, respectively (Mann-Whitney $U = 4143.50$, $P = 0.151$). The median age was 25.00 months and 26.00 months in SS subjects and AA controls, respectively. Ninety-six (49.5%) of the study subjects belonged to the upper socioeconomic strata (socioeconomic indices I and II), while 34.5% and 16.0% belong to the middle (socioeconomic index III) and lower (socioeconomic index IV and V) socioeconomic strata, respectively.

*3.1. Serum Iron, Serum Ferritin, Total Iron Binding Capacity, and Transferrin Saturation Profile of Study Subjects.* Comparisons of serum iron, serum ferritin, total iron binding capacity (TIBC), and transferrin saturation between SS subjects and AA controls are shown in Table 2. In both males and females, the mean serum iron values were higher among haemoglobin genotype AA controls than their SS counterparts but the observed difference was not significant ($P = 0.872$ and 0.166 for males and females, resp.). The mean TIBC values of males and females were also not significantly different for Hb AA subjects and their counterparts with Hb SS ($P > 0.05$).

Males and females with haemoglobin genotype AA had significantly lower serum ferritin when compared with their haemoglobin genotype SS counterparts ($P = 0.000$ for each gender). Irrespective of gender, the mean serum iron, mean serum ferritin TIBC and transferrin saturation was lower in subjects without history of blood transfusion prior

TABLE 1: Demographic characteristics of the study population.

| Characteristics | AA | SS | ALL |
|---|---|---|---|
| Gender | | | |
| Male | 49 (50.5) | 49 (50.5) | 98 (50.5) |
| Female | 48 (49.5) | 48 (49.5) | 96 (49.5) |
| Age group (years) | | | |
| 0-1 | 15 (15.5) | 6 (6.2) | 21 (10.8) |
| >1-2 | 33 (34.0) | 42 (43.3) | 75 (38.7) |
| >2-3 | 17 (17.5) | 11 (11.3) | 28 (14.4) |
| >3-4 | 18 (18.6) | 15 (15.5) | 33 (17.0) |
| >4-5 | 14 (14.4) | 23 (23.7) | 37 (19.1) |
| Socioeconomic index | | | |
| I | 18 (18.6) | 13 (13.4) | 31 (16.0) |
| II | 36 (37.1) | 29 (29.9) | 65 (33.5) |
| III | 27 (27.8) | 40 (41.2) | 67 (34.5) |
| IV | 15 (15.5) | 14 (14.9) | 29 (14.9) |
| V | 1 (1.0) | 1 (1.1) | 2 (1.0) |

TABLE 2: Serum iron, serum ferritin, total iron binding capacity, and transferrin saturation profile of study subjects.

| | SS Mean (SD) | AA Mean (SD) | M-W $U$-value | $P$ value |
|---|---|---|---|---|
| Serum iron ($\mu$g/dL) | | | | |
| Males | 67.4 (34.54) | 78.3 (64.28) | 960.50 | 0.872 |
| Female | 67.3 (47.44) | 85.8 (63.36) | 569.50 | 0.166 |
| Male and female | 67.4 (40.78) | 81.6 (63.61) | 2999.50 | 0.264 |
| Serum ferritin (ng/dL) | | | | |
| Male | 170.4 (107.53) | 62.0 (61.91) | 353.00 | 0.000* |
| Female | 211.5 (97.48) | 47.4 (42.30) | 87.00 | 0.000* |
| Male and female | 189.9 (104.28) | 55.5 (54.20) | 823.50 | 0.000* |
| Total iron binding capacity ($\mu$g/dL) | | | | |
| Male | 253.2 (86.73) | 274.6 | 851.50 | 0.496 |
| Female | 265.4 (81.99) | 293.5 (95.70) | 568.50 | 0.226 |
| Male and female | 259.0 (84.16) | 283.1 | 2817.00 | 0.18 |
| Transferrin saturation (%) | | | | |
| Male | 27.0 (12.14) | 29.1 (17.37) | 918.00 | 0.911 |
| Female | 24.9 (13.40) | 28.5 (16.55) | 614.00 | 0.474 |
| Male and female | 26.0 (12.70) | 28.8 (16.91) | 3089.50 | 0.697 |

M-W: Mann Whitney.
*Statistically significant.

to commencement of study but the difference was not statistically significant ($P > 0.05$).

Sixty-four of study subjects with haemoglobin genotype SS have never had blood transfusion prior to commencement of the study. Ten of the thirty-three sickle cell anaemia subjects who have a history of previous blood transfusions reported two or more transfusion episodes (nine had two episodes of previous blood transfusions while one reported blood transfusions on three different occasions). Comparisons of serum iron, serum ferritin, total iron binding capacity (TIBC), and transferrin saturation between sickle cell anaemia patients with past history of blood transfusion and those who have never been transfused are shown in Table 3. Irrespective of gender, the mean serum iron, mean

serum ferritin, TIBC, and transferrin saturation were lower in subjects with history of blood transfusion prior to commencement of study but the difference was not statistically significant ($P > 0.05$).

3.2. Comparison of Serum Ferritin and Transferrin Saturation between Sickle Cell Anaemia Patients with Past History of Blood Transfusion and Those Who Have Never Been Transfused. Table 4 shows the comparison of criteria for diagnosing iron deficiency among children with sickle cell anaemia with previous history of blood transfusion prior to commencement of study. The diagnosis of iron deficiency was established based on the following criteria: transferrin

TABLE 3: Serum iron, serum ferritin, total iron binding capacity, and transferrin saturation profile of sickle cell anaemia subjects according to history of blood transfusion.

| Variable | Past history of blood transfusion | | M-W $U$-Value | $P$ value |
| --- | --- | --- | --- | --- |
| | Yes Mean (SD) | No Mean (SD) | | |
| Serum iron ($\mu$g/dL) | 77.27 (48.28) | 62.08 (35.62) | 509.50 | 0.156 |
| Serum ferritin (ng/dL) | 202.85 (100.94) | 183.14 (106.35) | 574.00 | 0.045 |
| Total iron binding capacity ($\mu$g/dL) | 279.50 (97.00) | 248.69 (75.98) | 432.00 | 0.086 |
| Transferrin saturation (%) | 27.77 (13.33) | 25.11 (12.40) | 498.00 | 0.351 |

M-W: Mann Whitney.

TABLE 4: Serum ferritin and transferrin in subjects with sickle cell anaemia according to past history of blood transfusion.

| Variable | Past history of blood transfusion | | Total | $P$ value |
| --- | --- | --- | --- | --- |
| | Yes | No | | |
| Serum iron ($\mu$g/dL) | | | | 0.519[+] |
| <25 | 0 (0.0) | 3 (100.0) | 3 (100.0) | |
| ≥25 | 33 (35.1) | 61 (64.9) | 94 (100.0) | |
| Total | **33 (34.0)** | **64 (66.0)** | **97** | |
| Transferrin saturation (%) | | | | 0.613 |
| <16 | 6 (28.6) | 15 (71.4) | 21 (100.0) | |
| ≥16 | 27 (35.6) | 49 (64.4) | 76 (100.0) | |
| Total | **33 (34.0)** | **64 (66.0)** | **97** | |

Values in parenthesis are % of column total.
[+]Chi-square test ($\chi^2$).

saturation (Ts) < 16% [13, 14] or serum ferritin (SF) < 25 ng/dL [13, 14]. All the sickle cell anaemia subjects with serum ferritin <25 ng/dL reported no past history of blood transfusion while two-thirds of the sickle cell anaemia subjects with serum ferritin ≥25 ng/dL reported no past history of blood transfusion. Similarly, almost two-thirds and three-quarters of subjects with haemoglobin genotype SS with transferrin saturation ≥16% and <16%, respectively, had no blood transfusion prior to commencement of the study. However, these observed differences were not significant ($P$ = 0.864, $P$ = 0.085 for serum ferritin and transferrin saturation, resp.).

*3.3. Haemoglobin Concentration Distribution of Study Subjects.* The comparison of the mean haemoglobin concentration values between HbSS subjects and HbAA controls is shown in Table 5. Overall, the mean haemoglobin concentration was significantly higher among HbAA controls than their counterparts with sickle cell anaemia. This pattern was observed at all age groups except subjects >2 years to 3 years.

## 4. Discussion

Subjects with haemoglobin genotype SS had a somewhat lower mean serum iron concentration than haemoglobin genotype AA controls. This finding is consistent with that

of Jeyakumar et al. [13] in Ibadan, Nigeria. Serum iron concentration is a balance between intake on the one hand and excretion as well as increased utilization on the other. Since there is no empirical reason to believe that HbSS subjects had lower dietary intake of iron, attention will have to be focused on excretion. Thus it is attractive to agree with Jeyakumar et al. [13] that sickle cell anaemia patients lose excessive amounts of iron. The explanation may be found in the study by Koduri [14] in which it was stated that one-third of the haemolysis in sickle cell anaemia subjects takes place in the intravascular space and is associated with excessive urinary loss of iron. As far as the current study is concerned, however, these explanations remain conjectural because urinary loss of iron was not investigated.

The mean serum ferritin was significantly higher among SS subjects than AA controls. Serum ferritin is known to reflect mainly reticuloendothelial iron stores [5]. It is considered to be a sensitive indicator of body iron stores and thus elevated serum ferritin concentrations may reflect possible high body iron stores. A higher value of serum ferritin in children with sickle cell anaemia may be due to presence of increased iron in the reticuloendothelial cells resulting from the excessive breakdown of haemoglobin.

In absolute terms, the mean serum ferritin value of less than 220 $\mu$g/L in our HbSS subjects was lower than 367 $\mu$g/L reported by Hussain et al. [5] in London. The observed

TABLE 5: Haemoglobin concentration distribution of study subjects.

| Age group (years) | AA<br>Mean (SD) | SS<br>Mean (SD) | $t$-value | $P$ value |
| --- | --- | --- | --- | --- |
| 0-1 | 8.79 (1.24) | 6.62 (1.65) | 3.125 | 0.006* |
| >1-2 | 9.73 (2.21) | 6.60 (1.05) | 7.863 | 0.000* |
| >2-3 | 9.38 (0.80) | 7.72 (3.30) | 2.014 | 0.054 |
| >3-4 | 9.84 (1.05) | 6.55 (1.56) | 7.217 | 0.000* |
| >4-5 | 10.51 (0.90) | 6.85 (1.34) | 9.006 | 0.000* |
| ALL | 9.66 (1.58) | 6.79 (1.64) | 12.279 | 0.000* |

*Statistically significant.

difference is possibly an effect of age range of study subjects. It has been shown that serum ferritin levels may be modified by age [15]. Even within the relatively narrow age range involved in the current study, some positive correlation was demonstrated between age and serum ferritin levels. Thus the study by Hussain et al. [5] which included much older children (up to 15 years) would expectedly report higher ferritin levels. Serum ferritin may also be affected by genetic factors [16]. The current study recruited black children with sickle cell anaemia while Hussain et al. [5] recruited white children with conceivably different genetic composition. In addition, factors including overall nutrition could potentially affect ferritin levels.

In the present study, high serum ferritin level was accompanied by reduced serum iron in sickle cell anaemia subjects. The reason for this pattern of results was beyond the scope of the present study. It is however known that high iron stores as implied from high serum ferritin are associated with increased release of hepcidin which in turn leads to reduced serum iron [17]. Hepcidin is a 25 amino acid peptide made by hepatocytes [18]. Its production is enhanced by high iron stores and inflammation [17, 18]. It is, therefore, also attractive to speculate that sickle cell anaemia, being a state of chronic inflammation [19], would be associated with elevated hepcidin levels with consequent lower serum iron.

The TIBC measures the availability of iron binding sites [20]. Extracellular iron is transported in the body bound to transferrin, which is the primary iron-transport protein [20]. Hence, TIBC indirectly measures transferrin levels, which increase as stored iron decreases [20]. The present study showed that the mean TIBC was higher among AA controls than in SS subjects. The possible explanation may be the presence of high body iron stores among subjects with sickle cell anaemia revealed by higher serum ferritin values.

Similarly, we observed higher mean transferrin saturation among AA controls than in SS subjects irrespective of gender. Further, both haemoglobin SS subjects and haemoglobin AA controls had mean values within the normal range of 25% to 30% [21] but with haemoglobin SS in the lower band. The finding is consistent with the observation of slightly lower serum concentration of iron in sickle cell anaemia subjects in the current study. The explanation for the higher mean transferrin saturation among HbAA controls is not farfetched. The transferrin saturation is a measure of amount of iron bound to the protein transferrin and reflects iron transport. As the body iron stores are depleted, the transferrin saturation rises. It has been revealed in the current study that children with sickle cell anaemia have higher body iron stores potentially from increased red cell turnover and from blood transfusions.

Our centre does not have a chronic transfusion programme for sickle cell anaemia patients. Rather, blood transfusion is offered as needed when anaemia is severe. In consequence, the number of patients who had ever received transfusions was relatively small. Even then, very few of them had received enough units of blood transfusion to potentially affect their iron status. The ability of the study to test the influence of blood transfusion was therefore highly restricted.

Overall, the mean serum ferritin was significantly higher among children with sickle cell anaemia compared to haemoglobin AA controls which may be due to presence of increased iron in the reticuloendothelial cells because of the excessive breakdown of haemoglobin. Age had poor linear relationship with the transferrin saturation and serum ferritin. Further studies are needed to further explore the additional factors such as body composition that may influence iron status in children with sickle cell anaemia.

## Conflict of Interests

The authors declare that there is no conflict of interests regarding the publication of this paper.

## Authors' Contribution

The study was conceived by all the authors. Data was collected by all authors except O. A. Kehinde. S. O. Akodu and O. F. Njokanma analyzed the data while S. O. Akodu wrote the initial draft of the paper. All authors reviewed and approved the final paper for submission.

## References

[1] D. Mohanty, M. B. Mukherjee, R. B. Colah et al., "Iron deficiency anaemia in sickle cell disorders in India," *Indian Journal of Medical Research*, vol. 127, no. 4, pp. 366–369, 2008.

[2] M. E. Erlandson, B. Walden, G. Stern, M. W. Hilgartner, J. Wehman, and C. H. Smith, "Studies on congenital hemolytic syndromes, IV. Gastrointestinal absorption of iron," *Blood*, vol. 19, pp. 359–378, 1962.

[3] R. T. O'Brien, "Iron burden in sickle cell anaemia," *Journal of Pediatrics*, vol. 92, pp. 579–582, 1978.

[4] S. K. Ballas, "Iron overload is a determinant of morbidity and mortality in adult patients with sickle cell disease," *Seminars in Hematology*, vol. 38, no. 1, pp. 30–36, 2001.

[5] M. A. M. Hussain, L. R. Davis, M. Laulicht, and A. V. Hoffbrand, "Value of serum ferritin estimation in sickle cell anaemia," *Archives of Disease in Childhood*, vol. 53, no. 4, pp. 319–321, 1978.

[6] E. Vichinsky, K. Kleman, S. Embury, and B. Lubin, "The diagnosis of iron deficiency anemia in sickle cell disease," *Blood*, vol. 58, no. 5, pp. 963–968, 1981.

[7] G. M. Addison, M. R. Beamish, C. N. Hales, M. Hodgkins, A. Jacobs, and P. Llewellin, "An immunoradiometric assay for ferritin in the serum of normal subjects and patients with iron deficiency and iron overload," *Journal of Clinical Pathology*, vol. 25, no. 4, pp. 326–329, 1972.

[8] P. Ponka, "Cellular iron metabolism," *Kidney International, Supplement*, vol. 55, no. 69, pp. S2–S11, 1999.

[9] D. M. De Silva, C. C. Askwith, and J. Kaplan, "Molecular mechanisms of iron uptake in eukaryotes," *Physiological Reviews*, vol. 76, no. 1, pp. 31–47, 1996.

[10] O. Awotua-Efebo, E. A. Alikor, and K. E. Nkanginieme, "Malaria parasite density and splenic status by ultrasonography in stable sickle-cell anaemia (HbSS) children," *Nigerian Journal of Medicine*, vol. 13, no. 1, pp. 40–43, 2004.

[11] T. Higgins, E. Beutler, and B. T. Doumas, "Haemoglobin, iron and bilirubin," in *Textbook of Clinical Chemistry and Molecular Diagnostics*, C. A. Burtis, E. R. Ashwood, and D. E. Bruns, Eds., pp. 1186–1191, Elsevier, St. Louis, Mo, USA, 4th edition, 2006.

[12] G. A. Oyedeji, "Socio-economic and cultural background of hospitalized children in Ilesha," *Nigerian Journal of Paediatrics*, vol. 12, pp. 111–117, 1985.

[13] L. H. Jeyakumar, E. O. Akpanyung, A. A. Akinyemi, and G. O. Emerole, "An investigation into the iron status of children with sickle-cell disease in Western Nigeria," *Journal of Tropical Pediatrics*, vol. 33, no. 6, pp. 326–328, 1987.

[14] P. R. Koduri, "Iron in sickle cell disease: a review why less is better," *American Journal of Hematology*, vol. 73, no. 1, pp. 59–63, 2003.

[15] B. Mangosongo, F. M. Kalokola, E. K. Munubhi, and R. Mpembeni, "Iron deficiency in sickle cell anaemia patients in Dar es Salaam," *Tanzania Medical Journal*, vol. 19, pp. 5–8, 2004.

[16] J. L. Beard, "Iron biology in immune function, muscle metabolism and neuronal functioning," *Journal of Nutrition*, vol. 131, no. 2, pp. 568–579, 2001.

[17] E. Rossi, "Hepcidin—the iron regulatory hormone," *The Clinical Biochemist*, vol. 26, no. 3, pp. 47–49, 2005.

[18] T. Ganz, "Hepcidin, a key regulator of iron metabolism and mediator of anemia of inflammation," *Blood*, vol. 102, no. 3, pp. 783–788, 2003.

[19] O. S. Platt, "Sickle cell anemia as an inflammatory disease," *Journal of Clinical Investigation*, vol. 106, no. 3, pp. 337–338, 2000.

[20] A. C. Wu, L. Lesperance, and H. Bernstein, "Screening for iron deficiency," *Pediatrics in Review/American Academy of Pediatrics*, vol. 23, no. 5, pp. 171–178, 2002.

[21] R. T. Lagua and V. S. Claudio, "Dictionary terms," in *Textbook of Nutrition and Diet Therapy Reference Dictionary*, pp. 1–376, Chapman and Hall, New York, NY, USA, 4th edition, 1996.

# 4

# Role of Calcium in Phosphatidylserine Externalisation in Red Blood Cells from Sickle Cell Patients

**Erwin Weiss,[1] David Charles Rees,[2] and John Stanley Gibson[1]**

[1] Department of Veterinary Medicine, University of Cambridge, Madingley Road, Cambridge CB3 0ES, UK
[2] Department of Molecular Haematology, King's College School of Medicine, London SE5 9RS, UK

Correspondence should be addressed to John Stanley Gibson, jsg1001@cam.ac.uk

Academic Editor: Ferreira Costa

Phosphatidylserine exposure occurs in red blood cells (RBCs) from sickle cell disease (SCD) patients and is increased by deoxygenation. The mechanisms responsible remain unclear. RBCs from SCD patients also have elevated cation permeability, and, in particular, a deoxygenation-induced cation conductance which mediates $Ca^{2+}$ entry, providing an obvious link with phosphatidylserine exposure. The role of $Ca^{2+}$ was investigated using FITC-labelled annexin. Results confirmed high phosphatidylserine exposure in RBCs from SCD patients increasing upon deoxygenation. When deoxygenated, phosphatidylserine exposure was further elevated as extracellular $[Ca^{2+}]$ was increased. This effect was inhibited by dipyridamole, intracellular $Ca^{2+}$ chelation, and Gardos channel inhibition. Phosphatidylserine exposure was reduced in high $K^+$ saline. $Ca^{2+}$ levels required to elicit phosphatidylserine exposure were in the low micromolar range. Findings are consistent with $Ca^{2+}$ entry through the deoxygenation-induced pathway ($P_{sickle}$), activating the Gardos channel. $[Ca^{2+}]$ required for phosphatidylserine scrambling are in the range achievable *in vivo*.

## 1. Introduction

Patients with sickle cell disease (SCD) display a range of symptoms which include chronic anemia together with ischemic pain and organ damage [1]. The underlying cause is the presence in patients' red blood cells (RBCs) of the abnormal hemoglobin, HbS [2]. HbS polymerises into rigid rods on deoxygenation, changing RBC shape from biconcave disc into the characteristic sickle appearance [3]. RBC membrane permeability is markedly abnormal [4] whilst HbS is also unstable, representing an oxidative threat [5]. Altered behaviour of these HbS-containing RBCs (here termed HbS cells), other circulating cells, and the endothelium combine to reduce RBC lifespan (hence the anemia) and also result in microvascular occlusion (hence the ischemia) [6]. Although the exact pathogenesis remains unclear, an important feature is considered to be increased exposure of phosphatidylserine (PS) on the outer bilayer of the RBC membrane [7–10]. Externalised PS is prothrombotic, and also provides a potential adhesion site for both macrophages and activated endothelial cells, contributing to both reduced HbS cell lifespan and vascular occlusion [11–13].

Two membrane phospholipid transporters represent the major determinants of PS exposure in RBCs: the ATP-dependent aminophospholipid translocase (APLT or flippase) transports aminophospholipids (APs), including PS, from outer to inner leaflet, whilst the $Ca^{2+}$-dependent scramblase moves APs rapidly in both directions thus disrupting phospholipid asymmetry [14]. In normal RBCs, PS is largely confined to inner leaflet, through the dominant action of the flippase whilst the scramblase remains quiescent. A small, but variable, proportion of HbS cells from sickle cell patients, however, show exposure of PS ranging from about 2–10% [7, 9, 15, 16]. Both flippase inhibition and activation of the scramblase are probably involved [17]. Flippase inhibition could follow oxidative stress [18, 19], whilst scramblase activation could be caused by raised intracellular $Ca^{2+}$ (e.g., [19, 20]) or other stimuli (e.g., [21]). The exact mechanisms, however, remain uncertain.

It is also well established that deoxygenation of HbS *in vitro* results in increased PS exposure [22, 23] but, again, the mechanism is not clear. Possibilities include disruption of the spectrin cytoskeleton [24], ATP depletion [25], decrease in intracellular $Mg^{2+}$ [26], and also a rise in intracellular $Ca^{2+}$

[20, 26]. In many reports concerning PS exposure, however, $Ca^{2+}$ is not controlled or is present at unphysiological levels, making it difficult to assess its role definitively. In addition, whilst a more recent study correlated PS exposure in HbS cells with flippase inhibition, rather than elevation of intracellular $Ca^{2+}$, the effects of deoxygenation were not determined [9].

Deoxygenation of HbS cells as well as causing HbS polymerisation and shape change, also activates a permeability pathway termed $P_{sickle}$ [4, 27]. $P_{sickle}$ is often described as a deoxygenation-induced cation conductance, apparently unique to HbS-containing red cells. A major importance of $P_{sickle}$ is its permeability to $Ca^{2+}$ [28, 29]. Although $Ca^{2+}$ entry via this pathway represents an obvious link between HbS polymerisation and the deoxygenation-induced PS exposure, estimates suggest that the magnitude to which $Ca^{2+}$ may be elevated is still relatively modest (around 100 nM) [29], and several orders of magnitude below that required for scramblase activation (around 100 $\mu$M is usually cited [20, 30–32]). The present work is aimed at assessing the role of $Ca^{2+}$ in PS exposure in RBCs from sickle cell patients.

## 2. Materials and Methods

*2.1. Blood.* Anonymised, discarded, routine blood samples (taken into the anticoagulant EDTA) were collected from individuals homozygous for HbS (HbSS genotype, $n = 62$) with approval from the local Ethics committee. After withdrawal, blood samples were kept refrigerated until used. (RBCs from HbSS individuals are here termed HbS cells).

*2.2. Salines and Chemicals.* HbS cells were washed into low (LK) or high potassium- (HK-) containing saline, comprising (in mM) NaCl 140, KCl 4, glucose 5, HEPES 10 for LK saline, and NaCl 55, KCl 90, glucose 5 and HEPES 10 for HK saline, all pH 7.4 at 37°C, with different extracellular $[Ca^{2+}]$s ($[Ca^{2+}]_o$s) as indicated. When required, inhibitors (clotrimazole, DIDS, and dipyridamole) were added from stock solutions in DMSO. In these experiments, DMSO (final concentration 0.5%) was also added to controls. To investigate the effect of $Ca^{2+}$ chelation, MAPTAM (5 $\mu$M; Calbiochem, UK) was loaded into RBCs (5% haematocrit) for 60 min at 37°C with added pyruvate (5 mM) to prevent inhibition of glycolysis [33]. Extracellular chelator was removed by washing once with saline. Control RBCs without chelator were handled in the same way. FITC-labelled annexin V was obtained from Becton-Dickinson (Oxford, UK) in aqueous stock solutions (final concentration 0.3 $\mu$g·mL$^{-1}$). The calmodulin inhibitor $N$-(6-aminohexyl)-5-chloro-1-naphthalene sulphonamide (W-7) and the calcium fluorophore fluo-4-AM came from Invitrogen; all other reagents were obtained from Sigma (Poole, UK).

*2.3. Control of $O_2$ Tension, Measurement of PS Exposure and Intracellular $Ca^{2+}$.* Salines and HbS cell suspensions were first equilibrated with humidified air (oxygenated) or $N_2$ (deoxygenated) in Eschweiler tonometers (Eschweiler, Kiel, Germany). They were then placed in 24-well plates ($10^8$ cells·mL$^{-1}$, depth 3 mm) at 37°C in humidified incubators flushed with room air or 1% $O_2$ (using a Galaxy-R oxygen incubator, RS Biotech, Irvine, UK) for 3–18 hours. After incubation, RBCs were treated with vanadate (1 mM) to inhibit flippase activity. They were then immediately harvested, washed once, and resuspended at a concentration of $5 \times 10^6$ cells·mL$^{-1}$ in binding annexin buffer (composition in mM: 145 NaCl, 2.5 CaCl$_2$, 10 HEPES, pH 7.4) and incubated for 15 min at room temperature with FITC-labelled annexin (0.3 $\mu$g·mL$^{-1}$). Unattached annexin was then removed by washing once followed by resuspension in 5-times the initial volume of ice-cold binding buffer, after which samples were placed on ice. Percentage of RBCs with PS exposed on their external membrane was then measured in the FL-1 channel of a fluorescence-activated flow cytometer (FACSCalibur, BD), in which negative fluorescent gate was set using cells exposed to FITC-labelled annexin but in the absence of $Ca^{2+}$ (which prevents annexin binding). PS exposure here refers to the percentage of RBCs which fluoresce more brightly than the negative gate. To alter intracellular $[Ca^{2+}]$, RBCs at 1% Hct were exposed to the calcium ionophore bromo-A23187 (1–6 $\mu$M), vanadate (1 mM), EDTA (2 mM), and different $[Ca^{2+}]_o$s for 30 min to achieve the requisite final $[Ca^{2+}]_o$ [34]. This was multiplied by the square of Donnan ratio, $r^2([H^+]_i/[H^+]_o)^2 = 2.05$ [35, 36], to calculate $[Ca^{2+}]_i$. After 30 min, RBCs were treated with $Co^{2+}$ (0.4 mM, to block A23187) after which they were processed for annexin-labelling, as above. Annexin was used to label PS because it is important to compare findings with extensive reports in the literature using this PS marker (e.g., [8, 19, 37–39]). Bromo-A23187 (in preference to A23187 *per se*) was used because it does not fluoresce. These experiments were carried out in LK or HK saline, composition as above except for the addition of 0.15 mM MgCl$_2$ to keep intracellular $[Mg^{2+}]$ at physiological levels. Finally, to show $Ca^{2+}$-loading of RBCs, cells were loaded with fluo-4-AM (30 min at 37°C, 5 $\mu$M; then washed once) with fluo-4 fluorescence also then measured in the FITC channel by FACS.

*2.4. Statistics.* Unless otherwise stated, data are presented as means ± S.E.M. for blood samples from $n$ patients. Statistical significance of any differences was tested using paired Student's $t$-test (with $P < .05$ taken as significant).

## 3. Results

*3.1. The Effect of $Ca^{2+}$ on PS Exposure.* PS exposure in HbS cell samples taken from SCD patients and immediately labelled with FITC-annexin ranged from 0.4 to 16.0% with a mean of 2.3 ± 0.5% ($n = 36$). The effect of different $[Ca^{2+}]_o$s (0.1, 0.5, 1.1, 2 and 5 mM) on the percentage of HbS cells showing PS exposure was then investigated. In oxygenated (20% $O_2$) HbS cells, PS exposure was lower and although the extent of exposure was augmented when RBCs were incubated at higher $[Ca^{2+}]_o$s, the effect was small and not significant (Figure 1). When cells were deoxygenated (1% $O_2$), PS exposure was always higher than that observed in oxygenated HbS cells. There was also a marked increase in

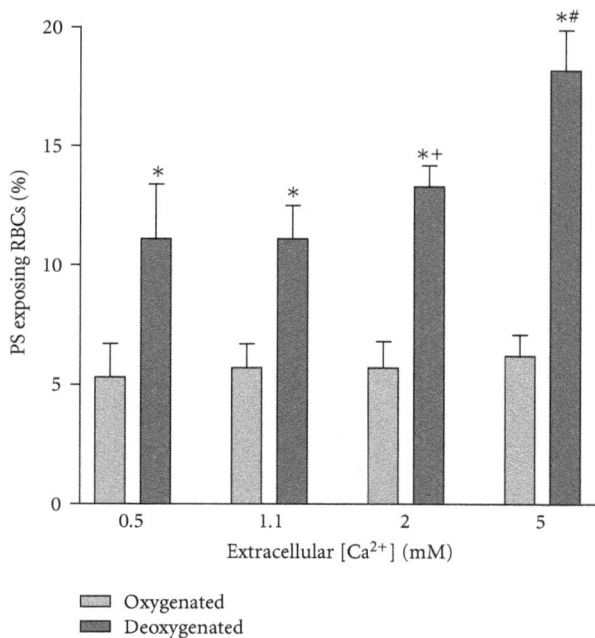

FIGURE 1: Effect of oxygen tension and extracellular $Ca^{2+}$ on phosphatidylserine (PS) exposure in red blood cells (RBCs) from sickle cell patients. RBCs were incubated for 18 hours at four extracellular $[Ca^{2+}]$'s (0.5, 1.1, 2.0 and 5.0 mM) after which they were labelled with FITC-annexin (as described in Section 2). Histograms representing mean percentage of positive RBCs $\pm$ S.E.M. for 5 different patients. *$P < .01$ deoxy compare to oxy; $^+P < .05$ cf 0.5 mM $Ca^{2+}$ deoxy; $^#P < .01$ cf 0.5 mM $Ca^{2+}$ deoxy.

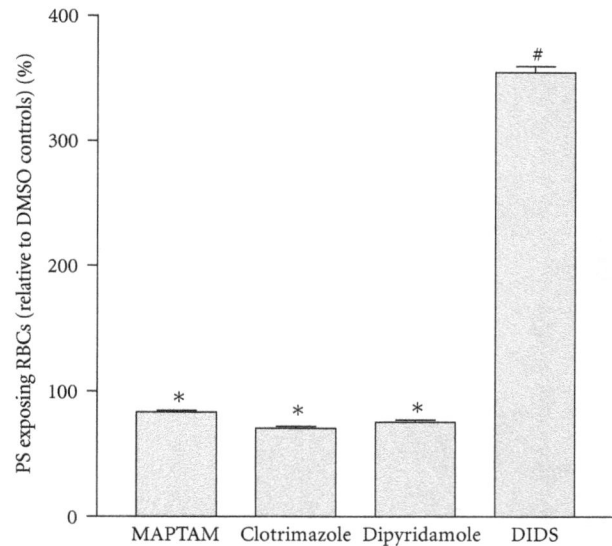

FIGURE 2: Effect of inhibitors on phosphatidylserine (PS) exposure in red blood cells (RBCs) from sickle cell patients. RBCs were incubated under deoxygenated conditions (1% $O_2$) for 3 hours (5 mM extracellular $[Ca^{2+}]$) after which they were labelled with FITC-annexin. Four conditions (all with 0.5% DMSO) are shown: MAPTAM-treated RBCs (loaded with 5 $\mu$M MAPTAM prior to deoxygenation), clotrimazole (10 $\mu$M), dipyridamole (50 $\mu$M), and DIDS (50 $\mu$M). Results are presented as percentage PS exposing RBCs relative to control RBCs exposed to 0.5% DMSO only. Histograms represent means $\pm$ S.E.M. ($n = 3$). *$P < .01$ and $^#P < .0001$ cf DMSO controls.

PS at the higher $[Ca^{2+}]_o$s (Figure 1). This effect was present within 30 min, with longer incubation periods increasing the effect. To determine whether $Ca^{2+}$ was acting extracellularly or intracellularly, HbS cells were loaded with the $Ca^{2+}$ chelator MAPTAM prior to deoxygenation (Figure 2). Over a 3 hour period, MAPTAM decreased the percentage of positive HbS cells ($P < .01$). This inhibitory effect did not persist over an 18 hour incubation, probably because the available cytoplasmic MAPTA becomes saturated with $Ca^{2+}$.

### 3.2. Effect of Partial $P_{sickle}$ Inhibitors on PS Exposure.

Although there are no specific inhibitors of $P_{sickle}$, dipyridamole is partially effective [40]. When present during deoxygenation, dipyridamole (50 $\mu$M) reduced PS exposure in deoxygenated HbS cells (Figure 2; $P < .01$), consistent with $Ca^{2+}$ entry via $P_{sickle}$ stimulating exposure. DIDS, although better known as a band 3 inhibitor, is also a partial $P_{sickle}$ inhibitor [41]. Addition of DIDS (50 $\mu$M), however, produced a marked increase in PS exposing RBCs with percentage of positive RBCs increasing several folds (Figure 2; $P < .01$). When DIDS was added to RBCs from normal HbAA individuals, PS exposure was also similarly increased: to $95.0 \pm 0.3\%$ in oxygenated conditions, and to $98.7 \pm 0.1\%$ in deoxygenated cells (both means $\pm$ S.E.M., $n = 3$). These findings suggest that annexin binding was caused

by DIDS reacting with its target on the RBC membrane. HbS cells exposed to DIDS, but not subsequently treated with FITC-annexin, did not fluoresce (e.g., 0% DIDS-treated without FITC-annexin cf 50% DIDS-treated with annexin), indicating that the high values were not due to fluorescence from DIDS itself.

### 3.3. PS Exposure and Red Cell Shrinkage.

Elevated intracellular $Ca^{2+}$ activates the Gardos channel and leads to $K^+$ loss with $Cl^-$ following through separate $Cl^-$ channels [4]. PS exposure could therefore be secondary to the ensuing cell shrinkage [37]. To investigate this possibility, HbS cells were suspended in high $K^+$-containing saline (90 mM) to remove any gradient for $K^+$ efflux. The deoxygenation-induced increase in PS exposure was abolished (Figure 3), with values reduced to those observed in oxygenated samples ($P < .001$ deoxy LK cf oxy LK; N.S. deoxy HK cf oxy LK). An estimate of RBC size is provided by FACS forward scatter measurement. Forward scatter was $487 \pm 8$ (means $\pm$ S.E.M., $n = 3$) in oxygenated LK saline, falling to $439 \pm 4$ in deoxygenated LK saline ($P < .005$). In deoxygenated HK saline a value of $497 \pm 3$ was obtained (N.S. cf. oxygenated LK saline). PS exposure following deoxygenation in LK saline was therefore accompanied by cell shrinkage. This was not observed during deoxygenation in high $K^+$ saline. A second method of inhibiting the Gardos channel, treatment with

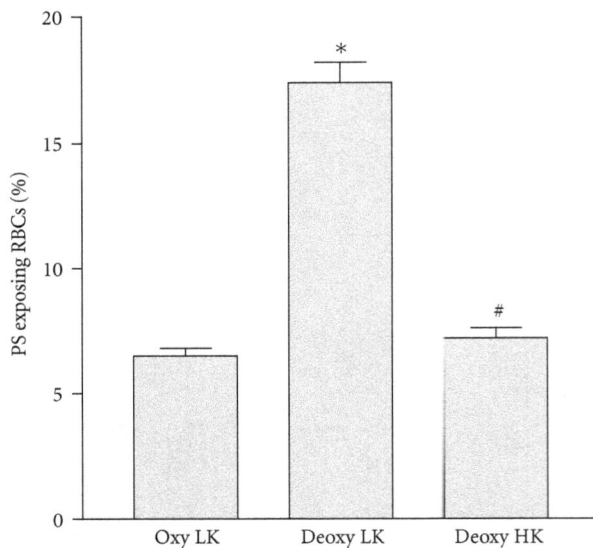

FIGURE 3: Effect of extracellular $K^+$ on phosphatidylserine (PS) exposure in red blood cells (RBCs) from sickle cell patients. RBCs were incubated for 18 hours with extracellular $[Ca^{2+}]$ of 5 mM under oxygenated (20% $O_2$) or deoxygenated (1% $O_2$) conditions in either low $K^+$-containing (extracellular $[K^+]$ of 5 mM) saline or high $K^+$-containing (90 mM $[K^+]$) saline. Histograms represent means ± S.E.M. ($n = 3$). *$P < .001$ compare to LK oxy; #N.S. cf. LK oxy.

clotrimazole (10 $\mu$M), was also tested. In this case, however, PS exposure was only partially prevented (Figure 2; $P < .01$).

### 3.4. PS Exposure and Direct Manipulation of Intracellular $[Ca^{2+}]$.

Treatment of RBCs with the divalent cation ionophore bromo-A23187 was used to alter intracellular $[Ca^{2+}]$ directly [34, 35]. RBCs were initially treated with vanadate (1 mM), to inhibit both the plasma membrane $Ca^{2+}$ pump and also the flippase. Following 30 min incubation with bromo-A23187 to alter $[Ca^{2+}]_i$, $Co^{2+}$ (0.4 mM) was then added to block $Ca^{2+}$ permeability via A23187 thereby keeping intracellular $[Ca^{2+}]$ constant during annexin labelling (for which 2.5 mM extracellular $[Ca^{2+}]$ is required). Results are shown in Figure 4. PS exposure is elicited as $[Ca^{2+}]_i$ increased above about 600 nM. A sigmoidal dependence of PS exposure with $[Ca^{2+}]$ was then apparent with an $EC_{50}$ of $1.31 \pm 0.84$ $\mu$M ($n = 6$). Peak exposures varied from 16–46%, mean $28 \pm 5$ ($n = 6$) with a plateau reached at about 10 $\mu$M and without further change at higher $[Ca^{2+}]_i$s ($[Ca^{2+}]$s up to 600 $\mu$M were tested).

### 3.5. Modulation of PS Exposure.

In the preceding section, although high affinity $Ca^{2+}$-induced scrambling was present, it was noticeable that nevertheless only a minority of all RBCs stained positively for PS using FITC-annexin—as is also found in many literature reports, for example, [39]. That $Ca^{2+}$ loading was complete and homogeneous was first ascertained using intracellular fluo-4 (Figure 5). It is apparent that the majority of RBCs were ($98 \pm 1$%, $n = 3$) $Ca^{2+}$-loaded. Uneven $Ca^{2+}$ loading can therefore be

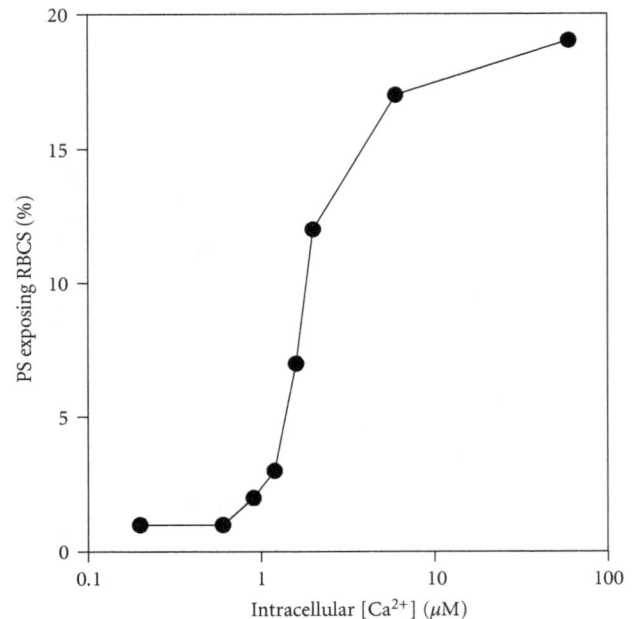

FIGURE 4: Effect of manipulation of intracellular $Ca^{2+}$ on phosphatidylserine (PS) exposure in red blood cells (RBCs) from sickle cell patients. RBCs were first treated with vanadate (1 mM) to inhibit the plasma membrane $Ca^{2+}$ pump and also the aminophospholipid translocase (flippase) before addition of bromo-A23187 (1.2 $\mu$M, 1% haematocrit) and requisite extracellular $[Ca^{2+}]$s for 30 min. They were then treated with $Co^{2+}$ (0.4 mM) before labelling with FITC-annexin. Intracellular $[Ca^{2+}]$ is calculated from extracellular $[Ca^{2+}] \times r^2$, where $r^2$ was taken as 2.05 [36]. Results presented are from a single experiment representative of 5 others.

discounted. As $K^+$ has been reported to inhibit PS scrambling [42], the effect of 30 min incubation in LK saline compared to HK was determined in the presence of bromo-A23187 and different $[Ca^{2+}]$. LK saline was found to increase the percentage of positive cells (Figure 6(a)), an effect again partially inhibited by clotrimazole (10 $\mu$M) which, for example, reduced percentage of positive cells from 44% to 28% at 10 $\mu$M $Ca^{2+}$. Finally, the effect of the calmodulin inhibitor W-7 was tested (Figure 6(b)). In this case, the percentage of positive RBCs increased. It was noticeable, however, that in all these manoeuvres, $Ca^{2+}$ affinity was unaffected (Figure 6).

## 4. Discussion

Whilst it is well known that RBCs from SCD patients show elevated levels of PS exposure and that these are increased upon deoxygenation, the mechanism is not clear. The present results explore more fully that the role of $Ca^{2+}$. $Ca^{2+}$ concentrations required for scrambling is considerably lower than previously appreciated. The $Ca^{2+}$ affinity of the scrambling process is not dissimilar to that associated with inhibition of flippase activity or activation of the $Ca^{2+}$-activated $K^+$ channel (Gardos channel). This important finding suggests coordination of these eryptotic events. Results also implicate a role for RBC shrinkage and shape change.

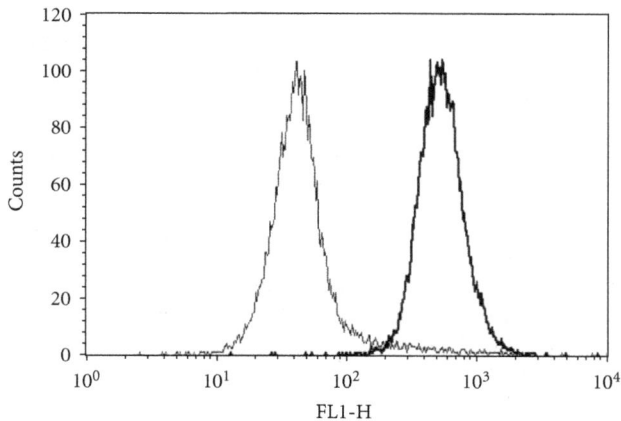

FIGURE 5: $Ca^{2+}$ loading of red blood cells (RBCs) from sickle cell patients. RBCs were loaded with the $Ca^{2+}$ fluorophore fluo-4 (see Methods). They were then incubated for 30 min in the absence (left—thin line) or presence (right—thick line) of bromo-A23187 at an extracellular $[Ca^{2+}]$ of 1 $\mu M$. Results are presented as histogram of fluorescence of a single experiment representative of 3.

### 4.1. Role of $Ca^{2+}$ and $P_{sickle}$ on PS Exposure.

Altering extracellular $Ca^{2+}$ levels had little effect on PS exposure in oxygenated HbS cells. Under deoxygenated conditions, however, PS exposure increased with $[Ca^{2+}]_o$. This effect was partially inhibited by dipyridamole [40] and by intracellular $Ca^{2+}$ chelation with MAPTAM treatment [34]. These findings are consistent with $Ca^{2+}$ entering via the deoxygenation-induced pathway $P_{sickle}$ [4, 27] and acting intracellularly. Intracellular $Ca^{2+}$ can have several actions. First, it will activate the Gardos channel leading to RBC shrinkage [43]. Second, it may stimulate the $Ca^{2+}$-dependent scramblase whilst inhibiting the ATP-dependent flippase [14]. Third, it may stimulate cysteine proteases [44]. Any of these events may lead to PS exposure [21]. Several manoeuvres were tested to separate these possibilities. The most effective way of inhibiting PS exposure was incubation in high $K^+$ saline. Removal of the electrochemical gradient for $K^+$ efflux abolished the deoxygenation-induced increase in PS exposure. The Gardos channel inhibitor clotrimazole also partially inhibited PS exposure. Findings are consistent with the hypothesis that activation of $P_{sickle}$, by deoxygenation mediates $Ca^{2+}$ entry, elevating $[Ca^{2+}]_i$ which then promotes PS exposure by Gardos channel activation, loss of intracellular solutes, and red cell shrinkage. Importantly, high $K^+$ salines were effective over all incubation times (up to 18 hours). Shrinkage has been shown previously to stimulate PS exposure in both normal RBCs and HbS cells [37, 45] and would appear to be involved in deoxygenation-induced PS exposure in sickle cells.

### 4.2. $Ca^{2+}$ Dependence of PS Exposure.

A major aim of this work was to determine unequivocally the intracellular $Ca^{2+}$ required to elicit PS exposure in HbS cells. This was investigated using RBCs loaded with different $[Ca^{2+}]$s using bromo-A23187. RBCs were first treated with vanadate (to inhibit both the plasma membrane $Ca^{2+}$ pump and

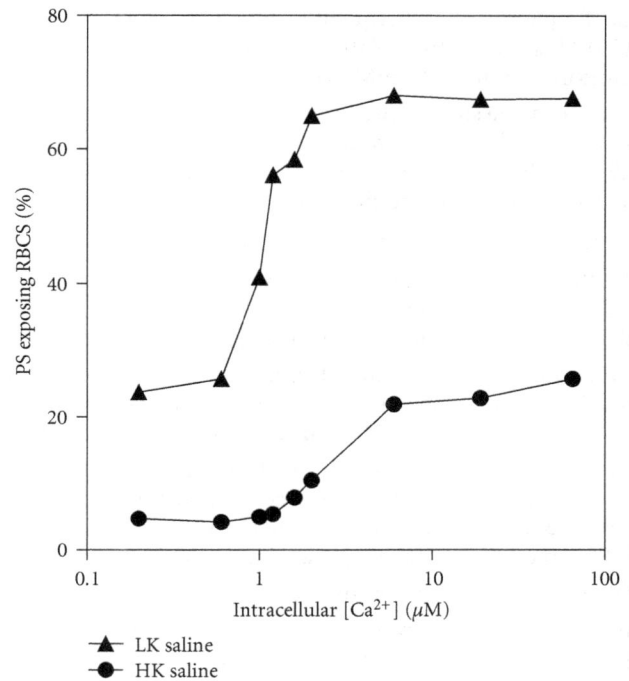

(a)

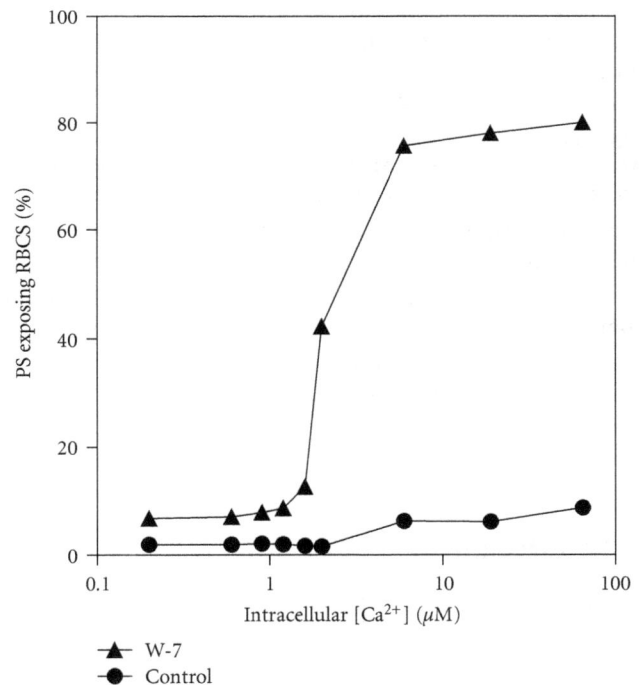

(b)

FIGURE 6: Effect of $K^+$ and calmodulin inhibition on $Ca^{2+}$-induced exposure of phosphatidylserine (PS) in red blood cells (RBCs) from sickle cell patients. Experimental details were as described in the legend to Figure 4, except that in (a) where incubation was carried out in either high $K^+$-(HK, $K^+$ = 90 mM) or low $K^+$-containing saline (LK, 4 mM), and, in (b) where HK saline was used in the absence or presence of W-7 (100 $\mu M$). Results are presented as single experiments representative of 3 others.

the flippase) and subsequently with $Co^{2+}$ (which blocks A23187 so that the relatively high $[Ca^{2+}]$ required for annexin binding, 2.5 mM, could not gain access to the cytoplasm). Results showed that PS exposure was stimulated by micromolar $Ca^{2+}$ concentrations with an $EC_{50}$ of about 1.2 $\mu$M. This concentration is similar, though slightly higher, compared with that required for half-maximal activation of the Gardos channel activation [46, 47] and for inhibition of the flippase [26]. A similar high affinity for $Ca^{2+}$ was also observed in RBCs incubated in LK saline indicating that high $K^+$ levels are not responsible for these observations. Calmodulin is known to interact with RBC cytoskeleton and influence PS exposure [48, 49]. Incubation with the calmodulin antagonist W-7 again showed a similar high $Ca^{2+}$ affinity for PS exposure. In this case, the percentage of positive cells was also increased so that the majority of RBCs became positive, showing that most RBCs are capable of PS scrambling at these low $Ca^{2+}$ levels. Previously reported values for activation of the scramblase are considerably higher than those given here, with values of 25–100 $\mu$M quoted [14, 32]. Previous measurements, however, were made largely on resealed RBC ghosts, inside-out vesicles, or purified PLSCR1 [30, 31, 50, 51], which may not in fact represent the RBC scramblase [52]. These preparations will also necessarily lack much of the cytoplasmic contents which may result in reduction in $Ca^{2+}$ affinity of the scrambling process. Furthermore, several previous reports were carried out in the presence of high concentrations of extracellular $Mg^{2+}$ (1 mM) [20, 30, 50], which with the ionophore A23187 would set intracellular $Mg^{2+}$ at over 2 mM, considerably in excess of the normal RBC $[Mg^{2+}]$ [53], and which might be expected to dampen any $Ca^{2+}$ driven process. We speculate that having a similar $Ca^{2+}$ level for Gardos channel activation, flippase inhibition and activation of scrambling would coordinate eryptotic events [21] and facilitate removal damaged RBCs in normal individuals, whilst in SCD patients, hyperactivity of these processes may contribute to disease pathogenesis.

## Acknowledgment

The authors thank the British Heart Foundation and the Medical Research Council Trust for financial support.

## References

[1] M. H. Steinberg, "Sickle cell anemia, the first molecular disease: overview of molecular etiology, pathophysiology, and therapeutic approaches," *TheScientificWorldJournal*, vol. 8, pp. 1295–1324, 2008.

[2] L. Pauling, H. A. Itano, S. J. Singer, and I. C. Wells, "Sickle cell anemia, a molecular disease," *Science*, vol. 110, no. 2865, pp. 543–548, 1949.

[3] H. F. Bunn and B. G. Forget, *Hemoglobin: Molecular, Genetic and Clinical Aspects*, Saunders, Philadelphia, Pa, USA, 1986.

[4] V. L. Lew and R. M. Bookchin, "Ion transport pathology in the mechanism of sickle cell dehydration," *Physiological Reviews*, vol. 85, no. 1, pp. 179–200, 2005.

[5] R. P. Hebbel, W. T. Morgan, J. W. Eaton, and B. E. Hedlund, "Accelerated autoxidation and heme loss due to instability of sickle hemoglobin," *Proceedings of the National Academy of Sciences of the United States of America*, vol. 85, no. 1, pp. 237–241, 1988.

[6] R. P. Hebbel, "Beyond hemoglobin polymerization: the red blood cell membrane and sickle disease pathophysiology," *Blood*, vol. 77, no. 2, pp. 214–237, 1991.

[7] J. F. Tait and D. Gibson, "Measurement of membrane phospholipid asymmetry in normal and sickle-cell erythrocytes by menas of annexin V binding," *Journal of Laboratory and Clinical Medicine*, vol. 123, no. 5, pp. 741–748, 1994.

[8] F. A. Kuypers, R. A. Lewis, M. Hua et al., "Detection of altered membrane phospholipid asymmetry in subpopulations of human red blood cells using fluorescently labeled annexin V," *Blood*, vol. 87, no. 3, pp. 1179–1187, 1996.

[9] K. De Jong, S. K. Larkin, L. A. Styles, R. M. Bookchin, and F. A. Kuypers, "Characterization of the phosphatidylserine-exposing subpopulation of sickle cells," *Blood*, vol. 98, no. 3, pp. 860–867, 2001.

[10] B. N. Y. Setty, S. Kulkarni, and M. J. Stuart, "Role of erythrocyte phosphatidylserine in sickle red cell-endothelial adhesion," *Blood*, vol. 99, no. 5, pp. 1564–1571, 2002.

[11] R. P. Hebbel, M. A. B. Boogaerts, J. W. Eaton, and M. H. Steinberg, "Erythrocyte adherence to endothelium in sickle-cell anemia. A possible determinant of disease severity," *New England Journal of Medicine*, vol. 302, no. 18, pp. 992–995, 1980.

[12] D. Chiu, B. Lubin, B. Roelofsen, and L. L. M. Van Deenen, "Sickled erythrocytes accelerate clotting in vitro: an effect of abnormal membrane lipid asymmetry," *Blood*, vol. 58, no. 2, pp. 398–401, 1981.

[13] B. N. Y. Setty and S. G. Betal, "Microvascular endothelial cells express a phosphatidylserine receptor: a functionally active receptor for phosphatidylserine-positive erythrocytes," *Blood*, vol. 111, no. 2, pp. 905–914, 2008.

[14] C. W. M. Haest, "Distribution and movement of membrane lipids," in *Red Cell Membrane Transport in Health and Disease*, I. Bernhardt and J. C. Ellory, Eds., pp. 1–25, Springer, Berlin, Germany, 2003.

[15] B. L. Wood, D. F. Gibson, and J. F. Tait, "Increased erythrocyte phosphatidylserine exposure in sickle cell disease: flow-cytometric measurement and clinical associations," *Blood*, vol. 88, no. 5, pp. 1873–1880, 1996.

[16] F. A. Kuypers, "Phospholipid asymmetry in health and disease," *Current Opinion in Hematology*, vol. 5, no. 2, pp. 122–131, 1998.

[17] L. A. Barber, M. B. Palascak, C. H. Joiner, and R. S. Franco, "Aminophospholipid translocase and phospholipid scramblase activities in sickle erythrocyte subpopulations," *British Journal of Haematology*, vol. 146, no. 4, pp. 447–455, 2009.

[18] P. F. Devaux and A. Zachowski, "Maintenance and consequences of membrane phospholipid asymmetry," *Chemistry and Physics of Lipids*, vol. 73, no. 1-2, pp. 107–120, 1994.

[19] K. De Jong, D. Geldwerth, and F. A. Kuypers, "Oxidative damage does not alter membrane phospholipid asymmetry in human erythrocytes," *Biochemistry*, vol. 36, no. 22, pp. 6768–6776, 1997.

[20] P. Williamson, A. Kulick, A. Zachowski, R. A. Schlegel, and P. F. Devaux, "Ca$^{2+}$ induces transbilayer redistribution of all major phospholipids in human erythrocytes," *Biochemistry*, vol. 31, no. 27, pp. 6355–6360, 1992.

[21] F. Lang, K. S. Lang, P. A. Lang, S. M. Huber, and T. Wieder, "Mechanisms and significance of eryptosis," *Antioxidants and Redox Signaling*, vol. 8, no. 7-8, pp. 1183–1192, 2006.

[22] D. Chiu, B. Lubin, and S. B. Shohet, "Erythrocyte membrane lipid reorganization during the sickling process," *British Journal of Haematology*, vol. 41, no. 2, pp. 223–234, 1979.

[23] B. Lubin, D. Chiu, and J. Bastacky, "Abnormalities in membrane phospholipid organization in sickled erythrocytes," *Journal of Clinical Investigation*, vol. 67, no. 6, pp. 1643–1649, 1981.

[24] P. F. H. Franck, E. M. Bevers, B. H. Lubin, et al., "Uncoupling of the membrane skeleton from the lipid bilayer. The cause of accelerated phospholipid flip-flop leading to an enhanced procoagulant activity of sickled cells," *Journal of Clinical Investigation*, vol. 75, no. 1, pp. 183–190, 1985.

[25] E. Middelkoop, B. H. Lubin, E. M. Bevers et al., "Studies on sickled erythrocytes provide evidence that the asymmetric distribution of phosphatidylserine in the red cell membrane is maintained by both ATP-dependent translocation and interaction with membrane skeletal proteins," *Biochimica et Biophysica Acta*, vol. 937, no. 2, pp. 281–288, 1988.

[26] M. Bitbol, P. Fellmann, A. Zachowski, and P. F. Devaux, "Ion regulation of phosphatidylserine and phosphatidylethanolamine outside-inside translocation in human erythrocytes," *Biochimica et Biophysica Acta*, vol. 904, no. 2, pp. 268–282, 1987.

[27] C. H. Joiner, "Cation transport and volume regulation in sickle red blood cells," *American Journal of Physiology*, vol. 264, no. 2, pp. C251–C270, 1993.

[28] M. D. Rhoda, M. Apovo, Y. Beuzard, and F. Giraud, "Ca$^{2+}$ permeability in deoxygenated sickle cells," *Blood*, vol. 75, no. 12, pp. 2453–2458, 1990.

[29] Z. Etzion, T. Tiffert, R. M. Bookchin, and V. L. Lew, "Effects of deoxygenation on active and passive Ca$^{2+}$ transport and on the cytoplasmic Ca$^{2+}$ levels of sickle cell anemia red cells," *Journal of Clinical Investigation*, vol. 92, no. 5, pp. 2489–2498, 1993.

[30] B. Verhoven, R. A. Schlegel, and P. Williamson, "Rapid loss and restoration of lipid asymmetry by different pathways in resealed erythrocyte ghosts," *Biochimica et Biophysica Acta*, vol. 1104, no. 1, pp. 15–23, 1992.

[31] F. Bassé, J. G. Stout, P. J. Sims, and T. Wiedmer, "Isolation of an erythrocyte membrane protein that mediates Ca$^{2+}$-dependent transbilayer movement of phospholipid," *Journal of Biological Chemistry*, vol. 271, no. 29, pp. 17205–17210, 1996.

[32] D. Kamp, T. Sieberg, and C. W. M. Haest, "Inhibition and stimulation of phospholipid scrambling activity. Consequences for lipid asymmetry, echinocytosis, and microvesiculation of erythrocytes," *Biochemistry*, vol. 40, no. 31, pp. 9438–9446, 2001.

[33] J. Garcia-Sancho, "Pyruvate prevents the ATP depletion caused by formaldehyde or calcium-chelator esters in the human red cell," *Biochimica et Biophysica Acta*, vol. 813, no. 1, pp. 148–150, 1985.

[34] T. Tiffert, Z. Etzion, R. M. Bookchin, and V. L. Lew, "Effects of deoxygenation on active and passive Ca$^{2+}$ transport and cytoplasmic Ca$^{2+}$ buffering in normal human red cells," *Journal of Physiology*, vol. 464, pp. 529–544, 1993.

[35] P. Flatman and V. L. Lew, "Use of ionophore A23187 to measure and to control free and bound cytoplasmic Mg in intact red cells," *Nature*, vol. 267, no. 5609, pp. 360–362, 1977.

[36] M. C. Muzyamba, E. H. Campbell, and J. S. Gibson, "Effect of intracellular magnesium and oxygen tension on K$^+$-Cl$^-$ cotransport in normal and sickle human red cells," *Cellular Physiology and Biochemistry*, vol. 17, no. 3-4, pp. 121–128, 2006.

[37] K. Lang, B. Roll, S. Myssina et al., "Enhanced erythrocyte apoptosis in sickle cell anemia, thalassemia and glucose-6-phosphate dehydrogenase deficiency," *Cellular Physiology and Biochemistry*, vol. 12, no. 5-6, pp. 365–372, 2002.

[38] Z. Yasin, S. Witting, M. B. Palascak, C. H. Joiner, D. L. Rucknagel, and R. S. Franco, "Phosphatidylserine externalization in sickle red blood cells: associations with cell age, density, and hemoglobin F," *Blood*, vol. 102, no. 1, pp. 365–370, 2003.

[39] K. de Jong and F. A. Kuypers, "Sulphydryl modifications alter scramblase activity in murine sickle cell disease," *British Journal of Haematology*, vol. 133, no. 4, pp. 427–432, 2006.

[40] C. H. Joiner, M. Jiang, W. J. Claussen, N. J. Roszell, Z. Yasin, and R. S. Franco, "Dipyridamole inhibits sickling-induced cation fluxes in sickle red blood cells," *Blood*, vol. 97, no. 12, pp. 3976–3983, 2001.

[41] C. H. Joiner, "Deoxygenation-induced cation fluxes in sickle cells: II. Inhibition by stilbene disulfonates," *Blood*, vol. 76, no. 1, pp. 212–220, 1990.

[42] J. L. N. Wolfs, P. Comfurius, O. Bekers et al., "Direct inhibition of phospholipid scrambling activity in erythrocytes by potassium ions," *Cellular and Molecular Life Sciences*, vol. 66, no. 2, pp. 314–323, 2009.

[43] G. Gárdos, "The function of calcium in the potassium permeability of human erythrocytes," *Biochimica et Biophysica Acta*, vol. 30, no. 3, pp. 653–654, 1958.

[44] D. R. Anderson, J. L. Davis, and K. L. Carraway, "Calcium-promoted changes of the human erythrocyte membrane. Involvement of spectrin, transglutaminase, and a membrane-bound protease," *Journal of Biological Chemistry*, vol. 252, no. 19, pp. 6617–6623, 1977.

[45] K. S. Lang, S. Myssina, V. Brand et al., "Involvement of ceramide in hyperosmotic shock-induced death of erythrocytes," *Cell Death and Differentiation*, vol. 11, no. 2, pp. 231–243, 2004.

[46] T. Tiffert, J. L. Spivak, and V. L. Lew, "Magnitude of calcium influx required to induce dehydration of normal human red cells," *Biochimica et Biophysica Acta*, vol. 943, no. 2, pp. 157–165, 1988.

[47] P. Bennekou and P. Christophersen, "Ion channels," in *Red Cell Membrane in Health and Disease*, I. Bernhardt and J. C. Ellory, Eds., pp. 139–152, Springer, Berlin, Germany, 2003.

[48] M. Strömqvist, Å. Berglund, V. P. Shanbhag, and L. Backman, "Influence of calmodulin on the human red cell membrane skeleton," *Biochemistry*, vol. 27, no. 4, pp. 1104–1110, 1988.

[49] Z. Wang, S. Li, Q. Shi, R. Yan, G. Liu, and K. Dai, "Calmodulin antagonists induce platelet apoptosis," *Thrombosis Research*, vol. 125, no. 4, pp. 340–350, 2010.

[50] L. A. Woon, J. W. Holland, E. P. W. Kable, and B. D. Roufogalis, "Ca$^{2+}$ sensitivity of phospholipid scrambling in human red cell ghosts," *Cell Calcium*, vol. 25, no. 4, pp. 313–320, 1999.

[51] J. G. Stout, Q. Zhou, T. Wiedmer, and P. J. Sims, "Change in conformation of plasma membrane phospholipid scramblase induced by occupancy of its $Ca^{2+}$ binding site," *Biochemistry*, vol. 37, no. 42, pp. 14860–14866, 1998.

[52] Q. Zhou, J. Zhao, T. Wiedmer, and P. J. Sims, "Normal hemostasis but defective hematopoietic response to growth factors in mice deficient in phospholipid scramblase 1," *Blood*, vol. 99, no. 11, pp. 4030–4038, 2002.

[53] P. W. Flatman, "The effect of buffer composition and deoxygenation on the concentration of ionized magnesium inside human red blood cells," *Journal of Physiology*, vol. 300, pp. 19–30, 1980.

# 5

# Integrating Interactive Web-Based Technology to Assess Adherence and Clinical Outcomes in Pediatric Sickle Cell Disease

**Lori E. Crosby,**[1,2] **Ilana Barach,**[3] **Meghan E. McGrady,**[2,3] **Karen A. Kalinyak,**[1,2] **Adryan R. Eastin,**[2] **and Monica J. Mitchell**[1,2,3]

[1] College of Medicine, University of Cincinnati, Cincinnati, OH 45221, USA
[2] Behavioral Medicine and Clinical Psychology, Cincinnati Children's Hospital Medical Center, Cincinnati, OH 45229, USA
[3] Department of Psychology, University of Cincinnati, Cincinnati, OH 45221, USA

Correspondence should be addressed to Lori E. Crosby, lori.crosby@cchmc.org

Academic Editor: Betty S. Pace

Research indicates that the quality of the adherence assessment is one of the best predictors for improving clinical outcomes. Newer technologies represent an opportunity for developing high quality standardized assessments to assess clinical outcomes such as patient experience of care but have not been tested systematically in pediatric sickle cell disease (SCD). The goal of the current study was to pilot an interactive web-based tool, the Take-Charge Program, to assess adherence to clinic visits and hydroxyurea (HU), barriers to adherence, solutions to overcome these barriers, and clinical outcomes in 43 patients with SCD age 6–21 years. Results indicate that the web-based tool was successfully integrated into the clinical setting while maintaining high patient satisfaction (>90%). The tool provided data consistent with the medical record, staff report, and/or clinical lab data. Participants reported that forgetting and transportation were major barriers for adherence to both clinic attendance and HU. A greater number of self-reported barriers ($P < .01$) and older age ($P < .05$) were associated with poorer clinic attendance and HU adherence. In summary, the tool represents an innovative approach to integrate newer technology to assess adherence and clinical outcomes for pediatric patients with SCD.

## 1. Introduction

Sickle cell disease (SCD) is a genetic red blood cell disorder characterized by the sickling of red blood cells resulting in pain episodes, organ damage, risk for infections, and decreased life expectancy [1]. Care guidelines for SCD recommend that patients attend routine clinic appointments one to two times per year and more frequently if there are complications or if clinical monitoring is needed to assess tolerance to medications and other treatments [1, 2]. Preventative care such as flu shots, immunizations, and monitoring labs is also essential to effectively manage sickle cell disease [3]. Hydroxyurea (HU), which is used to increase fetal hemoglobin (Hb F), has been shown to decrease morbidity and mortality in patients with SCD [4]. Studies have indicated that daily oral HU use is associated with reduced pain crises, hospitalizations, acute chest syndrome, and transfusions and improved growth and health-related quality of life [5–9]. Thus, the consequences of nonadherence to clinic attendance and HU treatments result in increased morbidity [10], healthcare costs [11], and decreased quality of life [12].

There is limited research available examining treatment nonadherence in pediatric SCD. A meta-analytic review found a nonadherence rate for clinic appointments in pediatric populations of approximately 40% [13]. Similarly, nonadherence rates for clinic appointments in SCD range between 36%–44% [14, 15]. On the surface, it would seem that patients who attend their appointments would demonstrate higher levels of adherence to their treatment regimen; however, the relationship between clinic attendance and treatment adherence appears to be complex. As an example, Finney et al. [16] found that the 48% of patients who kept their follow-up appointment had been nonadherent to their prescribed regimen. Thus, it is important to assess barriers to the treatment regimen even with patients who attend appointments regularly.

Research on medication adherence in SCD suggests higher rates for acute medications than daily medications. Dampier et al. [17] found that 85% of adolescents with SCD took analgesic medications on days when they experienced sickle-cell related pain. In contrast, studies found that 38%–60% of pediatric and adult patients were adherent to their prescribed days of home chelation therapy or deferoxamine usage [18, 19] and rates ranged from 12%–67% for young children with SCD taking prophylactic penicillin [20–22]. Studies of HU adherence in SCD have typically utilized small sample sizes or single measures of adherence (e.g., pill counts) [23]. Overall, these studies indicate variable rates of adherence and lower rates for long-term trials [23, 24]. For example, Zimmerman and colleagues discontinued HU in 12% of their participants due to nonadherence [24]. Data from our own clinic indicate that 30% of patients who were prescribed HU were discontinued due to nonadherence. Poor adherence with HU may have unintended consequences as the medication can be discontinued on the assumption that the patient is a nonresponder, while other patients may have their dose increased to a level that is toxic when they actually begin taking it. Standardized and multidimensional approaches to measuring adherence are needed to ensure that patients receive optimal benefits from the medication while also minimizing risks to patients.

Overall, research indicates low and variable adherence rates to different components of the SCD treatment regimen. Studies identifying barriers to adherence have indicated a clear link between adherence and poor clinical outcomes in pediatric populations [25]. In pediatric SCD samples, studies have identified the following as key barriers: competing activities, health status, patient-provider relationships, adverse clinical experiences, and forgetting [26]. Other studies have identified sociocultural barriers to adherence including developmental factors, transportation, and health literacy [27–29]. Multicomponent, behavioral, and educational interventions to promote adherence have been found to be well-established pediatric treatments, [30, 31]; however, a recent study indicates that the quality of the adherence assessment is one of the best predictors for improving clinical outcomes [25]. Newer technologies (e.g., computer-based, text messaging) represent an opportunity for developing high quality, standardized and cost-effective assessments of treatment adherence and clinical outcomes such as patient experience of care (e.g., communication with and responsiveness of staff, quality of information received, wait time, satisfaction, etc.), disease-specific outcomes (e.g., labs) and health-related quality of life [32]. These types of approaches have been used effectively in chronic illness populations including adults with hypertension, diabetes [33, 34], and pediatric asthma [35].

The current study represents a first step in integrating interactive web-based technologies in SCD clinical care. The aims of the current study were to pilot an interactive family-based web-based tool, the Take-Charge Program, to assess adherence and clinical outcomes including: (1) patient HU adherence, barriers to HU adherence, and potential solutions to improve HU adherence; (2) patient clinic attendance adherence, barriers to clinic attendance adherence, and potential solutions to improve clinic attendance; and (3) clinical outcomes (patient experience of care, sickle-related outcomes hemoglobin level, ANC, MCV, and percent fetal hemoglobin level for HU patients).

## 2. Participants and Methods

Data presented in this paper are from the baseline assessment of a larger longitudinal study being conducted at a tertiary urban pediatric medical center in the Midwest. Eligible participants were patients of a comprehensive SCD clinic, age 6 to 21 years (and their caregivers), and prescribed hydroxyurea (HU) therapy or referred by clinic staff for attendance problems. Patients who had significant health complications (e.g., acute illness, recent stroke) that would interfere with the completion of the study or significant cognitive or developmental disabilities were excluded due to the demand on participants to understand questions in the assessment. Of the 182 patients in the clinic, 98 were eligible based on the above criteria. To date, 47 patients have been enrolled in the study with 4 being withdrawn because they no longer met criteria; thus, data will be presented on the 43 participants in the sample. Potential participants were identified by the clinical staff and the research team confirmed eligibility criteria. All participants were approached during a scheduled clinic visit. After obtaining consent, data collection proceeded at that visit.

*2.1. Measures.* Patients and caregivers completed the following measures.

*2.1.1. Background Information Form.* This form summarized personal/family demographic information, including participant school/vocational history, parent education, family income, family transitions, and life events. In addition, self-report of pain frequency and intensity, and hospital and emergency room visits over the past year was collected for comparison with data collected from the medical record review.

*2.1.2. Barriers to Care Questionnaire [36].* This validated and reliable 40-item questionnaire measures parents' report of encounters or situations that may interfere with access to care, use of care, the patient-physician experience, or adherence with medical instructions. Barriers are conceptualized as multidimensional and include pragmatics (logistics, cost), expectations about care, health knowledge and beliefs, marginalization and health care navigation skills.

*2.1.3. The Take Charge Program (Web-Based Tool).* A voice-automated interactive web-based assessment tool was developed based on questions from the Disease Management

Interview [37] and consultation from clinic staff. Caregiver and child dyads complete the tool which takes approximately 15–20 minutes. The measure included questions and prompts that enabled patients and caregivers to identify barriers to adherence to clinic attendance and HU from a standard list [26, 37] and at least one strategy for improving adherence. The voice-automation increased the validity as literacy was not required to complete the measure. The initial development of the Take-Charge Program has been described elsewhere [38]. During the second phase of development, patients and caregivers matched barriers and potential solutions for HU. Cognitive interviewing was used to ensure that questions were being understood as intended [36, 38]. The web-based tool assessed clinic attendance, hydroxyurea adherence, and patient experience of care. The Clinic Attendance Module assessed self-reported adherence to clinic appointments on a 10-point Likert-type scale with 10 representing perfect adherence. The hydroxyurea module assessed self-reported HU adherence on a 10-point Likert-type scale with 10 representing perfect adherence. Both modules also asked participants to select applicable barriers and a potential solution to address these barriers. The Patient Experience of Care Module, an adapted version of Krahn et al.'s [39] questionnaire using a 4-point Likert scale and 2 open-ended questions assessed (1) wait time in clinic, (2) understanding of treatment recommendations by healthcare team, (3) time spent with healthcare team, and (4) helpfulness of web-based tool. Once participants identified a potential solution to try, clinic staff or a member of the research team utilized a standardized problem-solving intervention adapted from Behavioral Family Systems Therapy [40] to help participants develop a specific plan to implement the solution.

### 2.1.4. Medical Record Review.

Electronic medical records were reviewed to confirm participant's type of SCD and collect the following data: hemoglobin level, ANC, MCV, percent fetal hemoglobin, clinic attendance, ER visits, and hospitalizations. Information on the participant's prescribed treatment plan was also collected and verified with clinic staff.

### 2.2. Data Analysis.

Data collected from the web-based tool and electronic medical record (EMR) were integrated into a single database. Descriptive statistics and frequencies were utilized to summarize demographics, health characteristics, health care utilization, self-reported adherence, barriers, potential solutions, and patient experience of care. Pearson product-moment correlation coefficients were computed to conduct exploratory analyses to assess the relationship between adherence to clinic visits (e.g., self-reported barriers on the Take-Charge Program, number of barriers), adherence to HU (e.g., self-reported barriers on the Take-Charge Program, number of barriers), demographics, patient experience of care and sickle cell related outcomes. All analyses were conducted in IBM SPSS Statistics 19 (SPSS: An IBM Company).

## 3. Results

### 3.1. Participants.

Study participants included 43 youth with SCD ($M = 12.81 + 3.98$ years; 39.5% Male; 79.0% HbSS; 9.3% HbSC; 4.7% H$\beta^+$Thal; 7.0% other) and their primary caregivers (83.7% mothers; 7.0% fathers; 9.3% other). Additional demographic characteristics are reported in Table 1. This sample is representative of the total SCD clinic population, with the exception of hemoglobin type (fewer participants with HbSC) but is consistent with the fact that the majority of participants in the study were on HU therapy. With respect to clinical characteristics, 62.2% of the sample reported having six or less pain days in the past 12 months, and 61.5% reported missing 6 days of school for pain in the past 12 months. Emergency room (ER) visit and hospitalization data indicated that most participants had three or fewer ER visits (95.1%) or hospitalizations (90.5%) in the past 12 months (see Table 2).

### 3.2. Clinic Attendance.

According to the data, approximately half of participants (47.5%) indicate that they "always come" when describing their clinic attendance over the previous 12 months. This self-reported adherence was similar to data obtained from the EMR which indicated that 55% of patients never missed an appointment during this same period. Although about half of patients missed at least one appointment, a higher percent (75%) understood that their SCD providers recommended clinic appointments at least twice a year, and participants attended 84.5% of all scheduled appointments. Top-rated barriers on the Barriers to Care Questionnaire (BCQ) were related to pragmatics (i.e., logistics, cost) ($M = 76.1$; SD $= 15.7$) and healthcare navigation skills ($M = 79.4$, SD $= 22.4$). When asked specifically about barriers to clinic attendance on the Take-Charge Program, participants reported the following barriers: transportation difficulties (22.5%), inability to take off from work/school (17.5%), forgetting (10%), waiting too long (7.5%), competing activities (e.g., sports; 5%), feeling tired (5%); dislike of treatments (2.5%), feeling it is unnecessary (2.5%), and other (10%). Other barriers included getting appointment dates and times confused, not having transportation vouchers/setup, and not having appointments available at a time that works with the family's schedule. For potential solutions, 47.1% chose an individualized solution; 29.4% reported that they would try scheduling their appointment at a better/different time; and 5.9% reported that they would try setting an alarm (e.g., phone).

Participants were asked to rate their adherence on a scale of 0 to 10 with 10 being no problems with adherence. The mean rating for the sample was 8.9/10 ($N = 40$; SD : 2.1). They were also asked to rate how many visits they miss per year on average. The mean for missed visits was 1.0 ($N = 40$; SD $= 1.4$). Exploratory analyses showed that a greater percentage of no shows over the 12 month period prior to study enrollment was positively related to (1) more self-reported barriers to clinic attendance on the Take Charge Program $r = .550$, $n = 40$, $P < .001$; (2) the number of visits required $r = .455$, $n = 39$, $P < .01$; (3) age $r = .317$, $n = 41$,

TABLE 1: Patient demographics.

| | N (%) | Mean (SD) |
|---|---|---|
| Hemoglobin type | | |
|     HbSS | 34 (79.0) | |
|     HbSC | 4 (9.3) | |
|     Hb$^+$Thal | 2 (4.7) | |
|     Other | 3 (7.0) | |
| Gender | | |
|     Male | 17 (39.5) | |
|     Female | 26 (60.5) | |
| Age | | 12.81 (3.98) |
| Race | | |
|     African-American | 43 (100) | |
| Grade in school, median | | 6th |
| Primary caregiver | | |
|     Mother | 36 (83.7) | |
|     Father | 3 (7.0) | |
|     Other relative | 4 (9.3) | |
| Highest grade completed by caregiver | | |
|     High school | 15 (34.9) | |
|     Some college | 14 (32.6) | |
|     College degree | 13 (30.2) | |
|     Grad school | 1 (2.3) | |
| Family income | | |
|     < $10,000 | 14 (33.3) | |
|     $10,000–20,000 | 4 (9.5) | |
|     $21,000–30,000 | 6 (14.3) | |
|     $31,000–50,000 | 5 (11.9) | |
|     > $51,000 | 13 (31.0) | |

$P < .05$; and (4) marginally related to satisfaction with clinic visits $r = .323$, $n = 40$, $P < .052$.

3.3. *Hydroxyurea Adherence.* While less than a third of participants (26.7% saying "yes") reported that they "always took their HU," overall, participants rated themselves as an 8.8 on a 10-point scale for "how often do they take their medicines?" which converts to 88%. When asked about missing doses, participants reported that they missed an average of 1.3 doses of HU per week. Participants reported the following barriers to HU on the Take-Charge Program: forgetting (56.7%), not having the medication with me (26.7%), the medications running out (23.3%), yucky taste or smell (12.5%), upset stomach (12.5%), and being not sure why I take it (3.1%). Other barriers reported included not wanting to stop what the patient is doing to take medication and taking too many medications. For potential solutions, 20% chose to try putting the medication next to something they do every day (e.g., toothbrush, breakfast table); 15% chose to use an alarm clock or cell phone alarm; 15% chose to use a pill box; and 15% chose to use a calendar. Additional solutions selected were reminder calls, and coordinating better with child/caregiver. Also, clinic staff

rated that approximately 40% of participants were adherent to medications based on clinical data but staff felt that the clinical data of the other 60% indicated nonadherence or that further monitoring was needed. Number of missed doses of HU during the previous two weeks was related to age, with older age being related to greater nonadherence $r = .372$, $n = 31$, $P = .036$ and greater number of barriers reported on the Take-Charge Program $r = .421$, $n = 31$, $P = .023$.

3.4. *Clinic Integration.* Nearly all participants and their parents (41/43) completed the web-based assessment tool while waiting to see the care team for their appointment. The tool collected accurate and complete data with minimal missing data (3 participants due to technical errors). The majority of participants (64.9%) rated the web-based tool as very helpful and another twenty-five percent (24.3%) rated it as a little helpful.

3.5. *Clinical Outcomes*

*Patient Experience of Care.* The majority of patients (82%) reported a reasonable wait time (43% not at all; 29% short time) and only 18% reported that their wait time for the visit

TABLE 2: Patient clinical characteristics.

| | N (%) | Range |
|---|---|---|
| Pain days in past 12 months* | | 0–45 |
| 0 days | 5 (11.6) | |
| 1-2 days | 9 (20.9) | |
| 3–5 days | 6 (14.0) | |
| 6–10 days | 7 (16.3) | |
| >10 days | 16 (37.2) | |
| Missed school days due to pain in past 12 months+* | | 0–45 |
| 0 days | 8 (19.0) | |
| 1-2 days | 6 (14.3) | |
| 3–5 days | 7 (16.7) | |
| 6–10 days | 9 (21.4) | |
| >10 days | 12 (28.6) | |
| Hospitalizations in past 12 months+* | | 0–20 |
| 0 | 15 (35.7) | |
| 1-2 | 19 (45.2) | |
| 3 | 5 (11.9) | |
| 4 | 1 (2.4) | |
| 5 | 1 (2.4) | |
| 20 | 1 (2.4) | |
| ER visits in past 12 months+* | | 0–20 |
| 0 | 8 (19.0) | |
| 1-2 | 27 (64.3) | |
| 3 | 5 (11.9) | |
| 8 | 1 (2.4) | |
| 20 | 1 (2.4) | |

*$n = 37$
+*$n = 42$

was too long. With respect to the visit itself, approximately 79.5% of participants reported that they were satisfied with the amount of time the medical team spent with them during their visit. In addition, the majority of participants (82.1%) reported that what the medical team shared with them was very helpful. Specifically, participants reported that the medical information was helpful (16%), and they found discussions about the treatment plan (e.g., discussion around medicine dosage and test results; about steps she needs to take to stay healthy) very beneficial (12%). Some participants (38%) also reported that other things made the visit positive (e.g., toys, movies).

*Sickle Cell-Related Lab Values.* Lab values from the date of enrollment into the study (or within 30 days of enrollment) were obtained from an electronic portal that pulls data from the electronic medical record system. The mean hemoglobin level for participants was 9.7 ($N = 39$; SD = 1.28). For those participants on HU therapy, the mean percent fetal hemoglobin was 23.1 ($N = 26$; SD = 15.6), the MCV was 98.0 ($N = 28$; SD = 13.9), and the ANC was 4.2 ($N = 27$; SD = 2.44). There was not a significant relationship between lab values and patient satisfaction with the amount of time

spent with the medical team or the helpfulness of the medical information shared during the visit.

## 4. Discussion

This study highlights the potential to efficiently integrate interactive web-based technology in a clinic-based setting to assess treatment adherence, patient experience of care, and disease-specific outcomes in pediatric SCD. This study is significant as it piloted an innovative and high quality assessment process for capturing adherence data, including the barriers to adherence and potential solutions for addressing these barriers. The data from the tool showed a number of interesting trends. First, the tool proved to be a useful means for collecting data to understand adherence to clinic visits. Self-reported adherence to clinic visits was consistent with data from patients' EMR as both sources revealed a 12-month clinic attendance adherence rate ("always coming" and "attending all visits") of approximately 50%. It should be noted that the number of missed visits and adherence may be relative given that patients had 2 to 17 visits scheduled over the course of the year based on the complexity of treatments and disease-related complications (e.g., hospital discharge followup). Taken together, these findings suggest that nearly

85% of all scheduled clinic visits were attended by participants in this study. Understanding barriers to nonadherence was also important, especially given that adherence to clinic visits does not take into account cancellations, same day cancellations or rescheduled visits as a nonattended visit. Finally, data from the Take-Charge Program was integrated with patients' EMR data providing a wealth of data to inform clinical practice in "real time."

The barriers to clinic attendance endorsed by participants were multifaceted and included logistical (transportation, getting off work), health care navigation skills (using calendars to manage multiple appointments and medications), socioeconomic (lack of insurance), and disease-related barriers (did not feel well). BCQ mean scores for this sample were consistent with mean scores for other pediatric populations with similar challenges (e.g., asthma, children with special health care needs) [36, 41]. Participants also identified potential solutions for improving adherence and attendance (which is the basis for a larger longitudinal intervention study). Additional potential risk factors for no-shows emerged from exploratory analysis of the data which found that nonadherence to clinic visits increased with age, more required visits, and self-reported barriers to attendance. These findings, though preliminary, further highlight the richness of the data and provide meaningful trends and a basis for prioritizing patients who may be in need of additional clinical supports to ensure patient engagement and attendance.

The Take-Charge tool was also piloted to better understand the subset of patients on HU (74% of the sample). Anecdotally, nonadherence to HU is cited as a problem for many children and adolescents with SCD although developmentally-appropriate approaches for children and adolescents are very limited. The findings support that the Take-Charge tool was useful for assessing relevant information from participants on HU related to their perceptions of how they are to be taking their medications, concerns about side-effects and other barriers. Data from the tool highlighted that approaches to working with patients around medication management will need to address organizational issues [18, 19] such as helping patients and parents use calendars, phone alarms, and emerging innovative technologies (e.g., pill cases that glow in the dark and beep) to reduce the potential for "forgetting" to take medications, getting them refilled, and packing them when away from home.

Qualitative data from participants further highlight the importance of implementing family-based strategies and the need to tailor them appropriately to individual needs. Medication side-effects (e.g., taste, smell, upset stomach) and lack of awareness (i.e., to address patients who are not sure why they are taking medication) are other important barriers to address. Interestingly, some of the reasons that are commonly considered for nonadherence (e.g., the probability for loss of hair, stigma, fear of blood draws, and that the medicine would not make a difference) were not endorsed by these participants but still may be important for patients who do not agree to try the medication or who show early signs of nonadherence. Several participants noted that transportation and lack of insurance were barriers not only to clinic attendance, but also to HU adherence, highlighting the pervasiveness of income and access to health care on adherence. The barriers that are assessed in the tool appear to have some clinical utility as more barriers were related to a higher number of missed doses of medicine during the previous two weeks prior to the study. This study also supports previous research which suggests that age should also be considered as a target in the clinical evaluation, given the potential for nonadherence to medication increased with age [10, 34]. Data support the potential for the tool to reliably assess adherence and other health utilization outcomes while fostering individualized and family-based solutions for addressing barriers to adherence to clinic visits and medication. Patient experience of care data on the clinical integration of the tool showed positive trends with at least 90% of participants endorsing satisfaction/helpfulness of the tool. It was positive that satisfaction with the clinic visit was also not compromised with >90% also endorsing satisfaction with the clinic visit.

The limitations of the study should be noted. First, given the pilot/feasibility nature of the study, only patients who were engaged in our clinic were included in the study. It will be important in future clinical research to understand and address the barriers of patients (perhaps via the web or other engaging methods) who have lost contact or who are unable to attend clinic because of barriers and risks to determine if more significant intervention is needed. Second, the study included a range of participants across a broad developmental level. In addition, since this was a family-based assessment and intervention study, individual reports of barriers for patients and caregivers were not collected. This limitation should be overcome in future studies by insuring that older patients identify individual barriers to treatment adherence. Third, patients were diverse in income, disease severity, and other factors. Replicating this study with a larger sample to better understand adherence within developmental and disease-related subgroups will be important. Fourth, data collection from the EMR was a challenge in this study as corresponding lab values were not available for all study visits. It will be essential to better coordinate lab draws and study visits and to ensure study funds to pay for corresponding labs so that data can be tracked over time. Finally, the data reported here are cross-sectional and some are self-reported in nature. Future research is needed to monitor clinical outcome data longitudinally and to assess the relationship between adherence and clinical outcomes over time.

A next step in advancing our research is to refine the tool. There were a number of "other" responses that received a high endorsement which justify some additional revision of existing screens to include additional response options. While this program has the potential to be used as a tool to help improve adherence and clinical outcomes during follow-up visits, a goal and a challenge will be to maintain high patient satisfaction with the program. As the program becomes further standardized, another goal will be to streamline the clinic integration process and to pilot it in other SCD clinic settings. In spite of these limitations the study's overall goal was met which was to integrate the web-based tool within a clinic-based setting (rather than in a nonclinical research setting) and to assess adherence and clinical outcomes for pediatric patients with SCD.

## Conflict of Interests

All the authors declare that they have no conflicts of interests.

## Acknowledgments

The authors would like to acknowledge Heather Strong, Steven Lenzly, II, Annie Garner, and Keri Shiels for their assistance with data collection and data entry. The present study was funded by Grant #no.# U54HL070871, Comprehensive Sickle Cell Center, funded by the National Institutes of Health (NIH), National Heart, Lung, and Blood Institute (NHLBI).

## References

[1] National Institutes of Health: National Heart, and Blood Institute, "The management of sickle cell disease," NIH Publication No. 02-2117, 2002.

[2] S. Claster and E. P. Vichinsky, "Managing sickle cell disease," British Medical Journal, vol. 327, no. 7424, pp. 1151–1155, 2003.

[3] W. Y. Wong, "Prevention and management of infection in children with sickle cell anaemia," Paediatric Drugs, vol. 3, no. 11, pp. 793–801, 2001.

[4] O. S. Platt, D. J. Brambilla, W. F. Rosse et al., "Mortality in sickle cell disease. Life expectancy and risk factors for early death," The New England Journal of Medicine, vol. 330, no. 23, pp. 1639–1644, 1994.

[5] C. L. Edwards, M. T. Scales, C. Loughlin et al., "A brief review of the pathophysiology, associated pain, and psychosocial issues in sickle cell disease," International Journal of Behavioral Medicine, vol. 12, no. 3, pp. 171–179, 2005.

[6] S. Charache, F. B. Barton, R. D. Moore et al., "Hydroxyurea and sickle cell anemia: clinical utility of a myelosuppressive "switching" agent," Medicine, vol. 75, no. 6, pp. 300–326, 1996.

[7] S. Charache, M. L. Terrin, R. D. Moore et al., "Effect of hydroxyurea on the frequency of painful crises in sickle cell anemia," The New England Journal of Medicine, vol. 332, no. 20, pp. 1317–1322, 1995.

[8] W. C. Wang, K. H. Morales, C. D. Scher et al., "Effect of long-term transfusion on growth in children with sickle cell anemia: results of the stop trial," Journal of Pediatrics, vol. 147, no. 2, pp. 244–247, 2005.

[9] S. K. Ballas, F. B. Barton, M. A. Waclawiw et al., "Hydroxyurea and sickle cell anemia: effect on quality of life," Health and Quality of Life Outcomes, vol. 4, article 59, 2006.

[10] J. Dunbar-Jacob, J. A. Erlen, E. A. Schlenk, C. M. Ryan, S. M. Sereika, and W. M. Doswell, "Adherence in chronic disease," Annual Review of Nursing Research, vol. 18, pp. 48–90, 2000.

[11] S. D. Candrilli, S. H. O'Brien, R. E. Ware, M. C. Nahata, E. E. Seiber, and R. Balkrishnan, "Hydroxyurea adherence and associated outcomes among medicaid enrollees with sickle cell disease," American Journal of Hematology, vol. 86, no. 3, pp. 273–277, 2011.

[12] L. P. Barakat, M. Lutz, K. Smith-Whitley, and K. Ohene-Frempong, "Is treatment adherence associated with better quality of life in children with sickle cell disease?" Quality of Life Research, vol. 14, no. 2, pp. 407–414, 2005.

[13] W. M. Macharia, G. Leon, B. H. Rowe, B. J. Stephenson, and R. B. Haynes, "An overview of interventions to improve compliance with appointment keeping for medical services," Journal of the American Medical Association, vol. 267, no. 13, pp. 1813–1817, 1992.

[14] N. Robinson, H. Huber, P. Jenkins et al., "Improving access to medical care for children with sickle cell disease," in Proceedings of the 29th Annual Meeting of the National Sickle Cell Disease, Memphis, Tenn, USA, 2006.

[15] C. D. Thornburg, A. Calatroni, M. Telen, and A. R. Kemper, "Adherence to hydroxyurea therapy in children with sickle cell anemia," Journal of Pediatrics, vol. 156, no. 3, pp. 415–419, 2010.

[16] J. W. Finney, R. J. Hook, P. C. Friman, M. A. Rapoff, and E. R. Christophersen, "The overestimation of adherence to pediatric medical regimens," Children's Health Care, vol. 22, no. 4, pp. 297–304, 1993.

[17] C. Dampier, B. Ely, D. Brodecki, and P. O'Neal, "Characteristics of pain managed at home in children and adolescents with sickle cell disease by using diary self-reports," Journal of Pain, vol. 3, no. 6, pp. 461–470, 2002.

[18] M. J. Treadwell, A. W. Law, J. Sung et al., "Barriers to adherence of deferoxamine usage in sickle cell disease," Pediatric Blood and Cancer, vol. 44, no. 5, pp. 500–507, 2005.

[19] L. Weissman, M. Treadwell, and E. Vichinsky, "Evaluation of home desferal care in transfusion-dependent children with thalassemia and sickle cell disease," International Journal of Pediatric Hematology/Oncology, vol. 4, no. 1, pp. 61–68, 1997.

[20] M. Berkovitch, D. Papadouris, D. Shaw, N. Onuaha, C. Dias, and N. F. Olivieri, "Trying to improve compliance with prophylactic penicillin therapy in children with sickle cell disease," British Journal of Clinical Pharmacology, vol. 45, no. 6, pp. 605–607, 1998.

[21] V. Elliott, S. Morgan, S. Day, L. S. Mollerup, and W. Wang, "Parental health beliefs and compliance with prophylactic penicillin administration in children with sickle cell disease," Journal of Pediatric Hematology/Oncology, vol. 23, no. 2, pp. 112–116, 2001.

[22] S. J. Teach, K. A. Lillis, and M. Grossi, "Compliance with penicillin prophylaxis in patients with sickle cell disease," Archives of Pediatrics and Adolescent Medicine, vol. 152, no. 3, pp. 274–278, 1998.

[23] S. A. Zimmerman, W. H. Schultz, J. S. Davis et al., "Sustained long-term hematologic efficacy of hydroxyurea at maximum tolerated dose in children with sickle cell disease," Blood, vol. 103, no. 6, pp. 2039–2045, 2004.

[24] N. F. Olivieri and E. P. Vichinsky, "Hydroxyurea in children with sickle cell disease: impact on splenic function and compliance with therapy," Journal of Pediatric Hematology/Oncology, vol. 20, no. 1, pp. 26–31, 1998.

[25] M. R. DiMatteo, P. J. Giordani, H. S. Lepper, and T. W. Croghan, "Patient adherence and medical treatment outcomes: a meta-analysis," Medical Care, vol. 40, no. 9, pp. 794–811, 2002.

[26] L. E. Crosby, A. C. Modi, K. L. Lemanek, S. M. Guilfoyle, K. A. Kalinyak, and M. J. Mitchell, "Perceived barriers to clinic appointments for adolescents with sickle cell disease," Journal of Pediatric Hematology/Oncology, vol. 31, no. 8, pp. 571–576, 2009.

[27] A. Garcia-Gonzalez, M. Richardson, M. Garcia Popa-Lisseanu et al., "Treatment adherence in patients with rheumatoid

arthritis and systemic lupus erythematosus." *Clinical Rheumatology*, vol. 27, no. 7, pp. 883–889, 2008.

[28] D. Logan, N. Zelikovsky, L. Labay, and J. Spergel, "The Illness Management Survey: identifying adolescents' perceptions of barriers to adherence," *Journal of Pediatric Psychology*, vol. 28, no. 6, pp. 383–392, 2003.

[29] D. Schillinger, K. Grumbach, J. Piette et al., "Association of health literacy with diabetes outcomes," *Journal of the American Medical Association*, vol. 288, no. 4, pp. 475–482, 2002.

[30] M. M. Graves, M. C. Roberts, M. Rapoff, and A. Boyer, "The efficacy of adherence interventions for chronically ill children: a meta-analytic review," *Journal of Pediatric Psychology*, vol. 35, no. 4, pp. 368–382, 2010.

[31] S. Kahana, D. Drotar, and T. Frazier, "Meta-analysis of psychological interventions to promote adherence to treatment in pediatric chronic health conditions," *Journal of Pediatric Psychology*, vol. 33, no. 6, pp. 590–611, 2008.

[32] J. Stinson, R. Wilson, N. Gill, J. Yamada, and J. Holt, "A systematic review of internet-based self-management interventions for youth with health conditions," *Journal of pediatric psychology*, vol. 34, no. 5, pp. 495–510, 2009.

[33] D. L. Hunt, R. B. Haynes, R. S. A. Hayward, M. A. Pim, and J. Horsman, "Patient-specific evidence-based care recommendations for diabetes mellitus: development and initial clinic experience with a computerized decision support system," *International Journal of Medical Informatics*, vol. 51, no. 2-3, pp. 127–135, 1998.

[34] E. A. Walker, M. Molitch, M. K. Kramer et al., "Adherence to preventive medications: predictors and outcomes in the diabetes prevention program," *Diabetes Care*, vol. 29, no. 9, pp. 1997–2002, 2006.

[35] R. Shegog, L. K. Bartholomew, M. M. Sockrider et al., "Computer-based decision support for pediatric asthma management: description and feasibility of the stop asthma clinical system," *Health Informatics Journal*, vol. 12, no. 4, pp. 259–273, 2006.

[36] M. Seid, L. Opipari-Arrigan, L. R. Gelhard, J. W. Varni, and K. Driscoll, "Barriers to care questionnaire: reliability, validity, and responsiveness to change among parents of children with asthma," *Academic Pediatrics*, vol. 9, no. 2, pp. 106–113, 2009.

[37] A. C. Modi, L. E. Crosby, S. M. Guilfoyle, K. L. Lemanek, D. Witherspoon, and M. J. Mitchell, "Barriers to treatment adherence for pediatric patients with sickle cell disease and their families," *Children's Health Care*, vol. 38, no. 2, pp. 107–122, 2009.

[38] A. C. Modi, L. E. Crosby, J. Hines, D. Drotar, and M. J. Mitchell, "Feasibility of web-based technology to assess adherence to clinic appointments in youth with sickle cell disease," *Journal of Pediatric Hematology/Oncology*, vol. 34, no. 3, pp. e93–e96, 2012.

[39] G. L. Krahn, D. Eisert, and B. Fifield, "Obtaining parental perceptions of the quality of services for children with special health needs," *Journal of Pediatric Psychology*, vol. 15, no. 6, pp. 761–774, 1990.

[40] T. Wysocki, M. A. Harris, L. M. Buckloh et al., "Effects of behavioral family systems therapy for diabetes on adolescents' family relationships, treatment adherence, and metabolic control," *Journal of Pediatric Psychology*, vol. 31, no. 9, pp. 928–938, 2006.

[41] M. Seid, E. J. Sobo, L. R. Gelhard, and J. W. Varni, "Parents' reports of barriers to care for children with special health care needs: development and validation of the barriers to care questionnaire," *Ambulatory Pediatrics*, vol. 4, no. 4, pp. 323–331, 2004.

# 6

# Hospitalization Events among Children and Adolescents with Sickle Cell Disease in Basra, Iraq

**Zeina A. Salman[1] and Meaad K. Hassan[1,2]**

[1]Center for Hereditary Blood Diseases, Basra Maternity and Children Hospital, Basra, Iraq
[2]Department of Pediatrics, College of Medicine, University of Basra, Basra, Iraq

Correspondence should be addressed to Meaad K. Hassan; alasfoor_mk@yahoo.com

Academic Editor: Maria Stella Figueiredo

*Objectives.* Despite improvements in the management of sickle cell disease (SCD), many patients still experience disease-related complications requiring hospitalizations. The objectives of this study were to identify causes of hospitalization among these patients and factors associated with the length of hospital stay (LOS) and readmission. *Methods.* Data from 160 patients (<14 years old) with SCD who were admitted to the Basra Maternity and Children's Hospital from the first of January 2012 through July 2012 were analyzed. *Results.* The main causes of hospitalization were acute painful crises (73.84%), infections (9.28%), acute chest syndrome (8.02%), and acute splenic sequestration crisis (6.32%). The mean LOS was $4.34 \pm 2.85$ days. The LOS for patients on hydroxyurea ($3.41 \pm 2.64$ days) was shorter than that for patients who were not ($4.59 \pm 2.86$ days), $P < 0.05$. The readmission rate (23.1%) was significantly higher among patients with frequent hospitalizations in the previous year (OR 9.352, 95% CI 2.011–43.49), asthma symptoms (OR 4.225, 95% CI 1.125–15.862), and opioid use (OR 6.588, 95% CI 1.104–30.336). Patients on hydroxyurea were less likely to be readmitted (OR 0.082, 95% CI 0.10–0.663). *Conclusions.* There is a relatively high readmission rate among patients with SCD in Basra. The use of hydroxyurea significantly decreases the LOS and readmission rate.

## 1. Introduction

Sickle cell disease (SCD) is a multisystem disease associated with episodes of acute illness and progressive organ damage, and it represents a major public health problem because of its associated morbidity and mortality [1]. The prevalence of sickle hemoglobin (Hb S) in Basra is 6.48%, with a gene frequency of 0.0324% [2].

Patients with SCD have a chronic hemolytic anemia and can suffer from sudden, severe, and life-threatening complications caused by the acute sickling of red blood cells, with resultant pain or organ dysfunction. Repetitive sickling events can result in irreversible organ damage [3]. Children with SCD should be treated by experts, most often pediatric hematologists, for the management of this disease [4].

Comprehensive care and advances in clinical investigations have reduced the morbidity and mortality associated with SCD, especially in young children, and more patients are now surviving into adulthood. Most children with sickle cell anemia (93.9%) and nearly all children with milder forms of SCD (98.4%) now live to become adults [5, 6].

Severe complications of SCD often require hospitalization. The hospitalization of children with SCD constitutes a significant burden on their caregivers. The hospital admission pattern of children with SCD varies in different parts of the world.

Although acute, painful crises account for the majority of admissions in many countries. Infections are still the main cause of admissions in other areas, particularly in developing countries [7–10].

The average rate of painful crises prompting medical evaluation in sickle cell anemia (SCA) is 0.8 crises per year, although it is often treated inadequately in the emergency department [11, 12].

Approximately 40% of patients never seek medical attention for pain, while approximately 5% of patients account for one-third of all painful crises events requiring medical attention [11].

Acute chest syndrome (ACS), another important cause of morbidity and mortality among patients with SCD, refers to a constellation of findings that include a new radiodensity on chest radiograph, fever, respiratory distress, and pain that occurs often in the chest. Because of the clinical overlap between pneumonia and ACS, all episodes should be treated promptly with antimicrobial therapy including at least a macrolide and a 3rd-generation cephalosporin to treat the most common pathogens associated with ACS [4].

Many patients with SCD experience inpatient hospitalization for complications of the disease, with many who are also readmitted. Inpatient hospitalization for all children younger than 5 years was recommended by many centers because of the high risk of infection. In addition, all children, regardless of age, with the following high-risk features should be admitted: temperature above 38.5°C, marked lethargy, chest pain and/or shortness of breath, sudden onset of severe headache or seizures, sudden onset of pallor, abdominal distension, priapism, ill or toxic appearance, pain refractory to home treatment and joint pain, swelling, and redness [4, 11].

Identifying factors that can predict risk of readmission in SCD patients allows for the early diagnosis and treatment of groups particularly at risk, thus decreasing morbidity, improving quality of life, and reducing the SCD-related burden on health services [8].

The current study was conducted to identify the main causes of hospitalization among patients with SCD in Basra and to determine the factors associated with the length of hospitalization and with readmission of children and adolescents with SCD.

## 2. Patients and Methods

This descriptive study investigated children and adolescents with SCD who were admitted to the hereditary blood disease ward at the Basra Maternity and Children's Hospital for various reasons between the first of January 2012 and the end of July 2012. A total of 160 patients were recruited; their ages ranged from 9 months to 14 years.

The hospitalization event includes one or more than one admission during a period of more than 30 days from the primary admission [13]. According to this definition the total number of hospitalization events was 237.

Clinical data included age at presentation, sex, history of previous hospitalizations, the number of hospitalizations in the previous year, the number of blood transfusions in the previous year, and asthma symptoms. Disease severity was defined as ≥3 admissions and/or ≥3 blood transfusions in the previous year [13, 14].

The residence and educational level of the mother, the father, and the child (if of school age) were also reported. School attendance was assessed in school age children and was divided into regular, irregular, and left school [15].

Patient's medications like hydroxyurea (HU) and opioid, type of SCD according to the results of High Performance Liquid Chromatography (HPLC), diagnosis, and date of discharge were recorded.

Full clinical examinations were conducted for each patient, including a general examination, vital signs measurements, and a systemic examination.

Treatment, length of hospitalization, complications, outcome, and readmissions (if present) for the patient were recorded. Readmission was defined as a hospital admission occurring within 30 days of the primary admission [13].

In the Center for Hereditary Blood Diseases in Basra, we follow many strategies to reduce infections including penicillin prophylaxis for children ≤5 years old and vaccination (Haemophilus influenzae type b, meningococcus group C, and pneumococcal polysaccharide vaccine). It is worthy to mention that all aspects of management of these patients are free of charge. However, unfortunately we do not have neonatal screening program in Basra which enables early detection and when possible prevention of complications.

Informed consent was obtained from one or both parents for enrollment in the study. The study was approved by the Ethical Committee of the Basra Medical College.

2.1. Statistical Analysis. Statistical analysis was performed using SPSS program version (20) software. Data were expressed as the mean ± standard deviation (SD). Proportions were compared using cross-tabulations with chi-square tests. $t$-tests were used for quantitative comparisons and to compare the difference between two means. Comparisons between groups were made by using one-way analysis of variance (ANOVA) tests. A logistic regression analysis (Multinomial Logistic) was also performed using odds ratios (OR) with a 95% confidence interval (CI). For all tests, a $P$ value of <0.05 was considered to be statistically significant.

## 3. Results

The total number of patients admitted to the general pediatric wards and the hereditary blood diseases ward at the Basra Maternity and Children's Hospital during the study period was 4140. Of these patients, 160 had SCD, with a total of 237 hospitalization events (excluding patients who were readmitted within one month), which constituted 5.75% of the total admissions during the study period.

Of the 160 admitted patients with SCD during the study period, 91 (56.88%) were male, and 69 (43.12%) were female, Table 1. Their ages ranged from 9 months to 14 years, with a mean age (±SD) of 7.97 ± 3.65 years. The majority of admitted patients with SCD had S/β-Thalassemia (81.9%), and 41.25% were between 5 and 10 years old.

The majority of the mothers (68.75%) and 45.61% of the fathers either were illiterate or had received primary school education. One hundred (62.5%) hospitalized patients were of school age; however, only 13% of them regularly attended school.

Acute painful crisis was the most common cause of hospitalization events (73.84%), followed by infection (9.28%), ACS (8.02%), and acute splenic sequestration crisis (ASSC) in 6.32%, Table 2. However, when considering the causes of admission in relation to number of patients both infections and ACS were found to be the second cause of admission (11.8%).

TABLE 1: Selected sociodemographic characteristics of patients.

| Variable | SCA | | S/β-Thalassemia | | Total | |
|---|---|---|---|---|---|---|
| | Number | % | Number | % | Number | % |
| Age (years) | | | | | | |
| ≤5 | 10 | 6.24 | 34 | 21.26 | 44 | 27.5 |
| >5–10 | 14 | 8.74 | 52 | 32.51 | 66 | 41.25 |
| >10–14 | 5 | 3.12 | 45 | 28.13 | 50 | 31.25 |
| Sex | | | | | | |
| Male | 14 | 8.74 | 77 | 48.14 | 91 | 56.88 |
| Female | 15 | 9.36 | 54 | 33.76 | 69 | 43.12 |
| Residence | | | | | | |
| Urban | 13 | 8.11 | 70 | 43.76 | 83 | 51.87 |
| Rural | 16 | 9.99 | 61 | 38.14 | 77 | 48.13 |
| Educational level of father | | | | | | |
| Illiterate | 1 | 0.62 | 10 | 6.25 | 11 | 6.87 |
| Primary | 15 | 9.36 | 47 | 29.38 | 62 | 38.74 |
| Secondary | 6 | 3.75 | 54 | 33.75 | 60 | 37.5 |
| High education | 7 | 5.45 | 20 | 12.5 | 27 | 16.95 |
| Educational level of mother | | | | | | |
| Illiterate | 2 | 1.25 | 17 | 10.63 | 19 | 11.88 |
| Primary | 18 | 11.23 | 73 | 45.64 | 91 | 56.87 |
| Secondary | 7 | 4.37 | 30 | 18.75 | 37 | 23.12 |
| High education | 2 | 1.25 | 11 | 6.88 | 13 | 8.13 |
| Total | 29 | 18.1 | 131 | 81.9 | 160 | 100 |
| School attendance for children (number, 100) | | | | | | |
| Regular | 2 | 2 | 11 | 11 | 13 | 13 |
| Irregular | 15 | 15 | 49 | 49 | 64 | 64 |
| Left | 1 | 1 | 22 | 22 | 23 | 23 |

The extremities were the most common site of pain in both sexes (33.4% overall; 10.5% of female patients and 22.9% of male patients), followed by pain in more than one site (30.7%). The least common site of pain was joint pain (0.7%), Figure 1. There were no significant differences between the sexes concerning the site of pain, $P = 0.178$.

The presence of infections was also recorded. Urine cultures for patients with urinary tract infections (UTI) revealed *E. coli* in 5 cases, *Klebsiella* spp. in 2 cases, and *Proteus* spp. in 1 case. Two patients presented with fever, and all available investigations were negative, including a blood culture.

The pattern of admissions in relation to the type of SCD was studied and it was found that there is no significant difference except for ACS which was significantly higher among patients with Hb SS disease compared to those with S/β-Thalassemia, Table 3.

Forty-two (26.25%) patients had no history of blood transfusion. The mean frequency of blood transfusion was $4.43 \pm 0.54$/year; this frequency was significantly higher among patients with S/β-Thalassemia ($5.19 \pm 0.64$/year) compared to those with SCA ($1.00 \pm 0.21$/year), $P = 0.020$.

Compared to those patients with ASSC, patients with ACS stayed for a significantly longer time at the hospital, $P = 0.030$. The mean LOS for patients on HU was significantly shorter than the LOS for patients who did not receive this drug, $P = 0.032$. However, there was no statistically

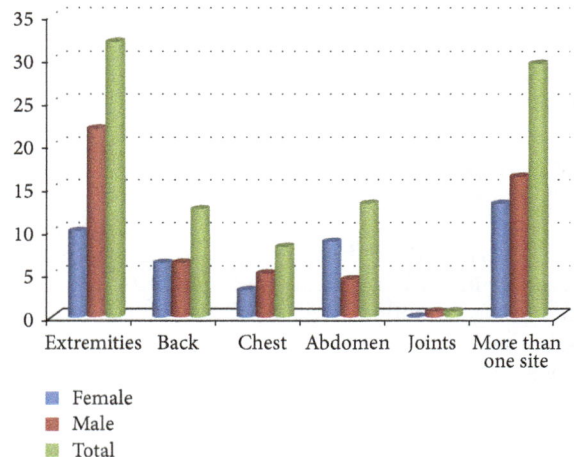

FIGURE 1: Frequency of sickle cell pain by body region and sex. $P$ value = 0.178 (chi-square test).

significant difference in LOS in relation to age, sex, or SCD type, Table 4.

Age, sex, type of SCD, LOS, clinical events, and main treatment modalities (blood transfusion, opioid, and HU) provided to children and adolescents with SCD who were

TABLE 2: Causes of hospital admission.

| Cause | Admitted patients | | Hospitalization events | |
|---|---|---|---|---|
| | Number | % | Number | % |
| Acute painful crisis | 104 | 65 | 175 | 73.84 |
| ACS/pneumonia | 19 | 11.88 | 19 | 8.02 |
| ASSC | 13 | 8.13 | 15 | 6.32 |
| Infection | | | | |
|   Urinary tract infection | 8 | 5 | 10 | 4.23 |
|   Hepatitis A | 4 | 2.5 | 4 | 1.69 |
|   Gastroenteritis | 3 | 1.88 | 4 | 1.69 |
|   Fever | 2 | 1.25 | 2 | 0.84 |
|   Cervical lymphadenitis | 2 | 1.25 | 2 | 0.84 |
| Bleeding due to hypersplenism | 2 | 1.25 | 3 | 1.27 |
| AVN | 1 | 0.63 | 1 | 0.42 |
| Stroke | 1 | 0.63 | 1 | 0.42 |
| Neuroblastoma | 1 | 0.63 | 1 | 0.42 |
| Total | 160 | 100 | 237 | 100 |

ACS: acute chest syndrome, ASSC: acute splenic sequestration crises, and AVN: avascular necrosis.

readmitted compared to those not readmitted were evaluated. The rate of readmissions among hospitalized patients was 23.1%. The mean LOS for readmitted patients was significantly longer than for patients who were not readmitted, $P = 0.022$, Table 5. A history of $\geq 3$ hospitalization in the previous year, asthma symptoms, and opioid use were significant risk factors for readmission, $P < 0.05$. Patients on HU were less likely to be readmitted, $P = 0.006$, Table 6.

## 4. Discussion

There is still a high utilization of medical resources by patients with SCD despite the reductions in morbidity and mortality associated with early screening and the use of prophylactic antibiotics. Interventions directed at the prevention of SCD complications and hospitalizations may reduce the significant economic burden of the disease [16].

In this study, the hospitalization of patients with SCD constituted about 6% of the total number of hospitalizations in the pediatric wards, excluding patients who were admitted to the Emergency Unit and discharged.

The current study showed that approximately two-thirds of school-aged, hospitalized patients have irregular school attendance and approximately one-fourth of hospitalized patients have left school, most likely because of their illness. Shapiro et al. found that, in the USA, approximately half of school absences of SD patients are associated with SCD-related pain. Other causes of school absences include minor infections, clinic visits, and other medical problems associated with SCD. In addition, families may perceive their

children as vulnerable and keep them out of school for problems that would not interfere with school attendance for most children. SCD-related pain and illness also have been shown to affect the psychosocial function and thus the school attendance of these patients [17].

Acute painful crisis was the most common cause of inpatient hospitalizations of SCD patients in this study. This finding supports results reported by Akar and Adekile in Kuwait (63.2%) [18], Jaiyesimi et al. in Oman (83%) [19], and Brown et al. in Nigeria (61.5%) [7].

Frequent acute painful crises requiring hospitalization are one of the characteristic features of SCD [20]. Individualized pain management in the emergency department is effective in improving the management quality of these crises and is associated with a high level of patient satisfaction and decreases in preventable hospitalizations [12, 20, 21].

In this study, the most common site of pain for both sexes was in the extremities. Similarly, Jaiyesimi et al. in Oman reported that 45% of hospitalized patients with SCD had pain in their extremities [19], and Fosdal and Wojner-Alexandrov in the USA found that the extremities were the most common site of pain. However, Fosdal and Wojner-Alexandrov also found that female patients were the most affected, in contrast with our findings [22].

Infections were found to be the second-leading cause of hospitalization among children and adolescents in Basra, followed by ACS then ASSC. Although infections contributed to a considerable percentage of in-patient hospitalizations, an earlier study in Basra reported a higher rate of infections (21%) among hospitalized children with SCD [23] compared to this study.

Despite the wide use of penicillin prophylaxis, the combination of suboptimal compliance and resistance to penicillin prophylaxis, nonvaccine serotypes of S. pneumoniae, and hyposplenism can all explain why children with SCD are still at an increased risk of bacterial infections [24].

ACS was an important cause of hospitalization among both types of SCD in this study. However, it was more common among patients with SCA compared to those with S/β-Thalassemia. This is consistent with research conducted by Hawasawi et al. in Saudi Arabia, who found that ACS was the third-leading cause of hospitalization events among patients with SCD [25], and by Tarer et al. in Guadeloupe, who found it to be the second-leading cause of hospitalization [26].

The LOS among hospitalized patients with SCD in relation to age and sex was not significantly different in Basra. Raphael et al. in the USA found that, after controlling for other factors, older age was the only sociodemographic variable associated with longer LOS [27]. In addition, there was no significant difference in the LOS for patients with both types of SCD, which is consistent with findings by Fosdal and Wojner-Alexandrov in the USA [22].

The mean LOS was longer for patients with ACS than for patients with ASSC. A similar finding was reported by Akar and Adekile in Kuwait, where the LOS for patients with ACS was 5.6 ± 3.3 days, and it was 3.2 ± 2.4 days for ASSC [18].

In this study, the LOS at the hospital was significantly shorter for SCD patients who were on HU compared with those who were not. Patients on HU were also less likely to be

TABLE 3: Causes of admission in relation to type of SCD.

| Causes of admission | SCA | | S/$\beta$-Thalassemia | | Total | |
|---|---|---|---|---|---|---|
| | Number | % | Number | % | Number | % |
| Acute painful crisis | 16 | 55.17 | 88 | 67.18 | 104 | 65 |
| ACS* | 8 | 27.59 | 11 | 8.4 | 19 | 11.88 |
| ASSC | 2 | 6.89 | 11 | 8.4 | 13 | 8.13 |
| Infection | | | | | | |
| UTI | | | 8 | 6.11 | 8 | 5 |
| Hepatitis A | 1 | 3.45 | 3 | 2.29 | 4 | 2.5 |
| Gastroenteritis | 1 | 3.45 | 2 | 1.53 | 3 | 1.88 |
| Fever | | | 2 | 1.53 | 2 | 1.25 |
| Cervical lymphadenitis | 1 | 3.45 | 1 | 0.76 | 2 | 1.25 |
| Bleeding due to hypersplenism | | | 2 | 1.53 | 2 | 1.25 |
| AVN | | | 1 | 0.76 | 1 | 0.63 |
| Stroke | | | 1 | 0.76 | 1 | 0.63 |
| Neuroblastoma | | | 1 | 0.76 | 1 | 0.63 |
| Total | 29 | 100 | 131 | 100 | 160 | 100 |

* $P$ value = 0.007 (chi-square).
ACS: acute chest syndrome, ASSC: acute splenic sequestration crises, AVN: avascular necrosis, and UTI: urinary tract infection.

TABLE 4: Length of hospital stay in relation to selected variables among patients with SCD.

| Variable | LOS (mean ± SD) | $P$ value |
|---|---|---|
| Age (year) | | |
| ≤5 | 3.81 ± 2.44 | |
| >5–10 | 4.63 ± 3.44 | 0.350 |
| >10 | 4.42 ± 2.25 | |
| Sex | | |
| Male | 4.18 ± 2.62 | |
| Female | 4.55 ± 3.14 | 0.421 |
| Type of SCD | | |
| SCA | 4.48 ± 2.16 | |
| S/$\beta$-Thalassemia | 4.31 ± 2.98 | 0.881 |
| HU | | |
| Not received | 4.59 ± 2.86 | |
| Received | 3.41 ± 2.64 | 0.032 |
| Final diagnosis | | |
| Acute painful crisis | 4.10 ± 2.75 | |
| ACS/pneumonia | 5.10 ± 2.44 | 0.030* |
| ASSC | 2.61 ± 0.96 | |

$P$ value calculated by ANOVA test for age and final diagnosis and by $t$-test for other variables.
* Significantly different between ACS and splenic sequestration in relation to length of stay.
ACS: acute chest syndrome, ASSC: acute splenic sequestration crises, HU: hydroxyurea, LOS: length of stay, SCD: sickle cell disease, and SCA: sickle cell anemia.

the SCD-related complications (mainly acute painful crises), the required hospitalizations, and the LOS [28, 29].

Of all the patients with SCD admitted to the hospital, 23.1% were readmitted within 30 days. This result is higher than that reported by Sobota et al. in the USA (17%) [30].

The readmission rate was significantly higher among patients with ≥3 hospitalizations in the previous year and among patients with asthma symptoms. These results are similar to those reported by Frei-Jones et al. in the USA [13] but in contrast to those reported by Sobota et al. in the USA, who found that asthma was not a risk factor for readmission [30].

Asthma is associated with an increase in SCD-related morbidity. Children with SCA and a clinical diagnosis of asthma had nearly twice as many episodes of ACS and more frequent painful episodes, which are 2 leading causes of hospitalization. Based on the pathogenesis of asthma and the prevalence of airway obstruction and airway liability, ventilation-perfusion mismatching may cause local tissue hypoxia, promote increased sickling of red blood cells, and initiate an ACS or a vasoocclusive pain episode [31].

The current study reported that patients with SCD who received opioids during their hospitalization were more likely to be readmitted, while patients who were on HU were less likely to be readmitted. This result could be because an increase in the levels of acute phase reactants that bind to opioids makes them unavailable to induce pain relief, the development of tolerance to opioids, or changes at the opioid receptor sites [21]. However, Loureiro et al. in Brazil did not find such an association; the only risk factors for readmission found in that study were previous vasoocclusive crises and renal failure [32].

readmitted within 30 days. This can be attributed to the fact that HU improves hematological parameters and decreases

TABLE 5: Readmission among hospitalized patients with SCD.

| Variable | Readmission | No readmission | P value |
|---|---|---|---|
| | Number (37) | Number (123) | |
| Mean age (year) ± SD* | 8.55 ± 3.53 | 7.80 ± 3.68 | 0.272 |
| Mean LOS ± SD* | 5.45 ± 3.45 | 4.01 ± 2.56 | 0.022 |
| | Number (%) | Number (%) | |
| Sex | | | |
|   Male | 19 (51.35) | 72 (58.54) | 0.431 |
|   Female | 18 (48.65) | 51 (41.46) | |
| Type of SCD | | | |
|   SCA | 6 (16.22) | 23 (18.70) | 0.732 |
|   S/β-Thalassemia | 31 (83.78) | 100 (81.30) | |
| Final diagnosis | | | |
|   Acute painful crisis | 21 (56.76) | 83 (67.48) | |
|   ACS | 2 (5.40) | 17 (13.82) | 0.572 |
|   ASSC | 3 (8.11) | 10 (8.13) | |
| Hospitalization in previous year | | | |
|   No | 2 (5.41) | 42 (34.15) | |
|   <3 | 9 (24.32) | 41 (33.33) | 0.000 |
|   ≥3 | 26 (70.27) | 40 (32.52) | |
| Blood transfusion in previous year | | | |
|   No | 5 (13.51) | 37 (30.10) | |
|   <3 | 13 (35.14) | 50 (40.70) | 0.027 |
|   ≥3 | 19 (51.35) | 36 (29.30) | |
| Blood transfusion during admission | | | |
|   Not received | 19 (51.35) | 64 (52.03) | 0.942 |
|   Received | 18 (48.65) | 59 (47.97) | |
| Asthma symptom | | | |
|   No | 16 (43.24) | 88 (71.54) | 0.002 |
|   Yes | 21 (56.75) | 35 (28.46) | |
| Opioid received | | | |
|   No | 19 (51.35) | 113 (91.87) | 0.000 |
|   Yes | 18 (48.65) | 10 (8.13) | |
| HU received | | | |
|   No | 33 (89.19) | 93 (75.61) | 0.077 |
|   Yes | 4 (10.81) | 30 (24.39) | |

*P values for age and LOS were assessed by t-test and for other variables by chi-square.
ACS: acute chest syndrome, ASSC: acute splenic sequestration crises, HU: hydroxyurea, LOS: length of stay, SCD: sickle cell disease, and SCA: sickle cell anemia.

Most patients were discharged in good health, and no deaths were reported in this study. This result could be related to the severity of the disease or to the short study period.

The main limitation of this study is its short duration. A longer duration may have revealed other causes of morbidity, and it would have enabled the assessment of mortality among these patients.

It can be concluded from this study that although acute painful crises were the most common cause of hospitalization and readmission among patients with SCD, infections were still reported in a significant proportion of patients with SCD. In addition, there was a relatively high rate of readmission, and the use of HU was associated with shorter LOS and fewer hospital readmissions.

## Disclaimer

The findings of this study are those of the authors and do not necessarily represent the official position of the Center for Hereditary Blood Diseases.

TABLE 6: Logistic regression analysis of different variables with readmission.

| Variable | OR | 95% (CI) | | P value |
|---|---|---|---|---|
| | | Lower | Upper | |
| Age (years) | 0.674 | 0.105 | 4.327 | 0.911 |
| LOS | 1.073 | 0.048 | 24.032 | 0.688 |
| Sex | 0.352 | 0.087 | 1.444 | 0.141 |
| Type of SCD | 0.431 | 0.076 | 2.445 | 0.350 |
| Acute painful crisis | 1.608 | 0.150 | 17.209 | 0.221 |
| Hospitalization in previous year ≥ 3 | 9.352 | 2.011 | 43.490 | 0.001 |
| Blood transfusion in previous year ≥ 3 | 3.325 | 0.477 | 23.163 | 0.393 |
| Asthma symptoms | 4.225 | 1.125 | 15.862 | 0.028 |
| Opioid received | 6.588 | 1.104 | 30.336 | 0.000 |
| HU received | 0.082 | 0.010 | 0.663 | 0.006 |

HU: hydroxyurea, LOS: length of stay, and SCD: sickle cell disease.

## Conflict of Interests

The authors declare no conflict of interests.

## Acknowledgments

The authors would like to thank Dr. Assad Yehia, Professor of Animal Production, College of Agriculture, and Dr. Narjis Abd-AL Hasan Ajeel, Professor of Community Medicine, College of Medicine, University of Basra, for their great help in the statistical analysis of the data.

## References

[1] R. D. Cançado, "Sickle cell disease: looking back but towards the future," *Revista Brasileira de Hematologia e Hemoterapia*, vol. 34, no. 3, pp. 175–177, 2012.

[2] M. K. Hassan, J. Y. Taha, L. M. Al-Naama, N. M. Widad, and S. N. Jasim, "Frequency of haemoglobinopathies and glucose-6-phosphate dehydrogenase deficiency in Basra," *Eastern Mediterranean Health Journal*, vol. 9, no. 1-2, pp. 45–54, 2003.

[3] A. M. Brandow and R. I. Liem, "Sickle cell disease in the emergency department: atypical complications and management," *Clinical Pediatric Emergency Medicine*, vol. 12, no. 3, pp. 202–212, 2011.

[4] M. R. De Baun, M. Frei-Jones, and E. Vichinsky, "Hemglobinobathies," in *Nelson TextBook of Pediatrics*, E. R. Behrman, R. M. Kliegman, and H. B. Jenson, Eds., pp. 1663–1670, Elsevier Saunders, Philadelphia, Pa, USA, 19th edition, 2011.

[5] R. Colombatti, M. Montanaro, F. Guasti et al., "Comprehensive care for sickle cell disease immigrant patients: a reproducible model achieving high adherence to minimum standards of care," *Pediatric Blood and Cancer*, vol. 59, no. 7, pp. 1275–1279, 2012.

[6] C. T. Quinn, Z. R. Rogers, T. L. McCavit, and G. R. Buchanan, "Improved survival of children and adolescents with sickle cell disease," *Blood*, vol. 115, no. 17, pp. 3447–3452, 2010.

[7] B. J. Brown, N. E. Jacob, I. A. Lagunju, and O. O. Jarrett, "Morbidity and mortality pattern in hospitalized children with sickle cell disorders at the University College Hospital, Ibadan, Nigeria," *Nigerian Journal of Paediatrics*, vol. 40, no. 1, pp. 34–39, 2013.

[8] G. Aljuburi, A. A. Laverty, S. A. Green, K. J. Phekoo, D. Bell, and A. Majeed, "Socio-economic deprivation and risk of emergency readmission and inpatient mortality in people with sickle cell disease in England: observational study," *Journal of Public Health*, vol. 35, no. 4, pp. 510–517, 2013.

[9] C. Booth, B. Inusa, and S. K. Obaro, "Infection in sickle cell disease: a review," *International Journal of Infectious Diseases*, vol. 14, no. 1, pp. e2–e12, 2010.

[10] A. N. Ikefuna and I. J. Emodi, "Hospital admission of patients with sickle cell anaemia pattern and outcome in Enugu area of Nigeria," *Nigerian Journal of Clinical Practice*, vol. 10, no. 1, pp. 24–29, 2007.

[11] P. Lanskowsky, S. Arkin, M. Atlas, B. Aygun, and D. Friedman, "Hemoglobin defects, sickle cell disease," in *Manual of Pediatric Hematology and Oncology*, P. Lanzkowsky, Ed., pp. 200–224, Academic Press, 5th edition, 2011.

[12] L. Krishnamurti, B. Smith-Packard, A. Gupta, M. Campbell, S. Gunawardena, and R. Saladino, "Impact of individualized pain plan on the emergency management of children with sickle cell disease," *Pediatric Blood and Cancer*, vol. 61, no. 10, pp. 1747–1753, 2014.

[13] M. J. Frei-Jones, J. J. Field, and M. R. DeBaun, "Risk factors for hospital readmission within 30 days: a new quality measure for children with sickle cell disease," *Pediatric Blood and Cancer*, vol. 52, no. 4, pp. 481–485, 2009.

[14] D. Jain, K. Italia, V. Sarathi, K. Ghoshand, and R. Colah, "Sickle cell anemia from central India: a retrospective analysis," *Indian Pediatrics*, vol. 49, no. 11, pp. 911–913, 2012.

[15] S. S. Al Arrayed and N. Haites, "Features of sickle cell disease in Bahrain," *Eastern Mediterranean Health Journal*, vol. 1, no. 1, pp. 112–119, 1995.

[16] T. L. Kauf, T. D. Coates, L. Huazhi, N. Mody-Patel, and A. G. Hartzema, "The cost of health care for children and adults with sickle cell disease," *American Journal of Hematology*, vol. 84, no. 6, pp. 323–327, 2009.

[17] B. S. Shapiro, D. F. Dinges, E. C. Orne et al., "Home management of sickle cell-related pain in children and adolescents: natural history and impact on school attendance," *Pain*, vol. 61, no. 1, pp. 139–144, 1995.

[18] N. A. Akar and A. Adekile, "Ten-year review of hospital admissions among children with sickle cell disease in Kuwait," *Medical Principles and Practice*, vol. 17, no. 5, pp. 404–408, 2008.

[19] F. Jaiyesimi, R. Pandey, D. Bux, Y. Sreekrishna, F. Zaki, and N. Krishnamoorthy, "Sickle cell morbidity profile in Omani children," *Annals of Tropical Paediatrics*, vol. 22, no. 1, pp. 45–52, 2002.

[20] Y. Lamarre, M. Romana, X. Waltz et al., "Hemorheological risk factors of acute chest syndrome and painful vaso-occlusive crisis in children with sickle cell disease," *Haematologica*, vol. 97, no. 11, pp. 1641–1647, 2012.

[21] S. K. Ballas, "Current issues in sickle cell pain and its management," *Hematology/the Education Program of the American Society of Hematology*, vol. 2007, no. 1, pp. 97–105, 2007.

[22] M. B. Fosdal and A. W. Wojner-Alexandrov, "Events of hospitalization among children with sickle cell disease," *Journal of Pediatric Nursing*, vol. 22, no. 4, pp. 342–346, 2007.

[23] I. A. Ali and M. K. Hassan, "Sickle cell syndrome in children in Basrah," *Medical Journal of Tikrit*, vol. 5, pp. 10–15, 1999.

[24] S. Chakravorty and T. N. Williams, "Sickle cell disease: a neglected chronic disease of increasing global health importance," *Archives of Disease in Childhood*, vol 100, no. 1, pp. 48–53, 2015.

[25] Z. M. Hawasawi, G. Nabi, M. S. F. Al Magamci, and K. S. Awad, "Sickle cell disease in childhood in Madina," *Annals of Saudi Medicine*, vol. 18, no. 4, pp. 293–295, 1998.

[26] V. Tarer, M. Etienne-Julan, J.-P. Diara et al., "Sickle cell anemia in Guadeloupean children: pattern and prevalence of acute clinical events," *European Journal of Haematology*, vol. 76, no. 3, pp. 193–199, 2006.

[27] J. L. Raphael, B. U. Mueller, M. A. Kowalkowski, and S. O. Oyeku, "Shorter hospitalization trends among children with sickle cell disease," *Pediatric Blood and Cancer*, vol. 59, no. 4, pp. 679–684, 2012.

[28] S. K. Ballas, R. L. Bauserman, W. F. McCarthy, O. L. Castro, W. R. Smith, and M. A. Waclawiw, "Hydroxyurea and acute painful crises in sickle cell anemia: effects on hospital length of stay and opioid utilization during hospitalization, outpatient acute care contacts, and at home," *Journal of Pain and Symptom Management*, vol. 40, no. 6, pp. 870–882, 2010.

[29] M. Mulaku, N. Opiyo, J. Karumbi, G. Kitonyi, G. Thoithi, and M. English, "Evidence review of hydroxyurea for the prevention of sickle cell complications in low-income countries," *Archives of Disease in Childhood*, vol. 98, no. 11, pp. 908–914, 2013.

[30] A. Sobota, D. A. Graham, E. J. Neufeld, and M. M. Heeney, "Thirty-day readmission rates following hospitalization for pediatric sickle cell crisis at freestanding children's hospitals: risk factors and hospital variation," *Pediatric Blood & Cancer*, vol. 58, no. 1, pp. 61–65, 2012.

[31] J. H. Boyd, E. A. Macklin, R. C. Strunk, and M. R. DeBaun, "Asthma is associated with acute chest syndrome and pain in children with sickle cell anemia," *Blood*, vol. 108, no. 9, pp. 2923–2927, 2006.

[32] M. M. Loureiro, S. Rozenfeld, M. S. Carvalho, and R. D. Portugal, "Factors associated with hospital readmission in sickle cell disease," *BMC Blood Disorders*, vol. 9, article 2, 2009.

# 7

# Relationship between Painful Crisis and Serum Zinc Level in Children with Sickle Cell Anaemia

**Edamisan Olusoji Temiye,[1] Edem Samuel Duke,[2] Mbang Adeyemi Owolabi,[3] and James Kweku Renner[1]**

[1] Department of Paediatrics, College of Medicine, University of Lagos (CMUL), P.M.B 12003, Lagos, Nigeria
[2] Critical Rescue International (CRI), Plot 144, Oba Akran Road, Ikeja, Lagos, Nigeria
[3] Department of Pharmaceutical Chemistry, Faculty of Pharmacy, College of Medicine, Idi-Araba, University of Lagos, P.M.B. 12003, Lagos, Nigeria

Correspondence should be addressed to Edamisan Olusoji Temiye, edatemiye2000@yahoo.co.uk

Academic Editor: Duran Canatan

Sickle cell anaemia (SCA) is associated with zinc deficiency; zinc supplementation may ameliorate some of its clinical manifestations including the relief of painful crisis. *Subjects and Methods.* Serum zinc levels were determined in 71 children with SCA and painful crisis and in equal numbers in steady state. Seventy-one children with AA genotype acted as controls. Qualitative assessment of zinc content of 24-hour dietary recall and the last meal consumed before blood was drawn was taken. Serum zinc was determined using atomic absorption spectrophotometer. Haemoglobin concentration and packed cell volume (PCV) were determined using standard methods. *Results.* The mean serum zinc concentration in the study was less than international reference range. The controls had significantly higher serum zinc concentrations than the SCA group (42.7 ± 13.6 versus 32.3 ± 14.0 $\mu$g/dL, $P < .000$); this difference was due to the significantly lower values of serum zinc in SCA with painful crisis compared with the remaining two groups $F = 30.9$, $P < .000$. There was a positive correlation between serum zinc and haemoglobin concentration only in the control group ($r = 0.4$; $P = .001$). *Conclusion.* The serum zinc levels in this study were low. Painful crisis in SCA may exert greater demand for zinc utilization in children with SCA thereby resulting in lower serum levels.

## 1. Introduction

Sickle cell anaemia is the most common inherited disorder of the black race. It affects red blood cells resulting in chronic haemolytic anaemia of varying severity and in some patients, periodic painful crisis caused by the occlusion of small blood vessels by spontaneous intravascular sickling with multiorgan affectation [1, 2].

Brewer and Oelshlegel discovered that calcium binding to red cell membrane is responsible for the formation of irreversible sickled cells and that the antisickling effect of zinc in sickle cell anaemia is due to its ability to antagonize calcium binding to red cell membrane [3]. In sickle cell anaemia, there is also increased oxidative stress and peroxidation as well as low antioxidant potential which predisposes the patients to vaso-occlusive crisis

[4–6]. Zinc exerts its antioxidant action by inhibition of lipid peroxidation which occurs in red blood cells and liver thereby stabilizing biomembranes and biostructures thus protecting the body against oxidative stress [5, 6]. These effects of zinc are believed to give zinc its ability to reduce vaso-occlusive crisis in sickle cell anaemia.

Various studies have shown that zinc deficiency may be common in SCA patients. This has been attributed to chronic haemolysis that occurs in these patients, increased demand and utilization, along with the secondary loss of zinc in the urine [1, 7, 8]. Furthermore, supplementation of zinc in sickle cell anaemia has been reported to improve wound healing, decrease incidence of infection, improve the age of attaining secondary sexual characteristics, reverse dark adaptation of the eyes, and accelerate growth [8–12].

Although it has been suggested that zinc therapy could reduce painful crisis [13, 14]; however, it has not been shown with certainty that zinc deficiency in sickle cell anaemia is directly related to the development or severity of vaso-occlusive crisis. Prasad et al. [15], in 1976 administered oral zinc sulfate to 10 adults who had severe painful crisis and found symptomatic improvement in 8 of the subjects, which they attributed to the antisickling effect of zinc. The significance of their findings may be limited because of the very small sample size and lack of control subjects in the study. In a placebo-controlled double-blind study, 145 sickle cell adult subjects were treated with either 220 mg of zinc sulphate 3 times daily or placebo [14]. After 18 months, the zinc-treated subjects had an average of 2.5 crises, compared to 5.3 in the placebo group; but the severity of painful crisis was not reduced. A study in Ibadan, Nigeria [16] found no relationship between serum zinc level and the different degrees of clinical severity of the disease in these subjects. They observed that the level of zinc in each patient, though significantly lower than the controls, had no correlation with the haematocrit, frequency of bone pain crisis, and susceptibility to infection. The sample size in their study was also small making it difficult to draw any valid inference.

It is probable that zinc deficiency may be associated with painful crisis. However, these authors are not aware of any previous work comparing zinc status in sickle cell anaemic patients in vaso-occlusive crisis with those in steady state. This study is therefore designed to assess the level of serum zinc in sickle cell anaemia children in painful state (vaso-occlusive crisis) as compared with those in steady state. We also relate the levels of serum zinc with diet and haemoglobin levels in the subjects.

## 2. Subjects and Methods

This was a case-controlled study of patients at the Lagos University Teaching Hospital (LUTH), Nigeria. The sample size for the study and the number of subjects for each arm were determined using standard formulae for population study [17], using the prevalence rate of SCA in western Nigeria [18] and the rate of deficient erythrocyte zinc level in sickle cell anaemia children in Zaria [19]. One hundred and forty-two paediatric subjects aged between one and 12 yrs who had haemoglobin genotype SS were studied. Of these, 71 were in had bone pain crisis and were recruited consecutively from both the haematology clinic and Children's Emergency Room (CHER) the remainder were in steady state recruited from the sickle cell clinic. The control group consisted of 71 apparently well subjects whose haemoglobin genotype was AA. They were recruited from the Well Baby and Children's Outpatient Clinic. Both the SCA in steady state subjects and the controls were selected such that they were matched for age and sex with the subjects who had painful crisis.

In this study, sickle cell anaemia in painful crisis was defined as subjects who had pains at the time of recruitment or within 48 hours before recruitment in any of the limbs [20], while steady state was defined as subjects who were apparently well without evidence of recent infection,

bone pain, or other problems for at least 4 weeks before recruitment [21]. The study, which was approved by the research and ethics committee of the hospital, lasted for a period of 12 months. Other inclusion criteria were that study population were not on any zinc-containing medications, they were fed at least 4 hours before blood collection, and had not been transfused with blood or blood products in the previous three months preceding study. Also included were subjects who did not have any symptoms or signs of infection such as fever (axillary temp $< 37.0°C$), acute respiratory infection, diarrhoea, or malaria. Additionally, controls had no evidence of chronic disease including protein energy malnutrition. The haemoglobin genotype of all the subjects was determined by haemoglobin cellulose electrophoresis.

After informed consent, a detailed history of each child from the care-giver was taken; these included the mother's and father's educational status and occupation, 24-hour meal recall, date of last blood transfusion, and the presence or absence of pain in the limbs. Physical examination including assessment for the presence or absence of fever (temp $> 37.0°C$), jaundice, pallor, finger clubbing, liver size, spleen size, and tenderness in the limbs, the weight, and length/height was done. Previous health status of each subject was obtained by examining the hospital records. Five mL of blood was collected from each subject by venepuncture after appropriate skin preparations with a 21-gauge stainless-steel needle with a polypropylene syringe (Norm-Ject; Henke Sass Wolf GMBH, Germany) [22]. Two mL of blood was transferred into a sodium ethylenediamine-tetra-acetate (EDTA) bottle for haemoglobin (Hb), Packed cell volume (PCV), and haemoglobin genotype determination using standard laboratory procedure. The remaining 3 mL was transferred into zinc free nonheparinized bottles previously washed clean of possible zinc contamination by leaving them soaked in 10% nitric acid for 24 hours and rinsed three times with deionised water. The clotted blood sample in the zinc-free bottles was centrifuged at 1500 rpm for 10 minutes and the serum removed with zinc free Pasteur Pipette prepared by previously washing with 10% nitric acid and thoroughly rinsed with deionised water as described for the bottles above [23]. The serum samples were then stored at $-20°C$ pending analysis [24]. All haemolysed samples were discarded. Before the analysis, the serum samples were allowed to come to room temperature and each mixed by gently inverting the tube four times. Serum zinc level was determined using an atomic absorption spectrophotometer (PU9100X, Philips, Holland) at the Food Technology laboratory of the Federal Institute of Industrial Research Oshodi (FIIRO) Lagos, Nigeria and following the method of Smith et al. [22]. The concentration of each sample, which was expressed in parts per million, was extrapolated from the calibration curve prepared from the standard zinc calibration curve and converted to µg/dL by calculation.

## 3. Classification of Zinc Content in 24-Hour Meal Recall

The zinc contents of 24-hour meal recall and the last meal consumed before blood was taken were classified based on

TABLE 1: Mean haematological parameters and serum zinc concentration in Cases and Controls.

| Parameter | Genotype (Mean ± 2SD) | | | $F$ | $P$-value |
| | Genotype AA ($n = 71$) | Sickle cell anaemia | | | |
| | | Steady state $n = 71$ | Painful crisis $n = 71$ | | |
|---|---|---|---|---|---|
| Age (mo) | 71.3 ± 34.3 | 67.2 ± 30.1 | 79.9 ± 31.7 | 2.9 | .06 |
| Weight (Kg) | 21.1 ± 8.0 | 17.9 ± 5.4 | 20.3 ± 6.3 | 4.6 | .01 |
| Height (cm) | 115.7 ± 21.1 | 108.4 ± 16.8 | 115.7 ± 17.8 | 3.6 | .03 |
| Hb (g/dL) | 11.3 ± 2.0 | 7.1 ± 1.1 | 7.6 ± 1.6 | 144.9 | .00 |
| PCV (%) | 33.1 ± 5.6 | 20.9 ± 3.4 | 22.3 ± 4.8 | 143.9 | .00 |
| Serum Zinc Conc ($\mu$g/dL) | 42.7 ± 13.6 | 38.4 ± 13.8 | 26.3 ± 11.3 | 30.9 | .00 |

$P < .05$ is significant.

the concentration of zinc in food items consumed by the subject. Thus each food item was classified as containing high, moderate, or low zinc [25, 26]. Meals which contain items such as plantain, red beef, sea foods, egg, milk, cocoa products, and fish were classified as high zinc content, while beans, cereals made out of maize and rice products contain moderate zinc. Cassava products were classified as having traces or low zinc content [25, 26]. For the purpose of this study, a subject who had more than 2 high zinc containing items with any 3 moderate zinc containing items or all high zinc containing items was classified as having high zinc diet. A subject who had one high zinc containing item and less than 3 moderate zinc containing items or had all moderate zinc containing items was classified as having moderate zinc, while a subject who had one moderate zinc or one high zinc containing item with low zinc containing item, or only low zinc containing items, was classified as having low zinc.

## 4. Data Analysis

Data generated was analysed using the SPSS statistical package version 11. Frequency distributions were generated for all categorical variables. The measures of location were determined for quantitative outcome such as age, zinc level, and haematocrit. Statistical significance between two means was assessed using Student $t$-test, while one-way analysis of variance was used where there were multiple means. Where there was significant difference within means, post hoc test was applied to determine where the level of significance occurred. Chi-square ($\chi^2$) test was applied for categorical variables and correlation analysis as applicable. Differences between values were accepted as statistically significant where probability was less than .05.

## 5. Results

Two hundred and thirteen children aged between one and 12 yrs were recruited into the study; seventy-one were controls with haemoglobin genotype AA, while one hundred and forty-two subjects had haemoglobin genotype SS. Seventy one of the subjects with sickle cell anaemia were in steady state while the rest had vaso-occlusive bone pain crisis. Eighty-two of the study subjects were males and 60 were

females giving a male : female ratio of 1.3 : 1. This difference was not statistically significant. Also, the male : female ratio for each of the subgroup was not significantly different.

The mean ages of the subjects in control group and those with sickle cell anaemia were 71.3 ± 34.3 months and 73.6 ± 31.4 months, respectively. The difference was not statistically significant. ($t = 0.5$, $P = .64$). Although the control subjects were heavier than the SCA subjects (weight (kg), 21.1 ± 8.0 versus 19.1 ± 6.0, $t = 2.1$, $P = .04$) and they were also taller, (height (cm) 115.7 ± 21.1 versus 112.1 ± 17.6, $t = 1.3$, $P = .2$), the differences were not statistically significant. However, the control subjects had a mean packed cell volume of 33.1 ± 5.6% and haemoglobin of 11.3 ± 2.0 g/dL which were significantly higher ($t = 16.9$, $P = .000$) than the SCA group with a mean packed cell volume of 21.6 ± 4.2% and haemoglobin concentration of 7.4 ± 1.4 g/dL, respectively. The mean serum zinc concentration in the control subjects was also significantly higher than the sickle cell anaemia group ($42.7 \pm 13.6$ versus $32.3 \pm 14.0$ $\mu$g/dL, $t = 5.2$, $P = .000$)

When the sickle cell anaemia group was subdivided into those in steady state and those with bone pain crisis, the mean age remained not significantly different although the mean age for subjects with painful crisis was higher than those of sickle cell anaemia in steady state and the control subjects. Sickle cell anaemia subjects in steady state were however significantly shorter than those with painful crisis and with haemoglobin AA. Similarly, sickle cell anaemia subjects in steady state were significantly lighter than the controls ($P = .01$) subjects and sickle cell anaemia subjects with painful crisis. The significant difference observed in the haemoglobin concentration and packed cell volume was found to be between the control group and the sickle cell anaemia in painful crisis and sickle cell anaemia in steady state. Although the sickle cell anaemia in painful crisis had higher haematological parameters than the steady state subjects, the difference was not statistically significant. The mean serum zinc concentration in subjects with haemoglobin genotype SS in steady state of 38.4 ± 13.8 $\mu$g/dL was significantly higher than in subjects with bone pain crisis of 26.3 ± 11.3 $\mu$g/dL ($P < .001$). The result also showed significantly higher mean serum zinc concentration levels ($P < .001$) in controls when compared with subjects in bone pain crisis. However, the differences between control and steady state subjects were not statistically significant, Table 1.

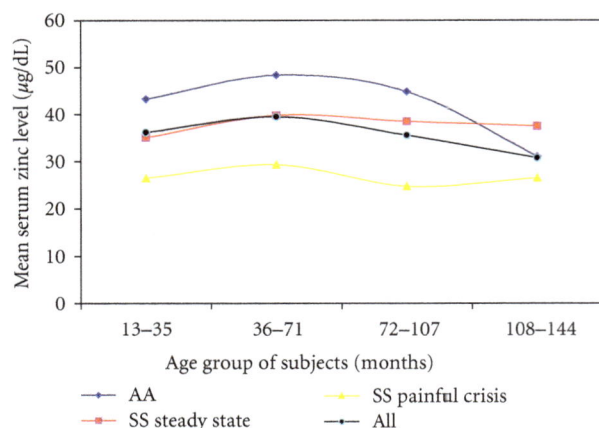

FIGURE 1: Mean zinc concentration by age groups in the three subgroups.

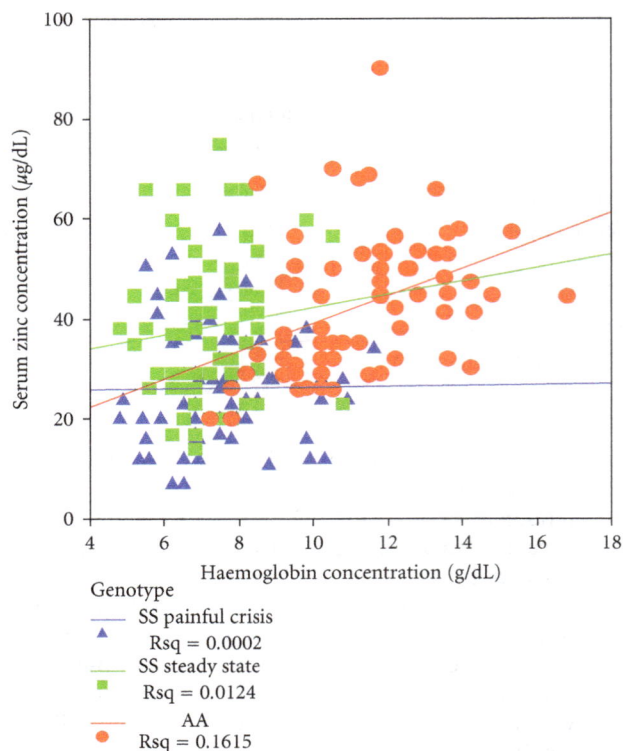

FIGURE 2: Linear relationship between haemoglobin concentration to serum zinc levels in Control, SCA in steady state, and SCA in painful crisis.

The subjects were arranged into four age groups. Thirty three subjects (15.5%) were between 13 and 35 months of age, 57 (26.7%) were in the age group of 36–71 months, the majority (83, 39.0%) were between 72 and 107 months of age and the remaining 40 (18.8%) were between 108–144 months of age. There were, however, no significant differences in the numbers of subjects in the different age groups ($P > .03$). The mean serum levels of zinc for the age groups for all the subjects ranged from $36.21 \pm 12.8\,\mu g/dL$ for age group of 13–35 months, $39.5 \pm 15.6\,\mu g/dL$ for age group of 36–71 months, $35.6 \pm 16.0\,\mu g/dL$, to $30.7 \pm 10.2\,\mu g/dL$, for age groups of 108–144 months. The differences in the values were statistically significant $F = 2.9, P = .04$.

When the subjects were grouped into controls, sickle cell steady state, and painful crisis, however, the control subjects had higher mean serum zinc levels than the sickle cell anaemia subgroups in all age groups except in the age group of 108–144 months where the steady state subjects had higher levels than the control group. These differences were statistically significant and the level of significance was between the controls and the sickle cell anaemia subjects in painful crisis except in the age group of 108–144 months where the level of significance was between the sickle cell anaemia in steady state and SCA in painful crisis. Among the controls, there was a significant fall in serum zinc levels as the subjects get older, $F = 5.0, P = .004$, but such decrease in zinc levels with age was not observed among the sickle cell subgroups; $F = 0.8, P = .3$ (in sickle cell anaemia in steady state and $F = 0.5, P = .7$ in sickle cell anaemia subjects in painful crisis). In all the age groups, the SCA in painful crisis had serum zinc levels significantly lower than those of controls and subject with SCA in steady state (Figure 1).

Figure 2 shows the correlation between haemoglobin and serum zinc concentrations. There is a positive correlation between haemoglobin concentration and zinc levels in the control group and this was significant ($r = 0.4, P < .001$). There was no correlation observed in the steady states subjects ($r = 0.01, P = .4$) and in subjects in bone pain crisis ($r = 0.01, P = .9$).

The effect of dietary intake of zinc-containing meals on serum zinc was assessed. Ten (4.7%) subjects were assessed to have consumed meals low in zinc content in the last 24 hours, 6 of these were SCA in steady state and 3 were SCA in painful crisis; the remaining subject in this category was the control. Ninety seven (45.5%) subjects, consisting of 18 controls, 31 SCA in steady state, and 48 SCA in painful crisis had food items with moderate zinc content. The remaining 106 (49.8%) subjects of whom 52 were in control group, 34 SCA in steady state, and 20 SCA with painful crisis had food items containing high level of zinc.

When the zinc content of food items consumed by subjects 24 hour prior to collection of blood for analysis were compared with mean serum zinc concentration, it was found that subjects in the control group whose meal were adjudged to contain moderate amount of zinc had mean serum zinc concentration of $41.1 \pm 17.2\,\mu g/dl$ compared to $43.3 \pm 12.5\,\mu g/dl$ in those whose food items contained high amount of zinc. This difference was however not statistically significant. In the SCA group, subjects in the steady state who consumed low zinc items in their meal had serum zinc concentration of $30.7 \pm 12.1\,\mu g/dL$, those that consumed moderate zinc levels had $40.8 \pm 14.0$ while those that

TABLE 2: Relationship between zinc content of 24-hour dietary recall and mean serum zinc level.

| Zinc content of meal | Mean serum zinc concentration $\mu$g/dL ($\pm$ SD) | | | F | P-value |
| --- | --- | --- | --- | --- | --- |
| | Genotype AA | Sickle cell anaemia | | | |
| | | Steady state | Painful crisis | | |
| Low | 45.0[††] | 30.7 (12.1) | 33.9 (20.7) | $t = 0.3$ | .8 |
| Moderate | 41.1 (17.2) | 40.8 (14.0) | 24.8 (10.5) | 18.4 | .000 |
| High | 43.3 (12.5) | 37.6 (13.7) | 28.5 (11.4) | 9.9 | .000 |

[††]Only one subject in the control group had low zinc item and was removed from the statistical analysis; therefore, student $t$-test was used to compare the mean zinc level between sickle cell anaemia subjects in steady state and painful crisis in the first row.

TABLE 3: Relationship between zinc content of last meal consumed before taking blood and mean serum zinc level.

| Zinc content of meal | Mean serum zinc concentration $\mu$g/dL ($\pm$ SD) | | | F | P-value |
| --- | --- | --- | --- | --- | --- |
| | Genotype AA $n = 71$ | Sickle cell anaemia | | | |
| | | Steady state $n = 71$ | Painful crisis $n = 71$ | | |
| Low | 46.7 (37.8) | 29.3 (10.8) | 20.0 (9.9) | 1.9 | .192 |
| Moderate | 40.6 (12.5) | 37.6 (13.0) | 25.7 (10.9) | 23.1 | .000 |
| High | 46.9 (10.8) | 55.4 (11.5) | 34.4 (11.5) | 6.6 | .004 |

consumed high zinc levels had a mean value of 37.6 ± 13.7. This difference was not statistically significant. SCA subjects with painful crisis who consumed low zinc containing meals had mean serum concentration of 33.9 ± 20.7 µg/dL. For those who consumed moderate zinc containing items had mean serum zinc level of 24.8 ± 10.5 µg/dL, and for those that took high zinc containing items their mean serum zinc concentration was 28.5 ± 11.4 µg/dL. Again this difference was not statistically significant. However, across the subgroups, control subjects had mean serum levels of zinc that were significantly higher than those in the SCA subgroups among subjects that consumed moderate to high zinc containing meals, Table 2.

When the zinc contents of the last meals consumed before blood was taken were considered, most subjects, 164 (77.0%) of whom 47, 59, and 58 were in the control, SCA steady state, and SCA painful crisis subgroups, respectively, consumed meals containing moderate zinc contents. Thirty-five (16.4%) subjects had food items containing high zinc content; 21 of these subjects were in control group while 6 and 8 subjects were in SCA in steady state and painful crisis, respectively. The remaining 14 (6.6%) (3 in control group, 6 SCA in steady state, and 5 in SCA painful crisis) had food items containing low zinc contents.

Using the content of the last meal consumed it was found that, except in the control groups, those that consumed high zinc containing meals had highest mean serum zinc levels. This was significant among the SCA in steady state, $F = 7.0$, $P = .002$, and just reached significant level in SCA in painful crisis, $F = 3.1, P = .05$. Within the subgroups, those with low zinc consumption had no significant difference, the mean serum zinc level was however significantly lower in SCA in painful crisis than those in controls and steady state who took food items with moderate zinc content. Similar trend was observed in those who consumed food items containing high zinc contents; again the mean serum level for SCA in

painful crisis was significantly lower than those of controls and SCA in steady state, Table 3.

## 6. Discussion

The serum zinc levels in this group of Nigerian children were found to be lower than the internationally acceptable normal values of 50–150 µg/dL {7.65–22.95 µmol/L} [27]. This is also true for the control group as well as those with sickle cell anaemia. Several studies have indicated that nutritional zinc deficiency is widespread all over the world. Akinkugbe and Ette [28] observed that low zinc levels are common in Nigerian children. Important risk factors related to zinc deficiency are common use of grain proteins and low content of zinc in breast milk of mothers and weaning food [27, 28]. These factors may be important in our subjects as more than 80% were on food containing low or moderate amount of zinc in their last meal before blood was drawn for analysis. This should reflect more accurately the nature of meal the child is taking than the 24-hour recall. Most of these food items contained high level of cassava- and grain-based diet which limits the quantity of zinc available for absorption due to their high phosphate and phytate content as zinc forms an unavailable complex with these compounds [27–29].

Although the subjects had low serum zinc levels, symptoms attributable solely to zinc deficiency were not found, especially in the control subjects. It is difficult to say at what level of serum zinc that symptoms of deficiency would appear, and the reasons for lack of symptoms in the control subjects is unclear. The significantly lower values of zinc observed in children older than 107 months in the control group probably reflect increased demand for zinc in already suboptimal zinc nutriture in these subjects at the commencement of pubertal growth [30].

In all age groups, the serum zinc levels were significantly lower in the SCA group than in the controls. This finding has been reported in several communications [6, 7, 15, 30] and has been attributed to several factors including the chronic haemolysis that characterizes sickle cell anaemia leading to loss of zinc from red blood cells which is an important storage site for zinc [6, 28]. Furthermore, there is a defective zinc homeostasis as a result of excessive excretion of zinc in urine or abnormal renal tubular reabsorption of zinc due to the sickling phenomena, increased demand and consumption due to increased oxidative stress and sickle cell redox imbalance [6, 8, 10]. The further lowering of serum zinc in SCA subjects with painful crisis in this study was an interesting finding. It could be postulated that SCA subjects who are more severely zinc-deficient would have more painful crisis. On the other hand, frequent painful crisis might interfere with nutrition and lead to more severe nutritional deficiencies [6].

Zinc is the most abundant intracellular element with 85% of total body zinc found in muscle and bone; less than 0.1% of total body zinc is in the plasma [31]. Plasma zinc is maintained by continuous shift from the intracellular sources and absorption from the intestine. Hence plasma zinc is a poor indicator of total body zinc. The retention time of zinc in the blood is estimated as 2.3 days [32]; however, metabolic stress, such as infection and acute illnesses which are more common in children with sickle cell disease compared to children with haemoglobin genotype AA, increases intracellular shift of zinc into the liver and lowers plasma level even when total body zinc level is unchanged [33]. As already noted above, the low plasma zinc level in this study in sickle cell anemia subjects with painful crisis may indicate the effects of stress in increasing the intracellular shifting of zinc into the liver from the plasma of these subjects rather than increased loss of zinc from the body.

This study showed a positive correlation between the serum zinc and haemoglobin in the control group. This is in conformity with the findings of Akinkugbe and Ette [28], whose study was on serum zinc and haemoglobin levels in children with common paediatric problems. However, there was no correlation between serum zinc and haemoglobin in the subjects with SCA; this is in conformity with the finding of Akenami et al. [16] in sickle cell anaemia children. The reason for this is not clear. It may be due to the chronic haemolytic state experienced by sickle cell anaemia subjects, leading to loss of zinc at it is storage site (red blood cell) and it is urinary loss. Further studies are required to explain this finding.

Zinc deficiency is associated with poor growth, among other clinical manifestations [8, 34]. In this study, the control group had significantly higher weight and height than the sickle cell anaemia group in steady state but not with the SCA group with painful crisis. This may be attributed to the growth retardation associated with zinc deficiency. However, one would have expected the SCA children with painful crisis who also had the lowest levels of serum zinc to be the most affected in growth, but this was not the case. The Haemoglobin concentration in the SCA with painful crisis was also higher than those without painful crisis. It is possible that the higher oxygen-carrying capacity of children with

painful crisis had a better effect on growth than the level of plasma zinc. Since there was also no significant difference in the quality of the meals consumed in terms of zinc content between these groups, it is possible that the lower serum zinc concentration in SCA subjects with painful crisis resulted from more severe disease with higher oxidative stress leading to higher utilization of zinc rather than a poorer serum zinc status.

Since this study was a cross-sectional one, it was important to observe whether the zinc status of these subjects improved several days after recovery from their painful episodes or whether zinc therapy would have aborted or shorten periods of painful episodes. These should form the basis for our next study in these children.

# References

[1] R. G. Hendrickse, "Disorders of the blood," in *Paediatrics in the Tropics*, R. G. Hendrickse, D. C. G. Barr, and T. S. Matthews, Eds., pp. 346–352, Oxford Blackwell Press, 1st edition, 1991.

[2] G. R. Serjeant, "Nomenclature and genetics of sickle cell disease, historical aspects," in *Sickle Cell Disease*, G. R. Serjeant, Ed., pp. 25–61, Oxford University Press, New York, NY, USA, 1st edition, 1988.

[3] G. J. Brewer and F. J. Oelshlegel Jr., "Antisickling effects of zinc," *Biochemical and Biophysical Research Communications*, vol. 58, no. 3, pp. 854–861, 1974.

[4] D. A. Adelekan, D. I. Thurnham, and A. D. Adekile, "Reduced antioxidant capacity in paediatric patients with homozygous sickle cell disease," *European Journal of Clinical Nutrition*, vol. 43, no. 9, pp. 609–614, 1989.

[5] C. K. Chow, "Nutritional influence on cellular antioxidant defense systems," *American Journal of Clinical Nutrition*, vol. 32, no. 5, pp. 1066–1081, 1979.

[6] R. M. W. Hasanato, "Zinc and antioxidant vitamin deficiency in patients with severe sickle cell anemia," *Annals of Saudi Medicine*, vol. 26, no. 1, pp. 17–21, 2006.

[7] M. B. Leonard, B. S. Zemel, D. A. Kawchak, K. Ohene-Frempong, and V. A. Stallings, "Plasma zinc status, growth, and maturation in children with sickle cell disease," *Journal of Pediatrics*, vol. 132, pp. 467–471, 1998.

[8] B. S. Zemel, D. A. Kawchak, E. B. Fung, K. Ohene-Frempong, and V. A. Stallings, "Effect of zinc supplementation on growth and body composition in children with sickle cell disease," *American Journal of Clinical Nutrition*, vol. 75, no. 2, pp. 300–307, 2002.

[9] W. J. Pories, J. H. Henzel, C. G. Rob, and W. H. Strain, "Acceleration of healing with zinc sulfate," *Annals of Surgery*, vol. 165, no. 3, pp. 432–436, 1967.

[10] A. S. Prasad, F. W. J. Beck, J. Kaplan et al., "Effect of zinc supplementation on incidence of infections and hospital admissions in sickle cell disease (SCD)," *American Journal of Hematology*, vol. 61, no. 3, pp. 194–202, 1999.

[11] A. S. Prasad, A. A. Abbasi, P. Rabbani, and E. DuMouchelle, "Effect of zinc supplementation on serum testosterone level in adult male sickle cell anemia subjects," *American Journal of Hematology*, vol. 10, no. 2, pp. 119–127, 1981.

[12] J. A. Warth, A. S. Prasad, F. Zwas, and R. N. Frank, "Abnormal dark adaptation in sickle cell anemia," *Journal of Laboratory and Clinical Medicine*, vol. 98, no. 2, pp. 189–194, 1981.

[13] A. S. Prasad and Z. T. Cossack, "Zinc supplementation and growth in sickle cell disease," *Annals of Internal Medicine*, vol. 100, no. 3, pp. 367–371, 1984.

[14] V. L. Gupta and B. S. Chaubey, "Efficacy of zinc therapy in prevention of crisis in sickle cell anemia: a double—blind, randomized controlled clinical trial," *The Journal of the Association of Physicians of India*, vol. 43, no. 7, pp. 467–469, 1995.

[15] A. S. Prasad, J. Ortega, G. J. Brewer, D. Oberleas, and E. B. Schoomaker, "Trace elements in sickle cell disease," *Journal of the American Medical Association*, vol. 235, no. 22, pp. 2396–2398, 1976.

[16] F. O. Akenami, Y. A. Aken'Ova, and B. O. Osifo, "Serum zinc, copper and magnesium in sickle cell disease at Ibadan, south western Nigeria," *African Journal of Medical Sciences*, vol. 28, no. 3-4, pp. 137–139, 1999.

[17] B. R. Kirkwood, "Calculation of required sample size," in *Medical Statistics*, B. R. Kirkwood, Ed., Blackwell Science Press, Oxford, UK, 1995.

[18] J. B. Familusi and A. A. Adeyokunnu, "Geographical distribution and pathogensis of the haemoglobinopathies," *DOKITA*, vol. 7, pp. 5–8, 1990.

[19] G. O. Ogunrinde, A. M. Yakubu, and O. O. Akinyanju, "Anthropometric measures and zinc status of children with sickle cell anaemia," *Nigerian Journal of Paediatrics*, vol. 27, pp. 64–69, 2000.

[20] O. O. Akinkugbe, "Sickle cell disease," in *Non Communicable Disease in Nigeria*, O. O. Akinkugbe, Ed., 1992.

[21] A. I. Juwah, E. U. Nlemadim, and W. Kaine, "Types of anaemic crises in paediatric patients with sickle cell anaemia seen in Enugu, Nigeria," *Archives of Disease in Childhood*, vol. 89, no. 6, pp. 572–576, 2004.

[22] J. C. Smith, G. P. Butrimovitz, and W. C. Purdy, "Direct measurement of zinc in plasma by atomic absorption spectroscopy," *Clinical Chemistry*, vol. 25, no. 8, pp. 1487–1491, 1979.

[23] R. C. Whitehouse, A. S. Prasad, P. I. Rabbani, and Z. T. Cossack, "Zinc in plasma, neutrophils, lymphocytes, and erythrocytes as determined by flameless atomic absorption spectrophotometry," *Clinical Chemistry*, vol. 28, no. 3, pp. 475–480, 1982.

[24] A. S. Prasad, D. Oberleas, and J. A. Halsted, "Determination of zinc in biological fluids by atomic absorption spectrophotometry in normal and cirrhotic subjects," *The Journal of Laboratory and Clinical Medicine*, vol. 66, no. 3, pp. 508–516, 1965.

[25] A. P. Balch, "Minerals," in *Prescription for Nutritional Healing*, P. A. Balch and J. F. Balch, Eds., New York Press, New York, NY, USA, 3rd edition, 2000.

[26] M. J. T. Norma, C. J. Pearson, and P. G. E. Searle, *Tropical Food Crops in Their Environment*, Cambridge University Press, Cambridge, UK, 2nd edition, 1996.

[27] S. M. Bahijri, "Serum zinc in infants and preschool children in the Jeddah area: effect of diet and diarrhea in relation to growth," *Annals of Saudi Medicine*, vol. 21, no. 5-6, pp. 324–329, 2001.

[28] F. M. Akinkugbe and S. I. Ette, "Role of zinc, copper, and ascorbic acid in some common clinical paediatric problems," *Journal of Tropical Pediatrics*, vol. 33, no. 6, pp. 337–342, 1987.

[29] A. Ploysangam, G. A. Falciglia, and B. J. Brehm, "Effect of marginal zinc deficiency on human growth and development," *Journal of Tropical Pediatrics*, vol. 43, no. 4, pp. 192–198, 1997.

[30] C. K. Phebus, B. J. Maciak, M. F. Gloninger, and H. S. Paul, "Zinc status of children with sickle cell disease: relationship to poor growth," *American Journal of Hematology*, vol. 29, no. 2, pp. 67–73, 1988.

[31] J. C. King, D. M. Shames, and L. R. Woodhouse, "Zinc homeostasis in humans," *Journal of Nutrition*, vol. 130, no. 5, pp. 1360S–1366S, 2000.

[32] R. Raghunath, R. M. Tripathi, R. N. Khandekar, and K. S. V. Nambi, "Retention times of Pb, Cd, Cu and Zn in children's blood," *The Science of the Total Environment*, vol. 207, no. 2-3, pp. 133–139, 1997.

[33] A. Lau and L. Chan, "Electrolytes, other minerals and trace elements," in *Basic Skills in Interpreting Laboratory Data*, M. Lee, Ed., pp. 119–150, Harvey Whitney Books, Bethesda, Md, USA, 4th edition, 2009.

[34] K. H. Brown, J. M. Peerson, J. Rivera, and L. H. Allen, "Effect of supplemental zinc on the growth and serum zinc concentrations of prepubertal children: a meta-analysis of randomized controlled trials1-3," *American Journal of Clinical Nutrition*, vol. 75, no. 6, pp. 1062–1071, 2002.

# 8

# Hematopoietic Stem Cell Function in a Murine Model of Sickle Cell Disease

**Elisabeth H. Javazon,[1] Mohamed Radhi,[2] Bagirath Gangadharan,[3] Jennifer Perry,[3] and David R. Archer[3]**

[1] Department of Biology, Morehouse College, 830 Westview Drive Southwest, Atlanta, GA 30314-3773, USA
[2] Department of Pediatrics, UI Hospitals and Clinics, University of Iowa, 2633 Carver Pavilion, 200 Hawkins Drive, Iowa City, IA 52242, USA
[3] Aflac Cancer and Blood Disorders Center, Emory University and Children's Healthcare of Atlanta, 2015 Uppergate Drive, Atlanta, GA 30322, USA

Correspondence should be addressed to David R. Archer, darcher@emory.edu

Academic Editor: Betty S. Pace

Previous studies have shown that the sickle environment is highly enriched for reactive oxygen species (ROS). We examined the oxidative effects of sickle cell disease on hematopoietic stem cell function in a sickle mouse model. *In vitro* colony-forming assays showed a significant decrease in progenitor colony formation derived from sickle compared to control bone marrow (BM). Sickle BM possessed a significant decrease in the KSL (c-kit$^+$, Sca-1$^+$, Lineage$^-$) progenitor population, and cell cycle analysis showed that there were fewer KSL cells in the $G_0$ phase of the cell cycle compared to controls. We found a significant increase in both lipid peroxidation and ROS in sickle-derived KSL cells. *In vivo* analysis demonstrated that normal bone marrow cells engraft with increased frequency into sickle mice compared to control mice. Hematopoietic progenitor cells derived from sickle mice, however, demonstrated significant impairment in engraftment potential. We observed partial restoration of engraftment by n-acetyl cysteine (NAC) treatment of KSL cells prior to transplantation. Increased intracellular ROS and lipid peroxidation combined with improvement in engraftment following NAC treatment suggests that an altered redox environment in sickle mice affects hematopoietic progenitor and stem cell function.

## 1. Introduction

Sickle cell disease (SCD) is one of the most common inherited hemoglobinopathies in the world. In the United States, approximately 1 in 600 African Americans have been diagnosed with SCD [1]. SCD is an autosomal recessive genetic disorder caused by a substitution of glutamic acid by valine in the beta subunit of the hemoglobin gene. This substitution results in the production of abnormal hemoglobin (HbS). Deoxygenated HbS polymerizes, resulting in intravascular hemolysis of the red blood cell and release of hemoglobin and other compounds into the plasma [2]. Repeating cycles of polymerization and hemolysis lead to vaso-occlusion and ischemia-reperfusion injury. Inherent in these processes are inflammatory responses and oxidant stress which result in pathological outcomes such as acute chest syndrome, pulmonary hypertension, and stroke in patients with SCD [3].

Oxidative stress is a result of increased production of reactive oxygen species (ROS) combined with decreased production or availability of antioxidants. Cellular metabolism of oxygen can lead to the production of ROS such as superoxide anion radicals, hydrogen peroxide, and hydroxyl radicals. ROS can impair the proper function of DNA, lipids, proteins, and carbohydrates [4]. An imbalance in the amount of pro-oxidants and antioxidants leads to an environment of oxidative stress, cell dysfunction, or cell death. Antioxidants such as nitric oxide (NO), superoxide dismutase (SOD), and reduced glutathione (GSH) function to neutralize excess ROS.

There is increasing evidence that oxidative stress and ROS play a pivotal role in the pathophysiology of numerous diseases including neurodegenerative diseases, cardiovascular diseases, cancers, and arthritis [5–10]. Oxidative stress has been linked to vascular defects leading to hypertension and atherosclerosis as well as cardiac defects leading to contractile dysfunction and dysrhythmias [11]. In addition to the ability to induce mutations in DNA, ROS play a key role in cell signaling and cell regulatory pathways and thus play a pivotal role in the development of tumors and malignancies [12–16].

In SCD, under low-oxygen conditions, HbS polymerizes leading to hemolysis and a significantly shortened lifespan [17]. Hemolysed RBCs release hemoglobin, iron, and arginase into the plasma resulting in decreased nitric oxide availability and leading to imbalanced vascular homeostasis and oxidative stress [17–19]. Sickle RBCs generate more superoxide, hydrogen peroxide, and lipid oxidation products compared to normal RBCs [20]. Increased ROS in platelets and polymorphonuclear neutrophils along with decreased glutathione levels has also been documented in patients with SCD [21]. In addition, endothelium exposed to sickled RBCs become activated, causing sickled RBCs and leukocytes to adhere to the activated endothelium, resulting in a release of cytokines and ROS [6, 22, 23]. In this study, we studied the effects of this pro-oxidant and proinflammatory environment on hematopoietic progenitor and stem cells in the Berkeley model of sickle cell disease.

## 2. Materials and Methods

*2.1. Animals.* Sickle mice, originally supplied by Dr. Pászty [24], express exclusively human $\alpha$-, $\beta^{sickle}$, and $\gamma$-globin and exist on a mixed genetic background (FVB/N, 129, DBA/2, C57BL/6, and Black Swiss). Breeding and pregnant sickle mice were fed TestDiet no. 0007573 (Purina). The colony is maintained by breeding female hemizygous mice with 2 copies of the transgene to homozygous male mice. The resulting pups are hemizygous, expressing one (H-1) or two (H-2) copies of the transgene, one copy of murine beta globin, but no expression of murine alpha globin. Homozygous "sickle" mice that only express human gamma, alpha, and beta$^{sickle}$ globins are easily distinguishable from wild type and the H-1 and H-2 hemizygotes by hemoglobin electrophoresis (Figure 1) [24, 25]. H-1 mice have ~28% sickle hemoglobin and H-2 mice have ~45%. Despite having only one copy of the sickle hemoglobin transgene, H-1 mice are hematologically more severe (Figure 1). H-2 and C57BL/6 were primarily used as control mice for the homozygous mice. All breeding and experimental procedures were performed at Emory University in accordance with the recommendations of the Institutional Animal Care and Use Committee (IACUC).

*2.2. Flow Cytometry.* Bone marrow was harvested and stained with the following fluorochrome-conjugated antibodies:

CD45.1-PE, CD45.2-APC, c-kit-FITC, Sca1-PE, and Lineage-APC (B220, CD3, CD11b, GR-1, and Ter119; BD Pharmingen, San Diego, CA), and KSL cells were sorted on a FACSAria. Cells from the peripheral blood were analyzed at various time points on an LSR II flow cytometer (BD Biosciences, San Jose, CA). Propidium iodide was used to exclude dead cells. For ROS analysis, cells were incubated in 160 $\mu$M Dichlorodihydrofluorescein diacetate (H$_2$DCFDA) (St. Louis, MO, Sigma-Aldrich) or 5 $\mu$M *N*-(fluorescein-5thiocarbamoyl)-1,2-dihexadecanoyl-*sn*-glycero-3-phosphoethanolamine, triethylammonium salt (DHPE) (Carlsbad, CA, Invitrogen) in HBSS for 15 min or 60 min, respectively, at 37°C shaking in the dark. Cells were washed and analyzed by flow cytometry. Absolute cell counts were performed using Trucount tubes (BD Biosciences).

*2.3. HPP Assay.* Twenty thousand freshly isolated bone marrow mononuclear cells were plated in methylcellulose medium (StemCell Technologies Inc., Vancouver) containing recombinant cytokines (100 ng rat steel factor, 1600U m-CSF, 75U IL-3, 5000U IL-1$\alpha$, 30 ng/mL EGF, and 30 ng/mL FGF) to analyze the colony-forming potential of stem cells derived from the bone marrow of sickle and control mice. Cells were cultured for 10 days, and colonies were counted using an inverted microscope.

*2.4. Hemoglobin Analysis.* Differential hemoglobin electrophoresis of peripheral blood from Berkeley sickle mice was performed to determine hetero- and homozygosity of the murine and human globin genes (Helena Titan III electrophoresis system, Helena Laboratories, Beaumont, TX) [26]. As shown in Figure 1, C57BL/6 mice express the murine beta globin "single" allele, the H-1 and H-2 hemizygotes express increasing amounts of human beta$^{sickle}$ globin in the presence of the murine allele expressing "diffuse" beta globin, and the mice homozygous for the deletions of murine alpha and beta globins express only human beta$^{sickle}$ globin.

*2.5. Transplants*

*2.5.1. The Effect of the Recipient Environment.* To test the effects of transplanting into the sickle microenvironment, $1 \times 10^7$ bone marrow cells from C57BL/6 mice (expressing CD45.2) were transplanted into homozygous sickle ($n = 8$) and B6.SJL-Ptprc$^a$ Pepc$^b$/BoyJ mice ($n = 10$; both expressing CD45.1) without ablation. While sickle and C57BL/6 share the MCH class I allele H-2K$^b$, their genetic backgrounds are not identical and therefore are unlikely to share the full haplotype. We have previously shown that T-cell costimulation blockade promotes engraftment across allo-barriers in this model, and it was therefore included in this protocol. Specifically, 500 $\mu$g each of hamster antimouse-CD40L (MR1; BioExpress, Lebanon, NH) and human CTLA4-immunoglobulin (generous gift from Dr. C. Larsen) was given intraperitoneally on days 0, 2, 4, and 7 relative to BMT.

*2.5.2. Competitive Repopulation Study.* To test the repopulation capacity of individual stem cell populations, three

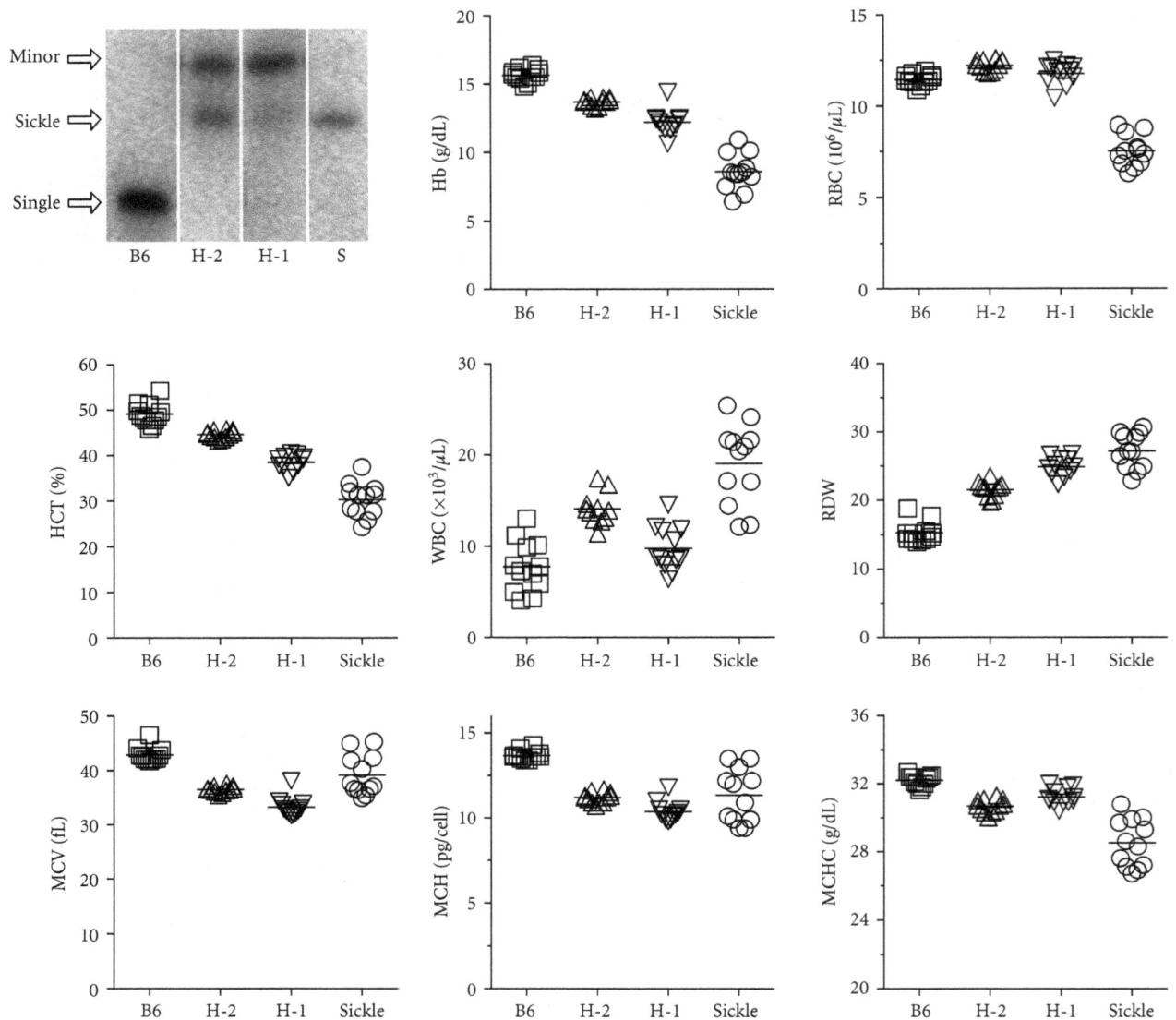

FIGURE 1: Hemoglobin and hematology profile of Berkeley sickle mice. Hemoglobin electrophoresis of RBC from C57BL/6, H-2, H-1, and homozygous sickle mice. C57BL/6 mice show a "single" hemoglobin band, whereas the H-2 and H-1 hemizygotes show beta-sickle globin resulting from two or one copy of the transgene, respectively, in combination with the minor band of diffuse beta-globins. Homozygous sickle mice only have the characteristic band of beta-sickle globin. The complete blood counts of C57BL/6 mice, H-2, H-1, and homozygous sickle mice ($n$ = 10 per genotype) are also shown with the hemizygous mice having intermediate values between C57BL/6 mice and homozygous sickle mice.

thousand KSL cells derived from homozygous H-2 sickle, or B6.SJL-Ptprc[a] Pepc[b]/BoyJ, were sorted using a FACSAria (BD Biosciences, San Jose, CA) and were cotransplanted with $2 \times 10^6$ competitive bone marrow cells derived from C57BL/6 mice. Due to the potential differences in background, F1 recipient mice were generated by breeding H-2 sickle mice (expressing CD45.1) to C57BL/6 mice (expressing GFP under the beta globin promoter and CD45.2). These recipient mice expressed GFP+, CD45.1, and CD45.2 double positive cells (F1 mice). All recipients ($n$ = 4 each group) were conditioned with two doses of 550 cGy total body irradiation on the day of BMT. To test the ability of the glutathione precursor to alleviate oxidant stress in the selected stem cell populations, groups of donor mice were also treated for four weeks with 0.163 g/L n-acetyl cysteine (NAC) in their drinking water (fresh NAC drinking water was made every two days). Mice were 12 weeks of age at the time of bone marrow harvest and transplantation.

## 3. Statistics

All statistical comparisons were performed using GraphPad Prism software utilizing one-way ANOVA with a Tukey posttest analysis unless otherwise stated (*$P < 0.05$; **$P < 0.01$; ***$P < 0.001$).

## 4. Results

*4.1. Stem Cell Number and Function.* Absolute cell counts were performed for stem/progenitor cells that were negative for markers of mature hematopoietic cells (T-cells, CD3; B-cells, B220; RBC, Ter-119; Myeloid cells, GR-1/Mac-1) while being positive for c-kit and Sca-1 (KSL, Figure 2(a)). Sickle mice had significantly fewer stem cells than control mice. We further quantified the number of a defined hematopoietic stem cell population (HSC; KSL/CD150+/CD48−) [27]. These cells were also significantly reduced in homozygous mice compared to controls (t-test, Figure 2(b)). As there were less stem cells in the bone marrow, we investigated the cell cycle status of HSC as a reduction in the number of quiescent cells ($G_0$ of the cell cycle) has been associated with mobilization of HSC in normal tissues, and HSCs are reported to be mobilized in sickle cell patients [28]. Figure 2(c) shows a reduced number of cycling KSL cells suggesting a reduced number of quiescent stem cells in the bone marrow. We then tested the functional capacity of KSL cells using the *in vitro* high proliferative potential (HPP) assay. Sickle-derived stem cells formed significantly fewer colonies compared to control ($P < 0.001$, Figure 2(d)).

*4.2. Oxidant Damage to Bone Marrow-Derived Cells.* Using flow cytometric analysis and DCF and DHPE dyes, we measured the intracellular content of ROS and lipid peroxidation, respectively, in KSL cells. $H_2DCFDA$ becomes deacetylated by intracellular esterases as it crosses the membrane and becomes brightly fluorescent once oxidized by ROS producing DCF [29]. DHPE loses its fluorescence upon reaction with peroxy radicals [29]. Sickle-derived KSL cells demonstrated significantly increased lipid peroxidation and ROS compared to those derived from normal and hemizygous mice ($P < 0.05$, Figures 2(e)–2(f)). Importantly, in all of the above assays, the hemizygous mice showed an intermediate phenotype that correlated to their hematological defect.

*4.3. Engraftment in the Sickle Microenvironment.* We then addressed the issue of whether the sickle bone marrow environment was more conducive to engraftment by donor cells. To compare the engraftment efficiency of bone marrow cells into control (C57BL/6) and homozygous sickle mice (sickle), we transplanted $1 \times 10^7$ control male bone marrow cells into mice receiving only costimulation blockade. As early as four weeks after transplantation, there was a significant increase in engrafted donor cells in the sickle mice compared to the control mice ($P > 0.001$, Figure 3(a)). This level of engraftment is remarkable considering the nonablative protocol, and the continued increase with time suggests that donor cells have a survival or proliferation advantage in the sickle environment. Peripheral RBC markers also showed correction of sickle hematology towards control levels indicating the survival advantage of normal over sickle RBC (Figures 3(b)–3(d)) [30].

*4.4. Engraftment Capacity of Sickle Hematopoietic Cells.* We then compared the engraftment potential of KSL cells derived from control, hemizygous, and homozygous sickle mice in a competitive repopulation assay to determine if sickle-derived KSL cells were functionally impaired. First, we bred male hemizygous sickle mice to female C57BL/6 mice to generate mice that expressed both CD45.1+ and CD45.2+ antigens on the surface of their cells (F1) allowing us to distinguish donor and host KSL as well as donor BM competitor cells. By HPLC, we confirmed that host F1 mice carried one copy of the human β sickle globin gene, as well as murine α and β globins (data not shown). For each experiment, KSL cells were derived from untreated, as well as NAC treated, control, hemizygous (H-2), and homozygous mice and transplanted into lethally irradiated F1 mice. Peripheral blood was analyzed at 4, 8, 12, 16, and 24 weeks after transplantation (Figure 4(a)). In two separate experiments, homozygous sickle-derived KSL cells demonstrated significantly reduced engraftment capabilities compared to control mice. NAC treatment improved engraftment of homozygous sickle KSL cells but did not fully correct the defect (Figure 4(b)).

## 5. Discussion

Despite the benefits of hydroxyurea, people with SCD have limited treatment options with the only curative treatment remaining hematopoietic stem cell transplant (HSCT). While the numbers of children receiving transplant have continued to grow and now total in the hundreds, the majority are still performed with myeloablative conditioning (recently reviewed in [31]). The outcomes of these transplants in children are generally good with high levels of disease-free survival. However [32], there are significant concerns regarding long-term toxicities and complications from the preparative regimen, especially with regard to continued CNS complications and gonadal toxicities [33].

The continued desire to be able to offer transplant to a much larger selection of patients, including adults, has driven a number of trials utilizing a variety of nonmyeloablative protocols [34–36]. Most recipients have not had sustained engraftment, but Hsieh et al. successfully transplanted a small group of adults with mobilized peripheral blood from matched sibling donors [37]. These limited successes, continued issues with posttransplantation immunosuppression, and the limited number of HLA-matched donors will drive alternative transplant protocols and techniques for therapy with genetically corrected autologous cells.

These are similar findings to those in the murine model of Ataxia telangiectasia (ATM), which also demonstrated significant impairment of stem cell populations at least partially due to ROS and oxidative stress [38, 39]. Ataxia telangiectasia is a rare, recessive genetic disorder that causes neurological degeneration. The *Atm* gene controls DNA repair, cell cycle, and redox homeostasis. Ito et al. found that bone marrow-derived stem cells from *Atm* knock-out mice possess increased ROS and activated p38 MAPK that resulted in a reduction in KSL number, decreased colony-forming potential, loss of quiescence, and defective self-renewal capacity [38]. Similarly, sickle bone marrow has reduced colony-forming potential, and fewer sickle HSCs are in $G_0$ suggesting

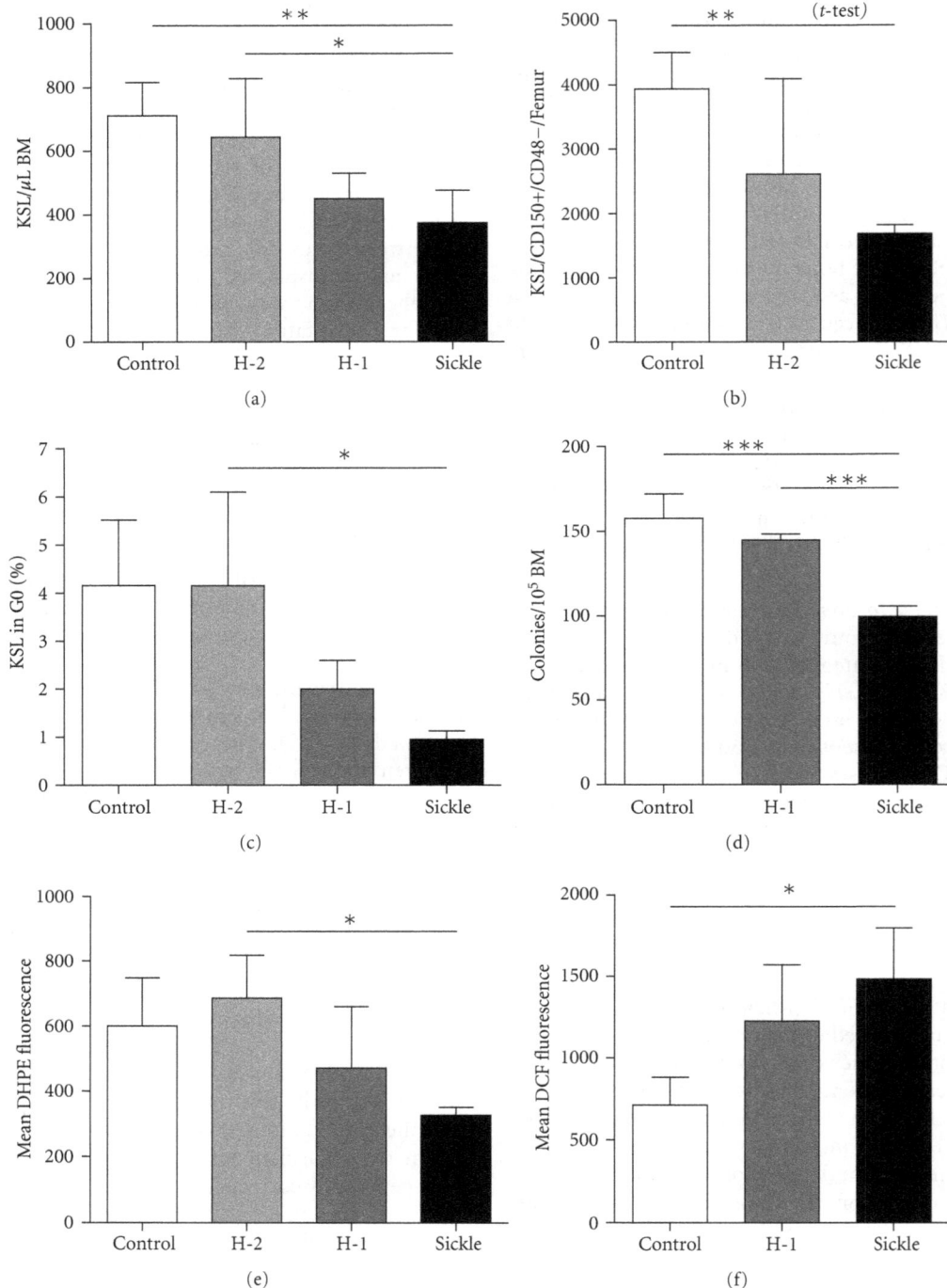

FIGURE 2: Stem cell number and oxidant state in Berkeley sickle mice. (a) Quantification of KSL progenitor cells in the bone marrow of control, hemizygous, and homozygous sickle mice showing a significant reduction in number in homozygous sickle mice. (b) Further examination of a phenotypically defined HSC population (KSL/CD150+/CD48−) also shows a reduction of HSC in sickle BM. (c) HSCs in the stem cell niche are known to be quiescent, and homozygous mice again show significant reduction in KSL cells in the $G_0$ phase of the cell cycle possibly indicating the mobilization of sickle progenitor cells. (d) The *in vitro* colony-forming, high proliferative potential assay (HPP) of stem/progenitor cells further indicates a significant reduction in colony-forming cells in homozygous mice. (e) To examine the effect of oxidant stress on hematopoietic progenitors, we measured lipid peroxidation using the fluorescent indicator DHPE. A reduction in fluorescence indicates increased activity of hydroxyl radicals. (f) Further quantification of reactive oxygen species was shown in sickle mice by the increased production of DCF (all graphs are presented as mean ± SD, $*P < 0.05$, $**P < 0.01$, $***P < 0.001$).

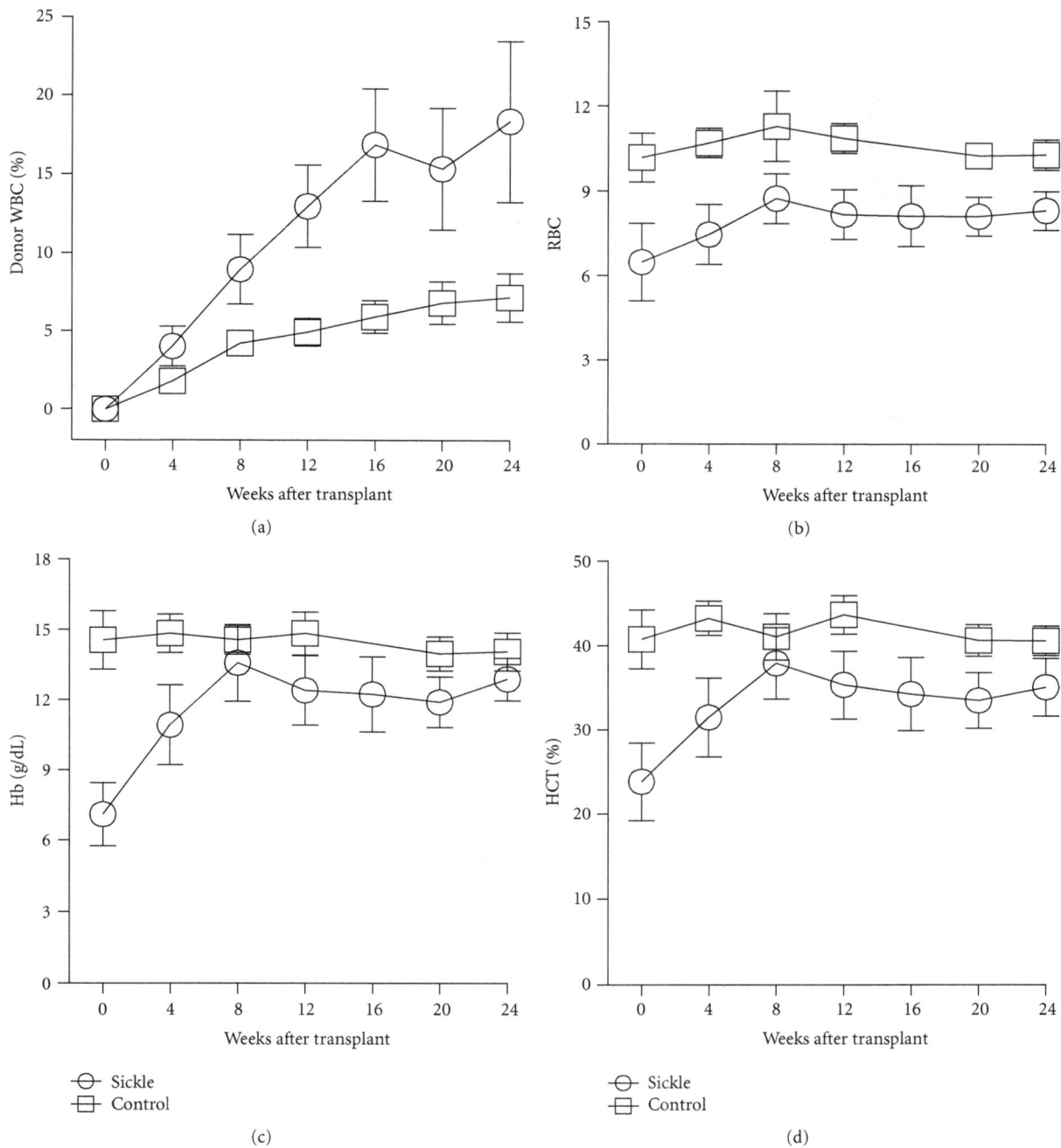

FIGURE 3: Preferential engraftment in sickle mice. (a) Peripheral WBC populations from normal mice engraft in homozygous sickle mice at a significantly ($P < 0.01$) faster rate than control mice when transplanted without ablation but in the presence of costimulation blockade. The levels of WBC engraftment coincide with (b)–(d) corresponding correction of RBC, hemoglobin, and hematocrit in recipient mice.

that stem cells are mobilized. This is consistent with the high peripheral WBC count in both mice and humans and previous reports of mobilization in SCD.

The oxidant damage of murine sickle HSC further translates into a functional defect in a reduced activity in a competitive repopulation assay. Interestingly, both hemizygote and homozygotes were affected. Antioxidant therapy in the form of NAC provided partial correction of the phenotype.

Similar results were found in the ATM model where six weeks of treatment with either NAC or catalase antioxidants restored Atm$^{-/-}$ HSC CFU ability to near normal levels [38]. In vivo full HSC engraftment was only achieved when recipient mice were also treated with NAC. Oxidant-mediated HSC dysfunction is commonly seen in number of other model systems including Fanconi anemia (Fancc$^{-/-}$) where ROS lead to increased apoptosis of Fancc$^{-/-}$ cells [40]. A lack

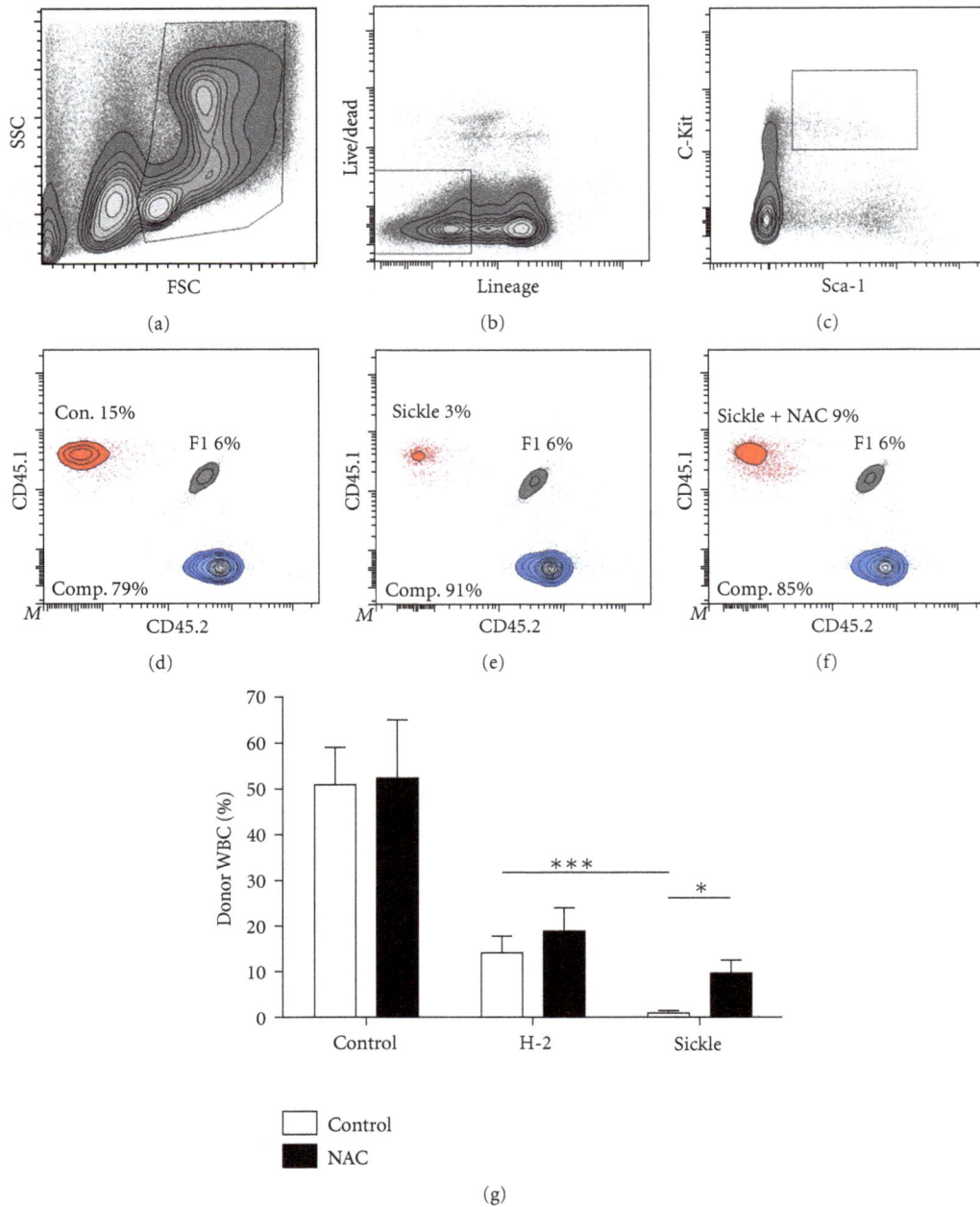

FIGURE 4: Functional defect of sickle hematopoietic stem cells in a competitive repopulation assay. Strategy for sorting KSL cells from whole bone marrow: mononuclear cells gated on FSC and SSC of whole BM (a), gated lineage and propidium iodide negative on mononuclear cells (b), and c-kit+, Sca1+, Lin− (KSL) cells (c). Peripheral blood engraftment after transplantation. Representative flow cytometry plots showing KSL cells from control mice engrafted at 15% (d), sickle KSL cells engrafted at 3% (e), and NAC- treated sickle KSL cells engrafted at 9% (f). Composite data showing a reduced capacity for engraftment between hemizygous and control mice and a further defect in KSL cells from homozygous mice 24 weeks after transplant (g). Graphical representation of the data from all mice: pretreatment of donor cells with NAC partially restored engraftment of KSL cells from homozygous sickle cell mice.

of FoxO family members also leads to an increase in ROS and a reduction in both HSC number and reconstitution ability [41]. In both of these models, antioxidant therapy with NAC is able to reverse or ameliorate the defects. Oxidant mediated stem cell damage is not limited to hematopoietic cells, for example, Kim and Wong demonstrated an oxidant-mediated defect in atm$^{-/-}$ neural stem cells that was responsive to NAC [42]. It is interesting to speculate that the high levels of oxidant stress could affect other organ-specific stem cell populations, and that this might be an important factor in the ongoing repair of sickle-related organ pathology. The HSC defects should also be considered when designing gene therapy protocols first, as there may be a reduced number of HSCs available for collection and secondly as the HSCs have a reduced engraftment potential prior to *ex-vivo* manipulation.

Clinically, patients with severe sickle disease, who would be a desirable target population for HSCT, are likely to encounter more complications during transplant due to ongoing disease-related pathology and inflammation. However, with successful immunomodulatory strategies our data would suggest that engraftment of HSC into the sickle environment itself should be successful, and donor cells may have a comparative advantage. This could be especially important if designing approaches based on mixed hematopoietic chimerism that have been successfully used in murine model systems [30, 43].

All of the major pathologic consequences of SCD such RBC lysis, endothelial activation, and vaso-occlusion either induce or exacerbate the production of ROS with subsequent effects being likely to contribute to further pathologic processes (recently reviewed in [3, 4]). Consequently, a number of investigators have studied the use of antioxidants in SCD, mostly focusing on RBC effects. Vitamins C and E and NAC have all been shown to reduce ROS and increase the levels of glutathione in sickle RBC and PMN *in vitro* [21]. Treatment of NAC reduced the formation of dense RBC and increased the levels of intracellular glutathione in RBC of patients with SCD; importantly this correlated with a reduction in the number of vaso-occlusive crises during the treatment period [44]. Similarly, treatment with NAC for 6 weeks reduced phosphatidyl serine exposure on the membrane of sickle RBC and the levels of cell-free hemoglobin [45] indicating a cellular effect for an oral antioxidant.

In summary, we describe the effects of sickle-mediated oxidant stress on the bone marrow environment and hematopoietic stem and progenitors and detail defects in HSC function that raise important concerns when designing future stem cell therapies for sickle cell disease.

## Acknowledgments

Flow cytometry was performed in the Emory-Children's Pediatric Research Center Flow Cytometry Core. Partial support was from HL073307 (D. R. Archer).

## References

[1] D. J. Weatherall and J. B. Clegg, "Inherited haemoglobin disorders: an increasing global health problem," *Bulletin of the World Health Organization*, vol. 79, no. 8, pp. 704–712, 2001.

[2] J. I. Malowany and J. Butany, "Pathology of sickle cell disease," *Seminars in Diagnostic Pathology*, vol. 29, pp. 49–55, 2012.

[3] E. Nur, B. J. Biemond, H. M. Otten, D. P. Brandjes, and J. J. B. Schnog, "Oxidative stress in sickle cell disease; pathophysiology and potential implications for disease management," *American Journal of Hematology*, vol. 86, no. 6, pp. 484–489, 2011.

[4] E. N. Chirico and V. Pialoux, "Role of oxidative stress in the pathogenesis of sickle cell disease," *IUBMB Life*, vol. 64, pp. 72–80, 2012.

[5] M. Aslan, D. Thornley-Brown, and B. A. Freeman, "Reactive species in sickle cell disease," *Annals of the New York Academy of Sciences*, vol. 899, pp. 375–391, 2000.

[6] R. P. Hebbel, R. Osarogiagbon, and D. Kaul, "The endothelial biology of sickle cell disease: inflammation and a chronic vasculopathy," *Microcirculation*, vol. 11, no. 2, pp. 129–151, 2004.

[7] D. K. Kaul, X. D. Liu, X. Zhang, L. Ma, C. J. C. Hsia, and R. L. Nagel, "Inhibition of sickle red cell adhesion and vasoocclusion in the microcirculation by antioxidants," *American Journal of Physiology*, vol. 291, no. 1, pp. H167–H175, 2006.

[8] A. Kyle Mack and G. J. Kato, "Sickle cell disease and nitric oxide: a paradigm shift?" *International Journal of Biochemistry and Cell Biology*, vol. 38, no. 8, pp. 1237–1243, 2006.

[9] S. S. Somjee, R. P. Warrier, J. L. Thomson, J. Ory-Ascani, and J. M. Hempe, "Advanced glycation end-products in sickle cell anaemia," *British Journal of Haematology*, vol. 128, no. 1, pp. 112–118, 2005.

[10] K. Ito, A. Hirao, F. Arai et al., "Regulation of oxidative stress by ATM is required for self-renewal of haematopoietic stem cells," *Nature*, vol. 431, no. 7011, pp. 997–1002, 2004.

[11] N. S. Dhalla, R. M. Temsah, and T. Netticadan, "Role of oxidative stress in cardiovascular diseases," *Journal of Hypertension*, vol. 18, no. 6, pp. 655–673, 2000.

[12] M. Valko, C. J. Rhodes, J. Moncol, M. Izakovic, and M. Mazur, "Free radicals, metals and antioxidants in oxidative stress-induced cancer," *Chemico-Biological Interactions*, vol. 160, no. 1, pp. 1–40, 2006.

[13] T. Finkel and N. J. Holbrook, "Oxidants, oxidative stress and the biology of ageing," *Nature*, vol. 408, no. 6809, pp. 239–247, 2000.

[14] S. Muhammad, A. Bierhaus, and M. Schwaninger, "Reactive oxygen species in diabetes-induced vascular damage, stroke, and Alzheimer's disease," *Journal of Alzheimer's Disease*, vol. 16, no. 4, pp. 775–785, 2009.

[15] K. Sugamura and J. F. Keaney Jr., "Reactive oxygen species in cardiovascular disease," *Free Radical Biology and Medicine*, vol. 51, pp. 978–992, 2011.

[16] C. L. Allen and U. Bayraktutan, "Oxidative stress and its role in the pathogenesis of ischaemic stroke," *International Journal of Stroke*, vol. 4, no. 6, pp. 461–470, 2009.

[17] Z. Y. Aliyu, A. R. Tumblin, and G. J. Kato, "Current therapy of sickle cell disease," *Haematologica*, vol. 91, no. 1, pp. 7–10, 2006.

[18] G. J. Kato, M. T. Gladwin, and M. H. Steinberg, "Deconstructing sickle cell disease: reappraisal of the role of hemolysis in the development of clinical subphenotypes," *Blood Reviews*, vol. 21, no. 1, pp. 37–47, 2007.

[19] M. T. Gladwin and G. J. Kato, "Cardiopulmonary complications of sickle cell disease: role of nitric oxide and hemolytic anemia," *Hematology*, pp. 51–57, 2005.

[20] R. P. Hebbel, J. W. Eaton, M. Balasingam, and M. H. Steinberg, "Spontaneous oxygen radical generation by sickle erythrocytes," *Journal of Clinical Investigation*, vol. 70, no. 6, pp. 1253–1259, 1982.

[21] J. Amer, H. Ghoti, E. Rachmilewitz, A. Koren, C. Levin, and E. Fibach, "Red blood cells, platelets and polymorphonuclear neutrophils of patients with sickle cell disease exhibit oxidative stress that can be ameliorated by antioxidants," *British Journal of Haematology*, vol. 132, no. 1, pp. 108–113, 2006.

[22] T. Dasgupta, R. P. Hebbel, and D. K. Kaul, "Protective effect of arginine on oxidative stress in transgenic sickle mouse models," *Free Radical Biology and Medicine*, vol. 41, no. 12, pp. 1771–1780, 2006.

[23] M. D. Brown, T. M. Wick, and J. R. Eckman, "Activation of vascular endothelial cell adhesion molecule expression by sickle blood cells," *Pediatric Pathology and Molecular Medicine*, vol. 20, no. 1, pp. 47–72, 2001.

[24] C. Pászty, C. M. Brion, E. Manci et al., "Transgenic knockout mice with exclusively human sickle hemoglobin and sickle cell disease," *Science*, vol. 278, no. 5339, pp. 876–878, 1997.

[25] C. T. Noguchi, M. Gladwin, B. Diwan et al., "Pathophysiology of a sickle cell trait mouse model: human $\alpha\beta$S transgenes with one mouse $\beta$-globin allele," *Blood Cells, Molecules, and Diseases*, vol. 27, no. 6, pp. 971–977, 2001.

[26] J. B. Whitney III, "Simplified typing of mouse hemoglobin (Hbb) phenotypes using cystamine," *Biochemical Genetics*, vol. 16, no. 7-8, pp. 667–672, 1978.

[27] M. J. Kiel, Ö. H. Yilmaz, T. Iwashita, O. H. Yilmaz, C. Terhorst, and S. J. Morrison, "SLAM family receptors distinguish hematopoietic stem and progenitor cells and reveal endothelial niches for stem cells," *Cell*, vol. 121, no. 7, pp. 1109–1121, 2005.

[28] H. Croizat, L. Ponchio, F. E. Nicolini, R. L. Nagel, and C. J. Eaves, "Primitive haematopoietic progenitors in the blood of patients with sickle cell disease appear to be endogenously mobilized," *British Journal of Haematology*, vol. 111, no. 2, pp. 491–497, 2000.

[29] J. Amer, A. Goldfarb, and E. Fibach, "Flow cytometric analysis of the oxidative status of normal and thalassemic red blood cells," *Cytometry Part A*, vol. 60, no. 1, pp. 73–80, 2004.

[30] L. S. Kean, E. A. Manci, J. Perry et al., "Chimerism and cure: hematologic and pathologic correction of murine sickle cell disease," *Blood*, vol. 102, no. 13, pp. 4582–4593, 2003.

[31] R. Khoury and M. R. Abboud, "Stem-cell transplantation in children and adults with sickle cell disease: an update," *Expert Review of Hematology*, vol. 4, no. 3, pp. 343–351, 2011.

[32] M. C. Walters, M. Patience, W. Leisenring et al., "Bone marrow transplantation for sickle cell disease," *New England Journal of Medicine*, vol. 335, no. 6, pp. 369–376, 1996.

[33] M. C. Walters, K. Hardy, S. Edwards et al., "Pulmonary, gonadal, and central nervous system status after bone marrow transplantation for sickle cell disease," *Biology of Blood and Marrow Transplantation*, vol. 16, no. 2, pp. 263–272, 2010.

[34] R. Iannone, J. F. Casella, E. J. Fuchs et al., "Results of minimally toxic nonmyeloablative transplantation in patients with sickle cell anemia and $\beta$-thalassemia," *Biology of Blood and Marrow Transplantation*, vol. 9, no. 8, pp. 519–528, 2003.

[35] J. T. Horan, J. L. Liesveld, P. Fenton, N. Blumberg, and M. C. Walters, "Hematopoietic stem cell transplantation for multiply transfused patients with sickle cell disease and thalassemia after low-dose total body irradiation, fludarabine, and rabbit anti-thymocyte globulin," *Bone Marrow Transplantation*, vol. 35, no. 2, pp. 171–177, 2005.

[36] L. Krishnamurti, S. Kharbanda, M. A. Biernacki et al., "Stable long-term donor engraftment following reduced-intensity hematopoietic cell transplantation for sickle cell disease," *Biology of Blood and Marrow Transplantation*, vol. 14, no. 11, pp. 1270–1278, 2008.

[37] M. M. Hsieh, E. M. Kang, C. D. Fitzhugh et al., "Allogeneic hematopoietic stem-cell transplantation for sickle cell disease," *New England Journal of Medicine*, vol. 361, no. 24, pp. 2309–2317, 2009.

[38] K. Ito, A. Hirao, F. Arai et al., "Reactive oxygen species act through p38 MAPK to limit the lifespan of hematopoietic stem cells," *Nature Medicine*, vol. 12, no. 4, pp. 446–451, 2006.

[39] K. Ito, K. Takubo, F. Arai et al., "Regulation of reactive oxygen species by Atm is essential for proper response to DNA double-strand breaks in lymphocytes," *Journal of Immunology*, vol. 178, no. 1, pp. 103–110, 2007.

[40] M. R. Saadatzadeh, K. Bijangi-Vishehsaraei, P. Hong, H. Bergmann, and L. S. Haneline, "Oxidant hypersensitivity of fanconi anemia type C-deficient cells is dependent on a redox-regulated apoptotic pathway," *Journal of Biological Chemistry*, vol. 279, no. 16, pp. 16805–16812, 2004.

[41] Z. Tothova, R. Kollipara, B. J. Huntly et al., "FoxOs are critical mediators of hematopoietic stem cell resistance to physiologic oxidative stress," *Cell*, vol. 128, no. 2, pp. 325–339, 2007.

[42] J. Kim and P. K. Y. Wong, "Loss of ATM impairs proliferation of neural stem cells through oxidative stress-mediated p38 MAPK signaling," *Stem Cells*, vol. 27, no. 8, pp. 1987–1998, 2009.

[43] L. S. Kean, M. M. Durham, A. B. Adams et al., "A cure for murine sickle cell disease through stable mixed chimerism and tolerance induction after nonmyeloablative conditioning and major histocompatibility complex-mismatched bone marrow transplantation," *Blood*, vol. 99, no. 5, pp. 1840–1849, 2002.

[44] B. S. Pace, A. Shartava, A. Pack-Mabien, M. Mulekar, A. Ardia, and S. R. Goodman, "Effects of N-acetylcysteine on dense cell formation in sickle cell disease," *American Journal of Hematology*, vol. 73, no. 1, pp. 26–32, 2003.

[45] E. Nur, D. P. Brandjes, T. Teerlink et al., "N-acetylcysteine reduces oxidative stress in sickle cell patients," *Annals of Hematology*. In press.

# 9

# Sickling Cells, Cyclic Nucleotides and Protein Kinases: The Pathophysiology of Urogenital Disorders in Sickle Cell Anemia

**Mário Angelo Claudino[1] and Kleber Yotsumoto Fertrin[2]**

[1] Laboratory of Multidisciplinary Research, São Francisco University (USF), 12916-900 Bragança Paulista, SP, Brazil
[2] Hematology and Hemotherapy Center, University of Campinas (UNICAMP), 13083-970 Campinas, SP, Brazil

Correspondence should be addressed to Mário Angelo Claudino, mario.claudino@gmail.com

Academic Editor: Solomon F. Ofori-Acquah

Sickle cell anemia is one of the best studied inherited diseases, and despite being caused by a single point mutation in the *HBB* gene, multiple pleiotropic effects of the abnormal hemoglobin S production range from vaso-occlusive crisis, stroke, and pulmonary hypertension to osteonecrosis and leg ulcers. Urogenital function is not spared, and although priapism is most frequently remembered, other related clinical manifestations have been described, such as nocturia, enuresis, increased frequence of lower urinary tract infections, urinary incontinence, hypogonadism, and testicular infarction. Studies on sickle cell vaso-occlusion and priapism using both *in vitro* and *in vivo* models have shed light on the pathogenesis of some of these events. The authors review what is known about the deleterious effects of sickling on the genitourinary tract and how the role of cyclic nucleotides signaling and protein kinases may help understand the pathophysiology underlying these manifestations and develop novel therapies in the setting of urogenital disorders in sickle cell disease.

## 1. Introduction

Sickle cell anemia (SCA) has been first described over a century ago [1] and has become one of the best studied inherited human diseases. Despite being caused by a single point mutation in the *HBB* gene, multiple pleiotropic effects of the abnormal hemoglobin S production range from vaso-occlusive crisis, stroke, and pulmonary hypertension to osteonecrosis and leg ulcers [2–4].

Genitourinary tract function is also affected in SCA, and although priapism is most frequently remembered, other related clinical manifestations have been described, such as nocturia, enuresis, increased frequency of lower urinary tract infections, urinary incontinence, hypogonadism, and testicular infarction. Sickle hemoglobin S (HbS) polymerizes when deoxygenated, resulting in a series of cellular alterations in red cell morphology and function that shorten the red cell life span and lead to vascular occlusion. Sickle cell disease (SCD) vaso-occlusion constitutes a complex multifactorial process characterized by oxidative stress and recurrent ischemia-reperfusion injury in a vicious circle contributing to reduced blood flow and results, eventually, in complete obstruction of the microcirculation and organic dysfunction [3–6]. The exact pathogenetic mechanisms that tie genitourinary complications to the fundamental event of HbS polymerization and hemolytic anemia in SCA have just about started to be unraveled.

This paper focuses on how previous, sometimes poorly explained, clinical observations of urogenital disorders in patients with SCD relate to more recent discoveries on the role of cyclic nucleotides and protein kinases in the pathophysiology of sickle vaso-occlusion.

## 2. Priapism

Priapism is defined as a prolonged and persistent penile erection, unassociated with sexual interest or stimulation, and is one of the complications associated with sickle cell anemia (SCA) since early in 1934 [7]. Priapism reaches a frequency of up to 45% in male patients with SCA, and the rate of resulting erectile dysfunction (ED) exceeds 30% [8–10].

Although this complication has been previously reviewed in depth in this journal [11], the main concepts behind its pathophysiology will be summarized here for better understanding of the mechanisms discussed throughout the paper, but readers are encouraged to read the previous review.

According to the American Urological Association Guidelines on the Management of Priapism, priapism can be subdivided into three categories: ischemic, stuttering, and nonischemic. Ischemic priapism (veno-occlusive, low flow) is a persistent erection marked by rigidity of the corpora cavernosa (CC) and little or no cavernous arterial inflow. In ischemic priapism, there are time-dependent changes in the corporal metabolic environment with progressive hypoxia, hypercarbia, and acidosis that typically generate penile pain. Penile sinusoids are regions prone to red blood cell sickling in SCD men because of blood stasis and slow flow rates, and ischemic priapism is thought to result from prolonged blockage of venous outflow by the vaso-occlusive process. Clinically, there is congestion and tenderness in the CC, sparing the glans and corpus spongiosum, usually with a prolonged course of over 3 hours, and frequently resulting in fibrosis and erectile dysfunction. Stuttering priapism (acute, intermittent, recurrent ischemic priapism) is characterized by a pattern of recurrence, but an increasing frequency or duration of stuttering episodes may herald a major ischemic priapism. Nonischemic priapism (arterial, high flow) is a persistent erection caused by unregulated cavernous arterial inflow. Typically, the corpora are tumescent but not rigid, the penis is not painful and is most frequently associated with trauma [12–16].

Conventional treatments are largely symptomatic, usually administered after the episode of priapism has already occurred, because the etiology and mechanisms involved in the development of priapism are poorly characterized [17, 18]. Preventive interventions have been proposed but, without a clear idea of the molecular mechanisms involved, they remain largely impractical to be applied in a regular basis in the clinic [17]. Due to the difficulty in exploring these mechanisms in patients, the use of animal models of priapism has become of utmost importance to decipher this devastating clinical challenge [19]. Animal models for priapism include dogs [20, 21], rabbits [22], rats [23–27], and mice [28–41].

Molecular biology and genetic engineering have been widely used in animal models to explore gene function in both human physiology and in the study of pathology of human priapism. Four major priapism animal models have been developed and have yielded greater knowledge on the intrinsic mechanisms underlying priapism: the intra-corporal opiorphins gene transfer rat model [42–45], the endothelial nitric oxide synthase (eNOS) with or without neuronal NOS (nNOS) knock-out (eNOS$^{-/-}$ ± nNOS$^{-/-}$) mouse models [28, 29, 31–33], the adenosine deaminase knock-out (Ada$^{-/-}$) mouse model [35, 36, 40, 41] and the transgenic sickle cell Berkeley mouse model [30, 33, 34, 37–39]. However, the Berkeley mouse is the only well-accepted animal model that displays clinical manifestations similar to those seen in humans with severe forms of SCD, including priapism [30, 34].

Priapism is essentially a derangement of normal erection. Penile erection is a hemodynamic event that is regulated by smooth muscle relaxation/contraction of corpora cavernosa and associated arterioles during sexual stimulation. The penile flaccidity (detumescence state) is mainly maintained by tonic release of norepinephrine through the sympathetic innervations of vascular and cavernosal smooth muscle cells [46]. During penile erection (tumescence state), vascular smooth muscle relaxation decreases vascular resistance, thereby increasing blood flow through cavernous and helicine arteries and filling sinusoids, which are expanded due to the relaxation of smooth muscle cells in the CC [47]. This physiological relaxation of penile smooth muscle is mainly, although not solely, mediated by the neurotransmitter nitric oxide (NO) that is produced by enzymes called NO synthases (NOS). NOSs are subdivided into three isoforms, endothelial NOS (eNOS or NOS3), neural NOS (nNOS or NOS1), and inducible NOS (iNOS or NOS2) [48, 49]. In the penile smooth muscle, NO is released from both nitrergic nerves and the sinusoidal endothelium [46, 50–52]. NO stimulates the soluble guanylyl cyclase (sGC) in the cavernosal smooth muscle, triggering increased synthesis of cyclic GMP (cGMP) that provides the main signal for smooth muscle relaxation [53]. cGMP levels in the CC are regulated by the rate of synthesis determined by sGC and the rate of cGMP hydrolysis mediated by phosphodiesterase type 5 (PDE5) [54, 55]. It has been reported that plasma hemoglobin released by intravascularly hemolysed sickle erythrocytes consumes NO, reducing its bioavailability in the erectile tissue, skewing the normal balance of smooth muscle tone towards vasoconstriction [17, 56, 57]. Champion and collaborators [33] showed that the penile smooth muscle of SCD transgenic mice presents with dysregulated PDE5A expression activity. Moreover, these mice had spontaneous priapism, amplified CC relaxation response mediated by the NO-cGMP signaling pathway, and increased intracavernosal pressure *in vivo* [37, 38].

Recent evidence has shown that another signaling pathway that may also contribute to the pathophysiology of priapism in SCD involves adenosine regulation. Similarly to NO, adenosine is a potent vasodilator produced by adenine nucleotide degradation. Adenosine is predominantly generated by adenosine monophosphate (AMP) dephosphorylation catalyzed by intracellular 5′-nucleotidase. Hydrolysis of s-adenosyl-homocysteine also contributes to intracellular adenosine formation [58, 59]. Extracellular adenosine may be generated by both adenine nucleotide degradation and dephosphorylation by ectonucleotidases [60]. Adenosine is then catabolized by two enzymes: adenosine kinase (ADK), which phosphorylates adenosine to AMP and is an important regulator of intracellular adenosine levels; and adenosine deaminase (ADA), which catalyzes the irreversible conversion of adenosine to inosine [58].

Several physiological processes may be affected by extracellular adenosine and this is mediated by four different receptors, referred to as $A_1$, $A_{2A}$, $A_{2B}$, and $A_3$. All four subtypes are members of the G protein-coupled receptor (GPCR) superfamily. The activation of the $A_1$ and $A_3$ adenosine receptors inhibits adenylyl cyclase activity and also results in increased activity of phospholipase C, while activation of the $A_{2A}$ and $A_{2B}$ subtypes increases adenylyl cyclase activity [58, 61]. Adenosine-induced vasodilation is mediated by increasing intracellular cyclic adenosine monophosphate (cAMP) levels in vascular smooth muscle cells via $A_2$ receptor signaling [62, 63]. cAMP activates protein kinase A (PKA) resulting in decreased calcium-calmodulin-dependent MLC phosphorylation and enhanced smooth muscle relaxation [64]. Its role in penile erection has been investigated in studies showing that intracavernous injection of adenosine resulted in tumescence and penile erection [36, 61, 65]. In addition, adenosine induces NO synthesis in endothelial cells through $A_2$ receptor signaling, and adenosine-mediated CC relaxation is partially dependent on endothelium-derived NO [36, 66–70].

A priapic phenotype in Ada$^{-/-}$ mice was identified and led to further investigation of the impact of adenosine in the pathophysiology of priapism [59]. Previous reports showed that high levels of adenosine caused prolonged corporal smooth muscle relaxation *in vitro*. However, this effect was quickly corrected by intraperitoneal injection of a high dose of polyethylene glycol-ADA (PEG-ADA), which effectively reduces adenosine levels systemically [36, 71]. Moreover, adenosine induced significant increases in cavernosal cAMP levels via $A_{2B}$ receptor activation. This demonstrated that $A_{2B}$ receptor signaling is required for adenosine-mediated stimulation of cAMP production in CC smooth muscle cells [36, 71]. Mi and collaborators [36] have studied adenosine levels in the penis of sickle cell mice and have found a significant increase in adenosine levels, suggesting that overproduction of adenosine may contribute to priapic activity in SCD [71, 72]. Sickle cell mice submitted to PEG-ADA treatment suffered significant reduction of force and duration of relaxation when compared with untreated mice [71]. In addition, increased adenosine levels contributed to the development of penile fibrosis in Ada$^{-/-}$ mice as well as in transgenic sickle cell mice [72]. These findings suggest a general contributory role of elevated adenosine in the pathophysiology of priapism associated with SCD.

Although the penile vascular endothelium and smooth muscle cells are sources of vasodilation factors such as NO and adenosine, there are vasoconstriction pathways important to the penile hemodynamics, such as the Rho-kinase (ROCK) pathway. The RhoA/ROCK signal transduction pathway has been shown to influence erectile function *in vivo* through an array of mechanisms, including vasoconstriction of the penile vasculature via smooth muscle contraction and regulation of eNOS [73–76]. This pathway is involved in the regulation of smooth muscle tone by modulating the sensitivity of contractile proteins to $Ca^{2+}$ [77]. RhoA regulates smooth muscle contraction by cycling between a GDP-bound inactive form (coupled to a guanine dissociation inhibitor, RhoGDI) and a GTP-bound active form [78–80]. Upstream activation of heterotrimeric G proteins leads to the exchange of GDP for GTP, an event carried out by the guanine exchange factors (GEFs) p115RhoGEF [81], PDZ-RhoGEF [82], and LARG (Leukemia-associated RhoGEF) [83], which are able to transduce signals from G protein-coupled receptors to RhoA [84–86]. ROCK is activated by RhoA and inhibits myosin phosphatase through the phosphorylation of its myosin-binding subunit, leading to an increase in $Ca^{2+}$ sensitivity. The RhoA/ROCK $Ca^{2+}$ sensitization pathway has been implicated in the regulation of penile smooth muscle contraction and tone both in humans and animals [77, 87]. ROCK exerts contractile effects in the penis by $Ca^{2+}$-independent promotion of myosin light chain (MLC) kinase or the attenuation of MLC phosphatase activity and reduction in endothelial-derived NO production [88]. RhoA activation, ROCK2 protein expression, as well as total ROCK activity decline in penile of SCD transgenic mice, highlighting that the molecular mechanism of priapism in SCD is associated with decreased vasoconstrictor activity in the penis [39]. Therefore, should impaired RhoA/ROCK-mediated vasoconstriction contribute to SCD-associated priapism, this pathway may become a novel therapeutic target in the management of this complication.

There has been no definite advance in the management of sickle cell-associated acute, severe priapism. Penile aspiration with or without saline intracavernosal injection and eventually performing surgical shunts remains mainstays of care, with no evident benefit of more common approaches, such as intravenous hydration, blood transfusions, and urinary alkalinization [89, 90]. Pharmacological interventions in such cases have been limited to intracavernosal use of sympathomimetic drugs, such as epinephrine, norepinephrine, and etilefrine, but there are anecdotal reports of acute use of PDE5 inhibitor sildenafil [91].

Nonetheless, most attempts to control SCD priapism have focused on its recurrent, stuttering form. Small case series of hormonal manipulation with diethylstilbestrol [92], gonadotropin-releasing hormone (GnRH) analogues [93], and finasteride [94] have been reported to successfully manage recurrent priapism. Increasing smooth muscle tone with oral $\alpha$-agonist etilefrine has also yielded only anecdotal evidence of benefit [95]. Unfortunately, a prospective study comparing etilefrine and ephedrine failed to demonstrate superiority or equivalence of both drugs in preventing recurrent priapism due to poor compliance and low recruitment reducing statistical power, but some evidence was obtained reassuring safety of the use of such strategies, and possibly indicating a lower severity of priapism attacks among compliant patients [96]. This favors off-label use of pseudoephedrine at bedtime advocated by some experts [57, 90]. Hydroxyurea has also been effective in preventing priapism recurrence in SCD in a small number of cases [97, 98]. Based on current knowledge of NO-dependent pathways, the use of PDE5 inhibitors has been studied. One clinical trial testing tadalafil in SCD patients has been terminated, but no outcome data have yet been published (ClinicalTrials.gov NCT00538564), and one ongoing trial aims at the effect of sildenafil in the same setting (ClinicalTrials.gov NCT00940901). Despite these efforts, scientists have become less optimistic concerning the tolerability of this approach, ever since the premature termination of the sildenafil trial for pulmonary hypertension in SCD patients, in which subjects on PDE5 inhibitor were more likely to have severe pain crises requiring hospitalization [99]. Therefore, novel therapies for preventing and treating priapism in SCD are still warranted if the incidence of impotence among these patients is expected to be reduced in the long term.

## 3. Infertility

Progress in the therapy of SCD, particularly the use of hydroxyurea, has considerably improved the prognosis of patients with SCD [100, 101], with their mean life expectancy reaching much over 40 years [102–104], rendering infertility an important issue. Nevertheless, long before hydroxyurea became a standard of care in SCD, seminal fluid parameters of SCD males had been reported to fall within the subfertile range due to decreased sperm concentration, total count, motility, and altered morphology [105–107], and a more recent study reported over 90% of patients had at least one abnormal sperm parameter [108].

Hydroxyurea (HU) has been reported to impair spermatogenesis, causing testicular atrophy, reversible decrease in sperm count, as well as abnormal sperm morphology and motility [108–114], and its current or previous use should be among the first probable causes to be considered in SCD patients complaining of infertility. Moreover, sperm abnormalities prior to HU have been attributed to variable effects of hypogonadism induced by SCD itself, and lack of appropriate testosterone production seems to be exacerbated by HU use in a mouse SCD model [115].

Considering that male fertility does not rely solely on the quality of the seminal fluid, other causes that may also render male patients with SCD prone to suffer from infertility include sexual problems, such as loss of libido, premature ejaculation, frequent priapism, and priapism-related impotence [105–107, 116–121].

Finding a single main cause for male infertility in a particular SCD patient is highly unlikely and probably will involve some degree of endocrinological impairment. A broader understanding of how hypogonadism takes place in SCD is necessary to explain fertility problems and requires knowledge of the complexity of sex hormone production regulation.

## 4. Hypogonadism

The etiology of hypogonadism in SCD patients is multifactorial, as several mechanisms have been suggested to contribute to its occurrence, such as primary gonadal failure [117, 122, 123], associated with or caused by repeated testicular infarction [124], zinc deficiency [125, 126], and partial hypothalamic hypogonadism [127].

Physical and sexual development are affected in both male and female SCD patients, with onset of puberty (menarche) and appearance of secondary sexual characteristics (pubic and axillary hair and beard) being usually delayed. The delay is greater in homozygous SCA and S-$\beta^0$-thalassemia than in SC disease and S-$\beta^+$-thalassemia [128–130]. Moreover, studies in male patients with SCD reported reduction of ejaculate volume, spermatozoa count, motility, and abnormal sperm morphology [106, 115].

Biochemical analyses have demonstrated low levels of testosterone and dihydrotestosterone and variable levels of follicle-stimulating hormone (FSH) and luteinizing hormone (LH) in patients with SCD [105–107, 118, 119, 121, 131]. The comparison between patients and controls matched according to stage of development of secondary sexual characteristics showed higher levels of LH in sickle cell disease, favoring some role for hypergonadotropic hypogonadism.

Leydig cells of the testes and other steroidogenic tissues produce hormones by a multienzymatic process, in which free cholesterol from intracellular stores is transferred to the outer and then to the inner mitochondrial membrane. Leydig cells produce androgens under the control of LH or its placental counterpart human chorionic gonadotropin (hCG), as well as in response to numerous intratesticular factors [114, 132]. LH/hCG receptors belong to the sGC-coupled seven-transmembrane-domain receptor family, whose activation leads to stimulation of adenylyl cyclase [133]. The resulting accumulation of intracellular cyclic adenosine monophosphate (cAMP) levels and the concomitant activation of the cAMP-dependent protein kinase (PKA) lead to the phosphorylation of numerous proteins, including the steroidogenic acute regulatory (StAR) protein [134, 135]. StAR localizes predominantly to steroid hormone-producing tissues and consists of a 37 kDa precursor containing an NH2-terminal mitochondrial targeting sequence and several isoelectric 30 kDa mature protein forms [136–138]. Steroid production in gonadal and adrenal cells requires both *de novo* synthesis and PKA-dependent phosphorylation of StAR-37 protein [139]. The newly synthesized StAR is functional and plays a critical role in the transfer of cholesterol from the outer to the inner mitochondrial membrane, whereas mitochondrial import and processing to 30 kDa StAR protein terminate this action [140–142].

HbS polymerization is mediated by upstream activation of adenosine receptor A$_{2B}$R by hypoxia, and hemolysis of irreversibly sickled red blood cells increases adenosine bioavailability through conversion of ATP by ectonucleotidases CD39 and CD73, thus predisposing patients with SCD to sustained high levels of cAMP [143, 144]. From this point of view, steroidogenesis could be expected to be increased in these patients.

Although Leydig cell steroidogenesis is predominantly regulated by cAMP/PKA, other pathways also influence this process [145], including the NO-cGMP signaling pathway [146]. NO promotes a biphasic modulation in the androgen production, stimulatory at low concentrations, and inhibitory at high concentrations [49, 147, 148]. SCA causes NO depletion, and in low levels, NO stimulates Leydig cell steroidogenesis by activating sGC [48, 49, 149] and promotes the formation of low levels of cGMP, albeit enough to activate the cGMP-dependent protein kinase (PKG) and phosphorylate StAR [49, 150]. This signaling is controlled by phosphodiesterases (PDEs) [151] and active transport systems that export cyclic nucleotides (multidrug-resistance proteins) from the cell [152]. In zona glomerulosa cells, activation of PKG II by cGMP regulates basal levels of aldosterone production and phosphorylation of StAR

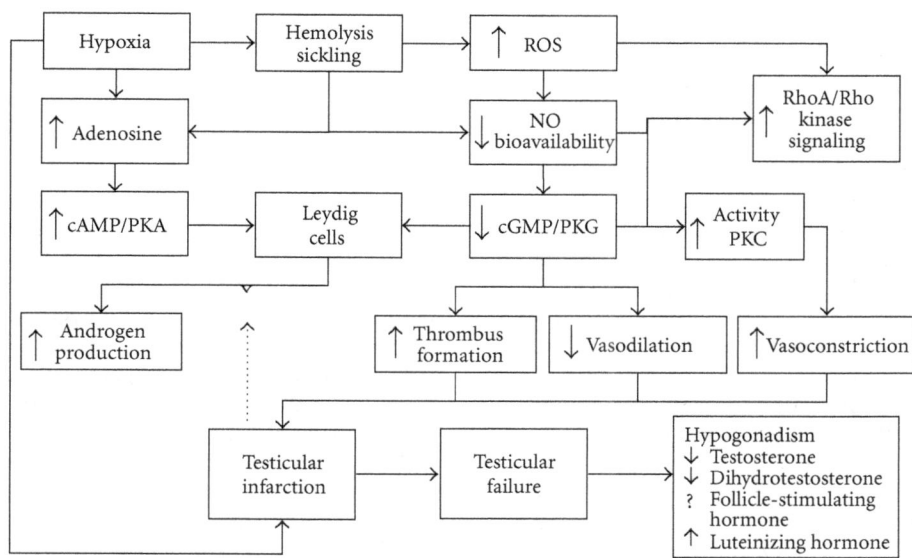

FIGURE 1: Schematic pathophysiology of hypogonadism and testicular infarction in sickle cell disease. The dashed arrow represents the blocking effect of gonadal failure over cyclic nucleotide-stimulated androgen production.

protein [150], but whether there is a role for cGMP in the zona reticularis, where adrenal androgenesis takes place, is unknown.

Hypogonadism observed in patients with SCD with lower circulating testosterone and higher LH levels suggests that, at least in this setting, despite the reduced cGMP- and elevated cAMP-mediated stimuli on androgen production, gonadal failure with Leydig cell impairment predominates in sex hormone production dysfunction (Figure 1). This further highlights that primary hypogonadism is possibly largely underdiagnosed and elicits more studies on the pathogenesis of testicular infarction.

## 5. Testicular Infarction

Segmental testicular infarction is an infrequent cause of acute scrotum and is rarely reported, with fewer than 40 cases published at the time of this paper. Its etiology is not always well defined, and it may be, at first, clinically mistaken for a testicular tumour [153, 154]. Common causes for testicular infarction are torsion of the spermatic cord, incarcerated hernia, infection, trauma, and vasculitis [131]. The usual presentation is a painful testicular mass unresponsive to antibiotics [155]. This testicular disorder has been associated with epididymitis, hypersensitivity angiitis, intimal fibroplasia of the spermatic cord arteries, polycythemia, anticoagulant use, benign testicular tumors and, in the interest of this review, sickle cell trait and sickle cell disease [124, 131, 155–158].

Testicular infarction related to sickling has been very rarely reported with only five individual cases found retrospectively, three associated with sickle cell disease and two with sickle cell trait [124, 155–157, 159]. Holmes and Kane reported the first testicular infarction in a patient with

SCD who presented with testicular swelling unresponsive to antibiotics. Physical examination revealed that a lesion suspicious for malignancy and ultrasonography demonstrated a hyperechoic mass with an anechoid rim and normal blood flow in the surrounding parenchyma. Radical orchiectomy revealed hemorrhagic infarction with sickle blood red cells. In another case report, SCA patient presented with acute scrotum and history of acute chest syndrome, splenic infarction, osteomyelitis, and hemolysis. Physical examination demonstrated an erythematous, tender, swollen testicle and ultrasound once again revealed normal echotexture and blood flow. Surgical exploration and pathological examination diagnosed segmental testicular infarction with vascular congestion and sickled red blood cells [124]. In the last testicular infarction case report in a patient with SCD presented with increased testicular volume, scrotal ultrasonography showed both echogenic and hypoechogenic regions and Doppler ultrasonography revealed vascular changes compatible with testicular infarction. Radical orchiectomy was performed 10 days after the initial presentation and microscopic evaluation showed necrotic seminiferous tubules devoid of nuclear debris, congestion, or acute inflammatory infiltrate, consistent with coagulative necrosis of ischemic origin [131].

Testicular blood flow is dependent on the internal spermatic, cremasteric, and deferential arteries. Obstruction of venous outflow may create venous thrombosis, testicular engorgement, and subsequent hemorrhagic infarction. In SCD, low oxygen tensions in erythrocytes lead to sickling cells that lose pliability in the microcirculation. Consequently, capillary flow becomes obstructed, worsening local tissue hypoxia, perpetuating the cycle of sickling, and promoting testicular infarction [124, 131, 157].

The cyclic nucleotides and protein kinases may play an important role in the pathophysiology of testicular infarction in SCD. Enhanced hemolysis and oxidative stress contribute to a reduction in nitric oxide (NO) bioavailability due to NO scavenging by free hemoglobin and reactive oxygen species (ROS) generation [160, 161]. As mentioned before, testicular NO signaling pathway is involved in the regulation of Leydig cell steroidogenesis [48, 49, 147–149, 162–164] but may also influence testicular circulation. We suggest that the reduction of NO bioavailability and consequent reduction of GMPc levels and of activity of PKG may decrease the vasodilation process in the testes. Moreover, reduced NO levels in patients with sickle cell disease contribute to the development of thrombus formation in the vascular system and could further enhance local ischemia [165, 166]. Furthermore, the cGMP-dependent protein kinase signaling pathway would normally inhibit RhoA-induced $Ca^{2+}$ sensitization, RhoA/ROCK signaling, and protein kinase C (PKC) activity that mediate contraction in vascular smooth muscle [167–171]. Thus, reduced NO levels may decrease cGMP-dependent protein kinase activity and promote increasing RhoA-induced $Ca^{2+}$ sensitization and PKC activity, favoring vasoconstriction in the testes. Therefore, tissue hypoxia, sickling of red blood cells, reduced levels of NO, possible thrombus formation, increased RhoA-induced $Ca^{2+}$ sensitization, and PKC activity may all lead to capillary and venous flow obstruction promoting testicular infarction (Figure 1).

Although testicular infarction in SCD has been very rarely reported, it has been speculated that silent testicular infarctions are much more common but generally overlooked clinically. Testicular biopsy in patients is rarely performed and additional studies are necessary to establish the true incidence of testicular infarction in patients with SCD or even sickle cell trait.

## 6. Urinary Bladder Dysfunction

The urinary bladder has two important functions: urine storage and emptying. Urine storage occurs at low pressure, implying that the bladder relaxes during the filling phase. Disturbances of the storage function may result in lower urinary tract symptoms (LUTSs), such as urgency, increased frequency, and urge incontinence, the components of the hypoactive or overactive bladder syndromes [172, 173]. The passive phase of bladder filling allows an increase in volume at a low intravesical pressure. The bladder neck and urethra remain in a tonic state to prevent leakage, thus maintaining urinary continence. Bladder emptying is accompanied by a reversal of function in which detrusor smooth muscle (DSM) contraction predominates in the bladder body that is accompanied by a concomitant reduction in outlet resistance of the bladder neck and urethra [174–176]. The bladder filling and emptying are regulated by interactions of norepinephrine (sympathetic component released by hypogastric nerve stimulation), acetylcholine and ATP (parasympathetic components released by pelvic nerve stimulation) with activation of adrenergic, muscarinic, and purinergic receptors, respectively [175].

Urinary bladder dysfunction is rarely spontaneously reported by SCD patients to their caregivers. With increasing survival of these patients, physicians may expect that urinary complaints increase in association with classical urological disorders associated with advanced age, such as urinary stress incontinence in multiparous women and benign prostatic hyperplasia in men. Nonetheless, clinical observations of medical complaints involving the urinary bladder start as early as childhood, with enuresis, and continue onto adulthood with nocturia and urinary tract infections, to name a few, although frequently neglected.

Nocturia has long been attributed to constant increased urinary volumes in SCD. As part of the renal complications of sickling, renal medullary infarcts lead to decreased ability to concentrate urine, yielding higher daily urinary volumes [177], compensatory polydipsia, and eventually, the need for nocturnal bladder voiding.

For comparison, the effects of polyuria on bladder function have been better characterized in diabetic bladder dysfunction (DBD). Both SCD and diabetes mellitus cause increased urinary volume and, to some extent, the two diseases involve cellular damage by oxidative stress mediators; so data from previous studies on DBD may help shed some light on preliminary data on bladder function in SCD animal models by understanding a known model of bladder dysfunction.

It has been suggested that DBD comprehends so-called early and late phases of the disease, owing to cumulative effects of initial polyuria secondary to hyperglycemia, complicated by oxidative stress influence on the urothelium and nervous damage in the long term of the natural history of diabetes mellitus. In the early phase of DBD, the bladder is hyperactive, leading to LUTS comprised mainly by nocturia and urge incontinence. Later in the course of the disease, the detrusor smooth muscle becomes atonic, abnormally distended, and incontinence is mainly by overflow associated with a poor control of urethral sphincters, and voiding problems take over [178].

DSM physiology also involves cyclic nucleotides and activation of protein kinases. DSM contractions are a consequence of cholinergic-mediated contractions and decreased $\beta$-adrenoceptor-mediated relaxations [179]. DSM contains a heterogeneous population of muscarinic receptor subtypes [180, 181], with a predominance of the M2 subtype and a smaller population of M3 receptors. However, functional studies showed that M3 receptors are responsible for promotion of contraction in the DSM of several animal models [182–185] and in humans [186, 187]. Activation of M3 muscarinic receptors in the DSM promotes stimulation of phospholipase C, activates PKC, and increases formation of inositol trisphosphate (IP$_3$) and diacylglycerol (DAG) to release calcium from intracellular stores, leading to DSM contraction [87]. Moreover, activation of M2 receptors also induces a DSM contraction indirectly by inhibiting the production of cAMP, reducing PKA activity, and reversing the relaxation induced by $\beta$-adrenoceptors [179]. Hence, both mechanisms promote urinary bladder emptying.

There is evidence that the $Ca^{2+}$-independent RhoA/ROCK pathway is involved in the regulation of smooth muscle tone by altering the sensitivity of contractile proteins to $Ca^{2+}$ [77]. This pathway has been shown to influence erectile function *in vivo* through an array of mechanisms, including phosphorylation of the myosin-binding subunit of MLC phosphatase, resulting in increased myosin phosphorylation. RhoA, a member of the Ras (Rat Sarcoma) low molecular weight of GTP-binding proteins, mediates agonist-induced activation of ROCK. The exchange of GDP for GTP on RhoA and translocation of RhoA from the cytosol to the membrane are markers of its activation and enable the downstream stimulation of various effectors such as ROCK, protein kinase N, phosphatidylinositol 3-kinase, and tyrosine phosphorylation [77]. The RhoA/ROCK $Ca^{2+}$ sensitization pathway has been implicated in the regulation of bladder smooth muscle contraction and tone in humans and animals [77, 188–191]. Thus, alterations in the contraction or relaxation mechanisms of DSM during the filling and emptying phases may contribute to urinary bladder dysfunction. Patients with SCD have not been evaluated for bladder dysfunction in a systematic manner, but preliminary data have shown that Berkeley mice (homozygous SS) exhibit hypocontractile DSM *ex vivo*, due to a significant decrease of contractile responses to muscarinic agonist carbachol and electrical field stimulation [192]. This bladder dysfunction may contribute to the increased risk of urinary tract infections observed in SCD patients.

In an epidemiological study of 321 children with SCD, 7% had a documented urinary tract infection (UTI), one-third had recurrent infections, and two-thirds had had a febrile UTI [193]. As in normal children, there was a strong predominance of females, and gram-negative organisms, particularly *Escherichia coli*, were usually cultured. Most episodes of gram-negative septicemia in SCD are secondary to UTI [194]. Moreover, UTIs are more frequent during pregnancy in women with SCA or sickle cell trait [195–197]. The prevalence of UTI in women with SCA is nearly twofold that of unaffected black American women. This association appears to be directly related to HbS levels, since patients with sickle trait have an increased prevalence of bacteriuria, but to a lesser degree than those with SCA. More recently, a study detected that a group of SCD children and adolescents had more symptoms of overactive bladder than a control group [198]. This could be a first documentation of a clinically evident of an early phase of sickle cell bladder dysfunction, but whether there is a late, hypotonic bladder phase in older sickle cell adults remains to be demonstrated.

The presence of increased intracavernosal pressure associated with the amplified corpus cavernosum relaxation response (priapism) mediated by NO-cGMP signaling pathway, the lack of RhoA/ROCK-mediated vasoconstriction in sickle cell transgenic Berkeley mice, and the association of priapism with genitourinary infections and urinary retention further suggest the possibility that changes in the DSM reactivity may contribute to urogenital complications in SCD [36, 38–40, 192]. Despite advances in the understanding of urogenital disorders in the SCD, further studies should clarify the pathophysiological mechanisms that underlie genitourinary manifestations of SCD.

## 7. Conclusions

Urogenital disorders in SCD are the result of pleotropic effects of the production of the abnormal sickling hemoglobin S. While priapism still stands out as the most frequently encountered, current knowledge of the effects of cyclic nucleotide production and activation of protein kinases allows to suspect underdiagnosis of bladder dysfunction and hypogonadism secondary to testicular failure. Moreover, despite our growing understanding of these complications, adequate, efficacious, and well-tolerated treatments are still unavailable, and male patients continue to suffer from infertility and erectile dysfunction. Further work in, both clinical assessments and experimental studies in this field are promising and should help increase physicians' awareness of the importance of more accurate diagnoses, design improved therapeutic strategies, and eventually, achieve better quality of life for SCD patients.

## Abbreviations

ROS:   Reactive oxygen species
NO:   Nitric oxide
cAMP:   Cyclic adenosine monophosphate
PKA:   Cyclic adenosine monophosphate-dependent protein kinase
cGMP:   Cyclic Guanosine monophosphate;
PKG:   Cyclic Guanosine monophosphate protein kinase;
PKC:   Protein kinase C.

## References

[1] C. J. Herrick, "The evolution of intelligence and its organs," *Science*, vol. 31, no. 784, pp. 7–18, 1910.

[2] M. H. Steinberg, "Management of sickle cell disease," *The New England Journal of Medicine*, vol. 340, no. 13, pp. 1021–1030, 1999.

[3] G. J. Kato and M. T. Gladwin, "Evolution of novel small-molecule therapeutics targeting sickle cell vasculopathy," *Journal of the American Medical Association*, vol. 300, no. 22, pp. 2638–2646, 2008.

[4] N. Conran, C. F. Franco-Penteado, and F. F. Costa, "Newer aspects of the pathophysiology of sickle cell disease vaso-occlusion," *Hemoglobin*, vol. 33, no. 1, pp. 1–16, 2009.

[5] R. P. Hebbel, M. A. B. Boogaerts, J. W. Eaton, and M. H. Steinberg, "Erythrocyte adherence to endothelium in sickle-cell anemia. A possible determinant of disease severity," *The New England Journal of Medicine*, vol. 302, no. 18, pp. 992–995, 1980.

[6] R. B. Francis Jr. and C. S. Johnson, "Vascular occlusion in sickle cell disease: current concepts and unanswered questions," *Blood*, vol. 77, no. 7, pp. 1405–1414, 1991.

[7] L. W. Diggs and R. E. Ching, "Pathology of sickle cell anemia," *Southern Medical Journal*, vol. 27, pp. 839–845, 1934.

[8] A. B. Adeyoju, A. B. K. Olujohungbe, J. Morris et al., "Priapism in sickle-cell disease; incidence, risk factors and complications—an international multicentre study," *BJU International*, vol. 90, no. 9, pp. 898–902, 2002.

[9] V. G. Nolan, D. F. Wyszynski, L. A. Farrer, and M. H. Steinberg, "Hemolysis-associated priapism in sickle cell disease," *Blood*, vol. 106, no. 9, pp. 3264–3267, 2005.

[10] T. J. Bivalacqua and A. L. Burnett, "Priapism: new concepts in the pathophysiology and new treatment strategies," *Current Urology Reports*, vol. 7, no. 6, pp. 497–502, 2006.

[11] G. M. Crane and N. E. Bennett Jr., "Priapism in sickle cell anemia: emerging mechanistic understanding and better preventative strategies," *Anemia*, vol. 2011, Article ID 297364, 6 pages, 2011.

[12] American Foundation for Urologic Disease, "Thought leader panel on evaluation and treatment of priapism. Report of the American Foundation for Urologic Disease (AFUD) thought leader panel for evaluation and treatment of priapism," *International Journal of Impotence Research*, vol. 15, supplement, pp. S39–S43, 2001.

[13] F. Numan, M. Cantasdemir, M. Ozbayrak et al., "Posttraumatic nonischemic priapism treated with autologous blood clot embolization," *Journal of Sexual Medicine*, vol. 5, no. 1, pp. 173–179, 2008.

[14] A. L. Burnett and T. J. Bivalacqua, "Glucose-6-phosphate dehydrogenase deficiency: an etiology for idiopathic priapism?" *Journal of Sexual Medicine*, vol. 5, no. 1, pp. 237–240, 2008.

[15] D. S. Finley, "Glucose-6-phosphate dehydrogenase deficiency associated stuttering priapism: report of a case," *Journal of Sexual Medicine*, vol. 5, no. 12, pp. 2963–2966, 2008.

[16] Y. C. Jin, S. C. Gam, J. H. Jung, J. S. Hyun, K. C. Chang, and J. S. Hyun, "Expression and activity of heme oxygenase-1 in artificially induced low-flow priapism in rat penile tissues," *Journal of Sexual Medicine*, vol. 5, no. 8, pp. 1876–1882, 2008.

[17] A. L. Burnett, "Pathophysiology of priapism: dysregulatory erection physiology thesis," *Journal of Urology*, vol. 170, no. 1, pp. 26–34, 2003.

[18] T. J. Bivalacqua, B. Musicki, O. Kutlu, and A. L. Burnett, "New insights into the pathophysiology of sickle cell disease-associated priapism," *Journal of Sexual Medicine*, vol. 9, pp. 79–87, 2011.

[19] Q. Dong, S. Deng, R. Wang, and J. Yuan, "In vitro and in vivo animal models in priapism research," *Journal of Sexual Medicine*, vol. 8, no. 2, pp. 347–359, 2011

[20] K. K. Chen, J. Y. Chan, L. S. Chang, M. T. Chen, and S. H. Chan, "Intracavernous pressure as an experimental index in a rat model for the evaluation of penile erection," *Journal of Urology*, vol. 147, no. 4, pp. 1124–1128, 1992.

[21] M. Ul-Hasan, A. I. El-Sakka, C. Lee, T. S. Yen, R. Dahiya, and T. F. Lue, "Expression of TGF-beta-1 mRNA and ultrastructural alterations in pharmacologically induced prolonged penile erection in a canine model," *The Journal of Urology*, vol. 160, no. 6, pp. 2263–2266, 1998.

[22] R. Munarriz, K. Park, Y. H. Huang et al., "Reperfusion of ischemic corporal tissue: physiologic and biochemical changes in an animal model of ischemic priapism," *Urology*, vol. 62, no. 4, pp. 760–764, 2003.

[23] Y. Evliyaoglu, L. Kayrin, and B. Kaya, "Effect of allopurinol on lipid peroxidation induced in corporeal tissue by venoocclusive priapism in a rat model," *British Journal of Urology*, vol. 80, no. 3, pp. 476–479, 1997.

[24] Y. Evliyaoğlu, L. Kayrin, and B. Kaya, "Effect of pentoxifylline on veno-occlusive priapism-induced corporeal tissue lipid peroxidation in a rat model," *Urological Research*, vol. 25, no. 2, pp. 143–147, 1997.

[25] O. Sanli, A. Armagan, E. Kandirali et al., "TGF-$\beta$1 neutralizing antibodies decrease the fibrotic effects of ischemic priapism," *International Journal of Impotence Research*, vol. 16, no. 6, pp. 492–497, 2004.

[26] Y. C. Jin, S. C. Gam, J. H. Jung, J. S. Hyun, K. C. Chang, and J. S. Hyun, "Expression and activity of heme oxygenase-1 in artificially induced low-flow priapism in rat penile tissues," *Journal of Sexual Medicine*, vol. 5, no. 8, pp. 1876–1882, 2008.

[27] N. Uluocak, D. Atilgan, F. Erdemir et al., "An animal model of ischemic priapism and the effects of melatonin on antioxidant enzymes and oxidative injury parameters in rat penis," *International Urology and Nephrology*, vol. 42, no. 4, pp. 889–895, 2010.

[28] P. L. Huang, T. M. Dawson, D. S. Bredt, S. H. Snyder, and M. C. Fishman, "Targeted disruption of the neuronal nitric oxide synthase gene," *Cell*, vol. 75, no. 7, pp. 1273–1286, 1993.

[29] P. L. Huang, Z. Huang, H. Mashimo et al., "Hypertension in mice lacking the gene for endothelial nitric oxide synthase," *Nature*, vol. 377, no. 6546, pp. 239–242, 1995.

[30] C. Pászty, C. M. Brion, E. Manci et al., "Transgenic knockout mice with exclusively human sickle hemoglobin and sickle cell disease," *Science*, vol. 278, no. 5339, pp. 876–878, 1997.

[31] P. L. Huang, "Lessons learned from nitric oxide synthase knockout animals," *Seminars in Perinatology*, vol. 24, no. 1, pp. 87–90, 2000.

[32] L. A. Barouch, R. W. Harrison, M. W. Skaf et al., "Nitric oxide regulates the heart by spatial confinement of nitric oxide synthase isoforms," *Nature*, vol. 416, no. 6878, pp. 337–340, 2002.

[33] H. C. Champion, T. J. Bivalacqua, E. Takimoto, D. A. Kass, and A. L. Burnett, "Phosphodiesterase-5A dysregulation in penile erectile tissue is a mechanism of priapism," *Proceedings of the National Academy of Sciences of the United States of America*, vol. 102, no. 5, pp. 1661–1666, 2005.

[34] Hsu, "Hemolysis in sickle cell mice causes pulmonary hypertension due to global impairment in nitric oxide bioavailability," *Blood*, vol. 109, no. 7, pp. 3088–3098, 2007.

[35] J. H. Yuan, J. L. Chunn, T. J. Mi et al., "Adenosine deaminase knockout in mice induces priapism via A2b receptor," *Journal of Urology*, vol. 177, supplement, p. 227, 2007.

[36] T. Mi, S. Abbasi, H. Zhang et al., "Excess adenosine in murine penile erectile tissues contributes to priapism via A2B adenosine receptor signaling," *Journal of Clinical Investigation*, vol. 118, no. 4, pp. 1491–1501, 2008.

[37] T. J. Bivalacqua, B. Musicki, L. L. Hsu, M. T. Gladwin, A. L. Burnett, and H. C. Champion, "Establishment of a transgenic sickle-cell mouse model to study the pathophysiology of priapism," *Journal of Sexual Medicine*, vol. 6, no. 9, pp. 2494–2504, 2009.

[38] M. A. Claudino, C. F. Franco-penteado, M. A. F. Corat et al., "Increased cavernosal relaxations in sickle cell mice priapism are associated with alterations in the NO-cGMP signaling pathway," *Journal of Sexual Medicine*, vol. 6, no. 8, pp. 2187–2196, 2009.

[39] T. J. Bivalacqua, A. E. Ross, T. D. Strong et al., "Attenuated rhoA/rho-kinase signaling in penis of transgenic sickle cell mice," *Urology*, vol. 76, no. 2, pp. 510.e7–510.e12, 2010.

[40] J. Wen, X. Jiang, Y. Dai et al., "Adenosine deaminase enzyme therapy prevents and reverses the heightened cavernosal relaxation in priapism," *Journal of Sexual Medicine*, vol. 7, no. 9, pp. 3011–3022, 2010.

[41] J. Wen, X. Jiang, Y. Dai et al., "Increased adenosine contributes to penile fibrosis, a dangerous feature of priapism, via A2B adenosine receptor signaling," *The FASEB Journal*, vol. 24, no. 3, pp. 740–749, 2010.

[42] Y. Tong, M. Tar, F. Davelman, G. Christ, A. Melman, and K. P. Davies, "Variable coding sequence protein A1 as a marker

for erectile dysfunction," *BJU International*, vol. 98, no. 2, pp. 396–401, 2006.

[43] Y. Tong, M. Tar, V. Monrose, M. DiSanto, A. Melman, and K. P. Davies, "hSMR3A as a marker for patients with erectile dysfunction," *Journal of Urology*, vol. 178, no. 1, pp. 338–343, 2007.

[44] Y. Tong, M. Tar, A. Melman, and K. Davies, "The opiorphin gene (ProL1) and its homologues function in erectile physiology," *BJU International*, vol. 102, no. 6, pp. 736–740, 2008.

[45] N. D. Kanika, M. Tar, Y. Tong, D. S. R. Kuppam, A. Melman, and K. P. Davies, "The mechanism of opiorphin-induced experimental priapism in rats involves activation of the polyamine synthetic pathway," *American Journal of Physiology*, vol. 297, no. 4, pp. C916–C927, 2009.

[46] K. E. Andersson, "Pharmacology of penile erection," *Pharmacological Reviews*, vol. 53, no. 3, pp. 417–450, 2001.

[47] P. V. Phatarpekar, J. Wen, and Y. Xia, "Role of adenosine signaling in penile erection and erectile disorders," *Journal of Sexual Medicine*, vol. 7, no. 11, pp. 3553–3564, 2010.

[48] M. S. Davidoff, R. Middendorff, B. Mayer, J. DeVente, D. Koesling, and A. F. Holstein, "Nitric oxide/cGMP pathway components in the Leydig cells of the human testis," *Cell and Tissue Research*, vol. 287, no. 1, pp. 161–170, 1997.

[49] S. A. Andric, M. M. Janjic, N. J. Stojkov, and T. S. Kostic, "Protein kinase G-mediated stimulation of basal Leydig cell steroidogenesis," *American Journal of Physiology*, vol. 293, no. 5, pp. E1399–E1408, 2007.

[50] A. L. Burnett, C. J. Lowenstein, D. S. Bredt, T. S. K. Chang, and S. H. Snyder, "Nitric oxide: a physiologic mediator of penile erection," *Science*, vol. 257, no. 5068, pp. 401–403, 1992.

[51] K. E. Andersson and G. Wagner, "Physiology of penile erection," *Physiological Reviews*, vol. 75, no. 1, pp. 191–236, 1995.

[52] T. F. Lue, "Erectile dysfunction," *The New England Journal of Medicine*, vol. 342, pp. 1802–1813, 2000.

[53] K. A. Lucas, G. M. Pitari, S. Kazerounian et al., "Guanylyl cyclases and signaling by cyclic GMP," *Pharmacological Reviews*, vol. 52, no. 3, pp. 375–414, 2000.

[54] M. Boolell, M. J. Allen, S. A. Ballard et al., "Sildenafil: an orally active type 5 cyclic GMP-specific phosphodiesterase inhibitor for the treatment of penile erectile dysfunction," *International Journal of Impotence Research*, vol. 8, no. 2, pp. 47–52, 1996.

[55] V. K. Gopal, S. H. Francis, and J. D. Corbin, "Allosteric sites of phosphodiesterase-5 (PDE5). A potential role in negative feedback regulation of cGMP signaling in corpus cavernosum," *European Journal of Biochemistry*, vol. 268, no. 11, pp. 3304–3312, 2001.

[56] K. Ohene-Frempong and M. H. Steinberg, "Clinical aspects of sickle cell anemia in adults and children," in *Disorders of Hemoglobin: Genetics, Pathophysiology and Clinical Management*, M. H. Steinberg, B. G. Forget, D. R. Higgs, and R. L. Nagel, Eds., pp. 611–670, Cambridge University Press, Cambridge, UK, 2001.

[57] Z. R. Rogers, "Priapism in sickle cell disease," *Hematology/Oncology Clinics of North America*, vol. 19, pp. 917–928, 2005.

[58] B. B. Fredholm, A. P. Ijzerman, K. A. Jacobson, K. N. Klotz, and J. Linden, "International Union of Pharmacology. XXV. Nomenclature and classification of adenosine receptors," *Pharmacological Reviews*, vol. 53, no. 4, pp. 527–552, 2001.

[59] P. V. Phatarpekar, J. Wen, and Y. Xia, "Role of adenosine signaling in penile erection and erectile disorders," *Journal of Sexual Medicine*, vol. 7, no. 11, pp. 3553–3564, 2010.

[60] S. P. Colgan, H. K. Eltzschig, T. Eckle, and L. F. Thompson, "Physiological roles for ecto-5′-nucleotidase (CD73)," *Purinergic Signalling*, vol. 2, no. 2, pp. 351–360, 2006.

[61] R. C. Tostes, F. R. C. Giachini, F. S. Carneiro, R. Leite, E. W. Inscho, and R. C. Webb, "Determination of adenosine effects and adenosine receptors in murine corpus cavernosum," *Journal of Pharmacology and Experimental Therapeutics*, vol. 322, no. 2, pp. 678–685, 2007.

[62] R. A. Olsson and J. D. Pearson, "Cardiovascular purinoceptors," *Physiological Reviews*, vol. 70, no. 3, pp. 761–845, 1990.

[63] A. M. Tager, P. LaCamera, B. S. Shea et al., "The lysophosphatidic acid receptor LPA1 links pulmonary fibrosis to lung injury by mediating fibroblast recruitment and vascular leak," *Nature Medicine*, vol. 14, no. 1, pp. 45–54, 2008.

[64] C. S. Lin, G. Lin, and T. F. Lue, "Cyclic nucleotide signaling in cavernous smooth muscle," *Journal of Sexual Medicine*, vol. 2, no. 4, pp. 478–491, 2005.

[65] D. Prieto, "Physiological regulation of penile arteries and veins," *International Journal of Impotence Research*, vol. 20, no. 1, pp. 17–29, 2008.

[66] A. Vials and G. Burnstock, "A$_2$-purinoceptor-mediated relaxation in the guinea-pig coronary vasculature: a role for nitric oxide," *British Journal of Pharmacology*, vol. 109, no. 2, pp. 424–429, 1993.

[67] L. Sobrevia, D. L. Yudilevich, and G. E. Mann, "Activation of A$_2$-purinoceptors by adenosine stimulates L-arginine transport (system y$^+$) and nitric oxide synthesis in human fetal endothelial cells," *Journal of Physiology*, vol. 499, no. 1, pp. 135–140, 1997.

[68] J. M. Li, R. A. Fenton, H. B. Wheeler et al., "Adenosine A$_{2a}$ receptors increase arterial endothelial cell nritric oxide," *Journal of Surgical Research*, vol. 80, no. 2, pp. 357–364, 1998.

[69] P. H. Chiang, S. N. Wu, E. M. Tsai et al., "Adenosine modulation of neurotransmission in penile erection," *British Journal of Clinical Pharmacology*, vol. 38, no. 4, pp. 357–362, 1994.

[70] M. Faria, T. Magalhães-Cardoso, J. M. Lafuente-De-Carvalho, and P. Correia-De-Sá, "Corpus cavernosum from men with vasculogenic impotence is partially resistant to adenosine relaxation due to endothelial A$_{2B}$ receptor dysfunction," *Journal of Pharmacology and Experimental Therapeutics*, vol. 319, no. 1, pp. 405–413, 2006.

[71] Y. Dai, Y. Zhang, P. Phatarpekar et al., "Adenosine signaling, priapism and novel therapies," *Journal of Sexual Medicine*, vol. 6, no. 3, supplement, pp. 292–301, 2009.

[72] J. Wen, X. Jiang, Y. Dai et al., "Increased adenosine contributes to penile fibrosis, a dangerous feature of priapism, via A$_{2B}$ adenosine receptor signaling," *The FASEB Journal*, vol. 24, no. 3, pp. 740–749, 2010.

[73] K. Chitaley, C. J. Wingard, R. Clinton Webb et al., "Antagonism of Rho-kinase stimulates rat penile erection via a nitric oxide-independent pathway," *Nature Medicine*, vol. 7, no. 1, pp. 119–122, 2001.

[74] T. M. Mills, K. Chitaley, C. J. Wingard, R. W. Lewis, and R. C. Webb, "Effect of rho-kinase inhibition on vasoconstriction in the penile circulation," *Journal of Applied Physiology*, vol. 91, no. 3, pp. 1269–1273, 2001.

[75] T. J. Bivalacqua, H. C. Champion, M. F. Usta et al., "RhoA/Rho-kinase suppresses endothelial nitric oxide synthase in the penis: a mechanism for diabetes-associated erectile dysfunction," *Proceedings of the National Academy of Sciences of the United States of America*, vol. 101, no. 24, pp. 9121–9126, 2004.

[76] B. Musicki, A. E. Ross, H. C. Champion, A. L. Burnett, and T. J. Bivalacqua, "Posttranslational modification of constitutive nitric oxide synthase in the penis," *Journal of Andrology*, vol. 30, no. 4, pp. 352–362, 2009.

[77] A. P. Somlyo and A. V. Somlyo, "Ca$^{2+}$ sensitivity of smooth muscle and nonmuscle myosin II: modulated by G proteins, kinases, and myosin phosphatase," *Physiological Reviews*, vol. 83, no. 4, pp. 1325–1358, 2003.

[78] N. Wettschureck and S. Offermanns, "Rho/Rho-kinase mediated signaling in physiology and pathophysiology," *Journal of Molecular Medicine*, vol. 80, no. 10, pp. 629–638, 2002.

[79] K. Riento and A. J. Ridley, "Rocks: multifunctional kinases in cell behaviour," *Nature Reviews Molecular Cell Biology*, vol. 4, no. 6, pp. 446–456, 2003.

[80] M. Bhattacharya, A. V. Babwah, and S. S. G. Ferguson, "Small GTP-binding protein-coupled receptors," *Biochemical Society Transactions*, vol. 32, no. 6, pp. 1040–1044, 2004.

[81] M. J. Hart, S. Sharma, N. Elmasry et al., "Identification of a novel guanine nucleotide exchange factor for the Rho GTPase," *Journal of Biological Chemistry*, vol. 271, no. 41, pp. 25452–25458, 1996.

[82] S. Fukuhara, C. Murga, M. Zohar, T. Igishi, and J. S. Gutkind, "A novel PDZ domain containing guanine nucleotide exchange factor links heterotrimeric G proteins to Rho," *Journal of Biological Chemistry*, vol. 274, no. 9, pp. 5868–5879, 1999.

[83] P. J. Kourlas, M. P. Strout, B. Becknell et al., "Identification of a gene at 11q23 encoding a guanine nucleotide exchange factor: evidence for its fusion with MLL in acute myeloid leukemia," *Proceedings of the National Academy of Sciences of the United States of America*, vol. 97, no. 5, pp. 2145–2150, 2000.

[84] E. M. Ross and T. M. Wilkie, "GTPase-activating proteins for heterotrimeric G proteins: regulators of G Protein Signaling (RGS) and RGS-like proteins," *Annual Review of Biochemistry*, vol. 69, pp. 795–827, 2000.

[85] S. Fukuharaa, H. Chikumi, and J. Silvio Gutkind, "RGS-containing RhoGEFs: the missing link between transforming G proteins and Rho?" *Oncogene*, vol. 20, no. 13, pp. 1661–1668, 2001.

[86] A. Schmidt and A. Hall, "Guanine nucleotide exchange factors for Rho GTPases: turning on the switch," *Genes and Development*, vol. 16, no. 13, pp. 1587–1609, 2002.

[87] C. E. Teixeira, F. B. M. Priviero, and R. C. Webb, "Effects of 5-cyclopropyl-2-[1-(2-fluoro-benzyl)-1H-pyrazolo[3,4-b]pyridine-3-yl]pyrimidin-4-ylamine (BAY 41-2272) on smooth muscle tone, soluble guanylyl cyclase activity, and NADPH oxidase activity/expression in corpus cavernosum from wild-type, neuronal, and endothelial nitric-oxide synthase null mice," *Journal of Pharmacology and Experimental Therapeutics*, vol. 322, no. 3, pp. 1093–1102, 2007.

[88] A. V. Somlyo, "New roads leading to Ca$^{2+}$ sensitization," *Circulation Research*, vol. 91, no. 2, pp. 83–84, 2002.

[89] E. Mantadakis, D. H. Ewalt, J. D. Cavender, Z. R. Rogers, and G. R. Buchanan, "Outpatient penile aspiration and epinephrine irrigation for young patients with sickle cell anemia and prolonged priapism," *Blood*, vol. 95, no. 1, pp. 78–82, 2000.

[90] G. J. Kato, "Priapism in sickle-cell disease: a hematologist's perspective," *The Journal of Sexual Medicine*, vol. 9, no. 1, pp. 70–78, 2012.

[91] E. S. Bialecki and K. R. Bridges, "Sildenafil relieves priapism in patients with sickle cell disease," *American Journal of Medicine*, vol. 113, no. 3, p. 252, 2002.

[92] G. R. Serjeant, K. de Ceulaer, and G. H. Maude, "Stilboestrol and stuttering priapism in homozygous sickle-cell disease," *The Lancet*, vol. 2, no. 8467, pp. 1274–1276, 1985.

[93] L. A. Levine and S. P. Guss, "Gonadotropin-releasing hormone analogues in the treatment of sickle cell anemia-associated priapism," *Journal of Urology*, vol. 150, no. 2, pp. 475–477, 1993.

[94] D. Rachid-Filho, A. G. Cavalcanti, L. A. Favorito, W. S. Costa, and F. J. B. Sampaio, "Treatment of recurrent priapism in sickle cell anemia with finasteride: a new approach," *Urology*, vol. 74, no. 5, pp. 1054–1057, 2009.

[95] I. Okpala, N. Westerdale, T. Jegede, and B. Cheung, "Etilefrine for the prevention of priapism in adult sickle cell disease," *British Journal of Haematology*, vol. 118, no. 3, pp. 918–921, 2002.

[96] A. D. Seftel, "A prospective diary study of stuttering priapism in adolescents and young men with sickle cell anemia: report of an international randomized control trial; The priapism in sickle cell study (PISCES study)," *Journal of Urology*, vol. 185, no. 5, pp. 1837–1838, 2011.

[97] S. T. O. Saad, C. Lajolo, S. Gilli et al., "Follow-up of sickle cell disease patients with priapism treated by hydroxyurea," *American Journal of Hematology*, vol. 77, no. 1, pp. 45–49, 2004.

[98] A. Hassan, A. Jam'a, and I. A. Al Dabbous, "Hydroxyurea in the treatment of sickle cell associated priapism," *Journal of Urology*, vol. 159, no. 5, p. 1642, 1998.

[99] R. F. Machado, R. J. Barst, N. A. Yovetich et al., "Hospitalization for pain in patients with sickle cell disease treated with sildenafil for elevated TRV and low exercise capacity," *Blood*, vol. 118, no. 4, pp. 855–864, 2011.

[100] S. Charache, M. L. Terrin, R. D. Moore et al., "Effect of hydroxyurea on the frequency of painful crises in Sickle cell anemia," *The New England Journal of Medicine*, vol. 332, no. 20, pp. 1317–1322, 1995.

[101] S. M. Bakanay, E. Dainer, B. Clair et al., "Mortality in sickle cell patients on hydroxyurea therapy," *Blood*, vol. 105, no. 2, pp. 545–547, 2005.

[102] O. S. Platt, D. J. Brambilla, W. F. Rosse et al., "Mortality in sickle cell disease—life expectancy and risk factors for early death," *The New England Journal of Medicine*, vol. 330, no. 23, pp. 1639–1644, 1994.

[103] D. R. Powars, L. S. Chan, A. Hiti, E. Ramicone, and C. Johnson, "Outcome of sickle cell anemia: a 4-decade observational study of 1056 patients," *Medicine*, vol. 84, no. 6, pp. 363–376, 2005.

[104] C. D. Fitzhugh, N. Lauder, J. C. Jonassaint et al., "Cardiopulmonary complications leading to premature deaths in adult patients with sickle cell disease," *American Journal of Hematology*, vol. 85, no. 1, pp. 36–40, 2010.

[105] C. R. D. Nahoum, E. A. Fontes, and F. R. Freire, "Semen analysis in sickle cell disease," *Andrologia*, vol. 12, no. 6, pp. 542–545, 1980.

[106] D. N. Osegbe, O. Akinyanju, and E. O. Amaku, "Fertility in males with sickle cell disease," *The Lancet*, vol. 2, no. 8241, pp. 275–276, 1981.

[107] V. O. Agbaraji, R. B. Scott, S. Leto, and L. W. Kingslow, "Fertility studies in sickle cell disease: semen analysis in adult male patients," *International Journal of Fertility*, vol. 33, no. 5, pp. 347–352, 1988.

[108] I. Berthaut, G. Guignedoux, F. Kirsch-Noir et al., "Influence of sickle cell disease and treatment with hydroxyurea on sperm parameters and fertility of human males," *Haematologica*, vol. 93, no. 7, pp. 988–993, 2008.

[109] C. C. Lu and M. L. Meistrich, "Cytotoxic effects of chemotherapeutic drugs on mouse testis cells," *Cancer Research*, vol. 39, no. 9, pp. 3575–3582, 1979.

[110] G. Ficsor and L. C. Ginsberg, "The effect of hydroxyurea and mitomycin C on sperm motility in mice," *Mutation Research*, vol. 70, no. 3, pp. 383–387, 1980.

[111] H. Singh and C. Taylor, "Effects of Thio-TEPA and hydroxyurea on sperm production in Lakeview hamsters," *Journal of Toxicology and Environmental Health*, vol. 8, no. 1-2, pp. 307–316, 1981.

[112] D. P. Evenson and L. K. Jost, "Hydroxyurea exposure alters mouse testicular kinetics and sperm chromatin structure," *Cell Proliferation*, vol. 26, no. 2, pp. 147–159, 1993.

[113] R. Wiger, J. K. Hongslo, D. P. Evenson, P. De Angelis, P. E. Schwarze, and J. A. Holme, "Effects of acetaminophen and hydroxyurea on spermatogenesis and sperm chromatin structure in laboratory mice," *Reproductive Toxicology*, vol. 9, no. 1, pp. 21–33, 1995.

[114] J. M. Saez, "Leydig cells: endocrine, paracrine, and autocrine regulation," *Endocrine Reviews*, vol. 15, no. 5, pp. 574–626, 1994.

[115] K. M. Jones, M. S. Niaz, C. M. Brooks et al., "Adverse effects of a clinically relevant dose of hydroxyurea used for the treatment of sickle cell disease on male fertility endpoints," *International Journal of Environmental Research and Public Health*, vol. 6, no. 3, pp. 1124–1144, 2009.

[116] G. Friedman, R. Freeman, and R. Bookchin, "Testicular function in sickel cell disease," *Fertility and Sterility*, vol. 25, no. 12, pp. 1018–1021, 1974.

[117] A. A. Abbasi, A. S. Prasad, and J. Ortega, "Gonadal function abnormalities in sickle cell anemia; studies in male adult patients," *Annals of Internal Medicine*, vol. 85, no. 5, pp. 601–605, 1976.

[118] O. Modebe and U. O. Ezeh, "Effect of age on testicular function in adult males with sickle cell anemia," *Fertility and Sterility*, vol. 63, no. 4, pp. 907–912, 1995.

[119] O. A. Dada and E. U. Nduka, "Endocrine function and hemoglobinopathies: relation between the sickle cell gene and circulating plasma levels of testosterone, luteinizing hormone (LH) and follicle stimulating hormone (FSH) in adult males," *Clinica Chimica Acta*, vol. 105, no. 2, pp. 269–273, 1980.

[120] M. A. F. El-Hazmi, H. M. Bahakim, and I. Al-Fawaz, "Endocrine functions in sickle cell anaemia patients," *Journal of Tropical Pediatrics*, vol. 38, no. 6, pp. 307–313, 1992.

[121] E. K. Abudu, S. A. Akanmu, O. O. Soriyan et al., "Serum testosterone levels of HbSS (sickle cell disease) male subjects in Lagos, Nigeria," *BMC Research Notes*, vol. 17, no. 4, p. 298, 2011.

[122] D. N. Osegbe and O. O. Akinyanju, "Testicular dysfunction in men with sickle cell disease," *Postgraduate Medical Journal*, vol. 63, no. 736, pp. 95–98, 1987.

[123] O. O. Abdulwaheed, A. A. Abdulrasaq, A. K. Sulaiman et al., "The hormonal assessment of the infertile male in Ilorin, Nigeria," *African Journal of Clinical Endocrinology & Metabolism*, vol. 3, pp. 62–64, 2002.

[124] O. N. Gofrit, D. Rund, A. Shapiro, O. Pappo, E. H. Landau, and D. Pode, "Segmental testicular infarction due to sickle cell disease," *Journal of Urology*, vol. 160, no. 3, part 1, pp. 835–836, 1998.

[125] A. S. Prasad, E. B. Schoomaker, and J. Ortega, "Zinc deficiency in sickle cell disease," *Clinical Chemistry*, vol. 21, no. 4, pp. 582–587, 1975.

[126] A. S. Prasad and Z. T. Cossack, "Zinc supplementation and growth in sickle cell disease," *Annals of Internal Medicine*, vol. 100, no. 3, pp. 367–371, 1984.

[127] C. S. Landefeld, M. Schambelan, S. L. Kaplan, and S. H. Embury, "Clomiphene-responsive hypogonadism in sickle cell anemia," *Annals of Internal Medicine*, vol. 99, no. 4, pp. 480–483, 1983.

[128] C. T. Jiminez, R. B. Scott, W. L. Henry et al., "Studies in sickle cell anemia. XXVI. The effect of homozygous sickle cell disease on the onset of menarche, pregnancy, fertility, pubescent changes and body growth in Negro subjects," *American Journal Of Diseases Of Children*, vol. 111, pp. 497–503, 1966.

[129] O. S. Platt, W. Rosenstock, and M. A. Espeland, "Influence of sickle hemoglobinopathies on growth and development," *The New England Journal of Medicine*, vol. 311, no. 1, pp. 7–12, 1984.

[130] M. A. Zago, J. Kerbauy, H. M. Souza et al., "Growth and sexual maturation of Brazilian patients with sickle cell diseases," *Tropical and Geographical Medicine*, vol. 44, no. 4, pp. 317–321, 1992.

[131] M. Li, J. Fogarty, K. D. Whitney, and P. Stone, "Repeated testicular infarction in a patient with sickle cell disease: a possible mechanism for testicular failure," *Urology*, vol. 62, no. 3, p. 551, 2003.

[132] M. L. Dufau, "The luteinizing hormone receptor," *Annual Review of Physiology*, vol. 60, pp. 461–496, 1998.

[133] M. Ascoli, F. Fanelli, and D. L. Segaloff, "The lutropin/choriogonadotropin receptor, a 2002 perspective," *Endocrine Reviews*, vol. 23, no. 2, pp. 141–174, 2002.

[134] D. M. Stocco, "StAR protein and the regulation of steroid hormone biosynthesis," *Annual Review of Physiology*, vol. 63, pp. 193–213, 2001.

[135] J. J. Tremblay, F. Hamel, and R. S. Viger, "Protein kinase A-dependent cooperation between GATA and CCAAT/enhancer-binding protein transcription factors regulates steroidogenic acute regulatory protein promoter activity," *Endocrinology*, vol. 143, no. 10, pp. 3935–3945, 2002.

[136] L. F. Epstein and N. R. Orme-Johnson, "Acute action of luteinizing hormone on mouse Leydig cells: accumulation of mitochondrial phosphoproteins and stimulation of testosterone synthesis," *Molecular and Cellular Endocrinology*, vol. 81, no. 1–3, pp. 113–126, 1991.

[137] L. F. Epstein and N. R. Orme-Johnson, "Regulation of steroid hormone biosynthesis: identification of precursors of a phosphoprotein targeted to the mitochondrion in stimulated rat adrenal cortex cells," *Journal of Biological Chemistry*, vol. 266, no. 29, pp. 19739–19745, 1991.

[138] T. Seebacher, E. Beitz, H. Kumagami, K. Wild, J. P. Ruppersberg, and J. E. Schultz, "Expression of membrane-bound and cytosolic guanylyl cyclases in the rat inner ear," *Hearing Research*, vol. 127, no. 1-2, pp. 95–102, 1999.

[139] F. Arakane, S. R. King, Y. Du et al., "Phosphorylation of steroidogenic acute regulatory protein (StAR) modulates its steroidogenic activity," *Journal of Biological Chemistry*, vol. 272, no. 51, pp. 32656–32662, 1997.

[140] I. P. Artemenko, D. Zhao, D. B. Hales, K. H. Hales, and C. R. Jefcoate, "Mitochondrial processing of newly synthesized steroidogenic acute regulatory protein (StAR), but not total StAR, mediates cholesterol transfer to cytochrome P450 side chain cleavage enzyme in adrenal cells," *Journal of Biological Chemistry*, vol. 276, no. 49, pp. 46583–46596, 2001.

[141] C. Jefcoate, "High-flux mitochondrial cholesterol trafficking, a specialized function of the adrenal cortex," *Journal of Clinical Investigation*, vol. 110, no. 7, pp. 881–890, 2002.

[142] J. Liu, M. B. Rone, and V. Papadopoulos, "Protein-protein interactions mediate mitochondrial cholesterol transport and steroid biosynthesis," *Journal of Biological Chemistry*, vol. 281, no. 50, pp. 38879–38893, 2006.

[143] H. K. Eltzschig, J. C. Ibla, G. T. Furuta et al., "Coordinated adenine nucleotide phosphohydrolysis and nucleoside signaling in posthypoxic endothelium: role of ectonucleotidases and adenosine $A_{2B}$ receptors," *Journal of Experimental Medicine*, vol. 198, no. 5, pp. 783–796, 2003.

[144] Y. Zhang, Y. Dai, J. Wen et al., "Detrimental effects of adenosine signaling in sickle cell disease," *Nature Medicine*, vol. 17, no. 1, pp. 79–86, 2011.

[145] D. M. Stocco, X. Wang, Y. Jo, and P. R. Manna, "Multiple signaling pathways regulating steroidogenesis and steroidogenic acute regulatory protein expression: more complicated than we thought," *Molecular Endocrinology*, vol. 19, no. 11, pp. 2647–2659, 2005.

[146] M. L. Khurana and K. N. Pandey, "Receptor-mediated stimulatory effect of atrial natriuretic factor, brain natriuretic peptide, and C- type natriuretic peptide on testosterone production in purified mouse Leydig cells: activation of cholesterol side- chain cleavage enzyme," *Endocrinology*, vol. 133, no. 5, pp. 2141–2149, 1993.

[147] K. Del Punta, E. H. Charreau, and O. P. Pignataro, "Nitric oxide inhibits leydig cell steroidogenesis," *Endocrinology*, vol. 137, no. 12, pp. 5337–5343, 1996.

[148] J. G. Drewett, R. L. Adams-Hays, B. Y. Ho, and D. J. Hegge, "Nitric oxide potently inhibits the rate-limiting enzymatic step in steroidogenesis," *Molecular and Cellular Endocrinology*, vol. 194, no. 1-2, pp. 39–45, 2002.

[149] S. Valenti, C. M. Cuttica, L. Fazzuoli, G. Giordano, and M. Giusti, "Biphasic effect of nitric oxide on testosterone and cyclic GMP production by purified rat Leydig cells cultured in vitro," *International Journal of Andrology*, vol. 22, no. 5, pp. 336–341, 1999.

[150] S. Gambaryan, E. Butt, K. Marcus et al., "cGMP-dependent protein kinase type II regulates basal level of aldosterone production by zona glomerulosa cells without increasing expression of the steroidogenic acute regulatory protein gene," *Journal of Biological Chemistry*, vol. 278, no. 32, pp. 29640–29648, 2003.

[151] D. A. Kass, H. C. Champion, and J. A. Beavo, "Phosphodiesterase type 5: expanding roles in cardiovascular regulation," *Circulation Research*, vol. 101, no. 11, pp. 1084–1095, 2007.

[152] S. A. Andric, T. S. Kostic, and S. S. Stojilkovic, "Contribution of multidrug resistance protein MRP5 in control of cyclic guanosine 5′-monophosphate intracellular signaling in anterior pituitary cells," *Endocrinology*, vol. 147, no. 7, pp. 3435–3445, 2006.

[153] G. C. Fernández-Pérez, F. M. Tardáguila, M. Velasco et al., "Radiologic findings of segmental testicular infarction," *American Journal of Roentgenology*, vol. 184, no. 5, pp. 1587–1593, 2005.

[154] S. Madaan, S. Joniau, K. Klockaerts et al., "Segmental testicular infarction: conservative management is feasible and safe," *European Urology*, vol. 53, no. 2, pp. 441–445, 2008.

[155] D. P. Han, R. R. Dmochowski, M. H. Blasser, and J. R. Auman, "Segmental infarction of the testicle: atypical presentation of a testicular mass," *Journal of Urology*, vol. 151, no. 1, pp. 159–160, 1994.

[156] G. H. Urwin, N. Kehoe, S. Dundas, and M. Fox, "Testicular infarction in a patient with sickle cell trait," *British Journal of Urology*, vol. 58, no. 3, pp. 340–341, 1986.

[157] N. M. Holmes and C. J. Kane, "Testicular infarction associated with sickle cell disease," *Journal of Urology*, vol. 160, no. 1, p. 130, 1998.

[158] D. Bruno, D. R. Wigfall, S. A. Zimmerman, P. M. Rosoff, and J. S. Wiener, "Genitourinary complications of sickle cell disease," *Journal of Urology*, vol. 166, no. 3, pp. 803–811, 2001.

[159] P. S. Sarma, "Testis involvement in sickle cell trait," *The Journal of the Association of Physicians of India*, vol. 35, no. 4, p. 321, 1987.

[160] K. J. Hurt, B. Musicki, M. A. Palese et al., "Akt-dependent phosphorylation of endothelial nitric-oxide synthase mediates penile erection," *Proceedings of the National Academy of Sciences of the United States of America*, vol. 99, no. 6, pp. 4061–4066, 2002.

[161] K. C. Wood, L. L. Hsu, and M. T. Gladwin, "Sickle cell disease vasculopathy: a state of nitric oxide resistance," *Free Radical Biology and Medicine*, vol. 44, no. 8, pp. 1506–1528, 2008.

[162] M. L. Adams, E. R. Meyer, B. N. Sewing, and T. J. Cicero, "Effects of nitric oxide-related agents on rat testicular function," *Journal of Pharmacology and Experimental Therapeutics*, vol. 269, no. 1, pp. 230–237, 1994.

[163] D. B. Hales, "Testicular macrophage modulation of Leydig cell steroidogenesis," *Journal of Reproductive Immunology*, vol. 57, no. 1-2, pp. 3–18, 2002.

[164] C. Mondillo, R. M. Pagotto, B. Piotrkowski et al., "Involvement of nitric oxide synthase in the mechanism of histamine-induced inhibition of leydig cell steroidogenesis via histamine receptor subtypes in sprague-dawley rats," *Biology of Reproduction*, vol. 80, no. 1, pp. 144–152, 2009.

[165] A. Solovey, R. Kollander, L. C. Milbauer et al., "Endothelial nitric oxide synthase and nitric oxide regulate endothelial tissue factor expression in vivo in the sickle transgenic mouse," *American Journal of Hematology*, vol. 85, no. 1, pp. 41–45, 2010.

[166] L. De Franceschi, M. D. Cappellini, and O. Olivieri, "Thrombosis and sickle cell disease," *Seminars in Thrombosis and Hemostasis*, vol. 37, no. 3, pp. 226–236, 2011.

[167] R. Gopalakrishna, Zhen Hai Chen, and U. Gundimeda, "Nitric oxide and nitric oxide-generating agents induce a reversible inactivation of protein kinase C activity and phorbol ester binding," *Journal of Biological Chemistry*, vol. 268, no. 36, pp. 27180–27185, 1993.

[168] V. Sauzeau, H. Le Jeune, C. Cario-Toumaniantz et al., "Cyclic GMP-dependent protein kinase signaling pathway inhibits RhoA- induced $Ca^{2+}$ sensitization of contraction in vascular smooth muscle," *Journal of Biological Chemistry*, vol. 275, no. 28, pp. 21722–91729, 2000.

[169] N. Sawada, H. Itoh, J. Yamashita et al., "cGMP-dependent protein kinase phosphorylates and inactivates RhoA," *Biochemical and Biophysical Research Communications*, vol. 280, no. 3, pp. 798–805, 2001.

[170] N. L. Jernigan, B. R. Walker, and T. C. Resta, "Chronic hypoxia augments protein kinase G-mediated $Ca^{2+}$ desensitization in pulmonary vascular smooth muscle through inhibition of RhoA/Rho kinase signaling," *American Journal of Physiology*, vol. 287, no. 6, pp. L1220–L1229, 2004.

[171] F. B. M. Priviero, L. M. Jin, Z. Ying, C. E. Teixeira, and R. C. Webb, "Up-regulation of the RhoA/Rho-kinase signaling pathway in corpus cavernosum from endothelial Nitric-Oxide Synthase (NOS), but not neuronal NOS, null mice,"

*Journal of Pharmacology and Experimental Therapeutics*, vol. 333, no. 2, pp. 184–192, 2010.

[172] P. Abrams, "Describing bladder storage function: overactive bladder syndrome and detrusor overactivity," *Urology*, vol. 62, no. 5, supplement 2, pp. 28–37, 2003.

[173] M. C. Michel and M. M. Barendrecht, "Physiological and pathological regulation of the autonomic control of urinary bladder contractility," *Pharmacology and Therapeutics*, vol. 117, no. 3, pp. 297–312, 2008.

[174] K. E. Andersson, P. Hedlund, A. J. Wein, R. R. Dmochowski, and D. R. Staskin, "Pharmacologic perspective on the physiology of the lower urinary tract," *Urology*, vol. 60, no. 5, pp. 13–20, 2002.

[175] K. E. Andersson and A. Arner, "Urinary bladder contraction and relaxation: physiology and pathophysiology," *Physiological Reviews*, vol. 84, no. 3, pp. 935–986, 2004.

[176] S. L. M. Peters, M. Schmidt, and M. C. Michel, "Rho kinase: a target for treating urinary bladder dysfunction?" *Trends in Pharmacological Sciences*, vol. 27, no. 9, pp. 492–497, 2006.

[177] K. I. Ataga and E. P. Orringer, "Renal abnormalities in sickle cell disease," *American Journal of Hematology*, vol. 63, no. 4, pp. 205–211, 2000.

[178] F. Daneshgari, G. Liu, L. Birder, A. T. Hanna-Mitchell, and S. Chacko, "Diabetic bladder dysfunction: current translational knowledge," *Journal of Urology*, vol. 182, no. 6, pp. S18–S26, 2009.

[179] C. R. Chapple, T. Yamanishi, R. Chess-Williams, J. G. Ouslander, J. P. Weiss, and K. E. Andersson, "Muscarinic receptor subtypes and management of the overactive bladder," *Urology*, vol. 60, no. 5, pp. 82–89, 2002.

[180] S. S. Hegde and R. M. Eglen, "Muscarinic receptor subtypes modulating smooth muscle contractility in the urinary bladder," *Life Sciences*, vol. 64, no. 6-7, pp. 419–428, 1999.

[181] S. S. Hegde, A. Choppin, D. Bonhaus et al., "Functional role of M2 and M3 muscarinic receptors in the urinary bladder of rats in vitro and in vivo," *British Journal of Pharmacology*, vol. 120, no. 8, pp. 1409–1418, 1997.

[182] P. A. Longhurst, R. E. Leggett, and J. A. K. Briscoe, "Characterization of the functional muscarinic receptors in the rat urinary bladder," *British Journal of Pharmacology*, vol. 116, no. 4, pp. 2279–2285, 1995.

[183] A. Choppin, R. M. Eglen, and S. S. Hegde, "Pharmacological characterization of muscarinic receptors in rabbit isolated iris sphincter muscle and urinary bladder smooth muscle," *British Journal of Pharmacology*, vol. 124, no. 5, pp. 883–888, 1998.

[184] S. Mutoh, J. Latifpour, M. Saito, and R. M. Weiss, "Evidence for the presence of regional differences in the subtype specificity of muscarinic receptors in rabbit lower urinary tract," *Journal of Urology*, vol. 157, no. 2, pp. 717–721, 1997.

[185] D. J. Sellers, T. Yamanishi, C. R. Chapple, C. Couldwell, K. Yasuda, and R. Chess-Williams, "M3 muscarinic receptors but not M2 mediate contraction of the porcine detrusor muscle in vitro," *Journal of Autonomic Pharmacology*, vol. 20, no. 3, pp. 171–176, 2000.

[186] G. D'Agostino, M. L. Bolognesi, A. Lucchelli et al., "Prejunctional muscarinic inhibitory control of acetylcholine release in the human isolated detrusor: involvement of the M4 receptor subtype," *British Journal of Pharmacology*, vol. 129, no. 3, pp. 493–500, 2000.

[187] R. Chess-Williams, C. R. Chapple, T. Yamanishi, K. Yasuda, and D. J. Sellers, "The minor population of M3-receptors mediate contraction of human detrusor muscle in vitro,"

*Journal of Autonomic Pharmacology*, vol. 21, no. 5, pp. 243–248, 2001.

[188] L. O. S. Leiria, F. Z. T. Mónica, F. D. G. F. Carvalho et al., "Functional, morphological and molecular characterization of bladder dysfunction in streptozotocin-induced diabetic mice: eidence for a role for L-type voltage-operated $Ca^{2+}$ channels," *British Journal of Pharmacology*, vol. 163, no. 6, pp. 1276–1288, 2011.

[189] A. C. Ramos-Filho, F. Z. Mónica, C. F. Franco-Penteado et al., "Characterization of the urinary bladder dysfunction in renovascular hypertensive rats," *Neurourology and Urodynamics*, vol. 30, no. 7, pp. 1392–402, 2011.

[190] K. Nakanishi, T. Kamai, T. Mizuno, K. Arai, and T. Yamanishi, "Expression of RhoA mRNA and activated RhoA in urothelium and smooth muscle, and effects of a Rho-kinase inhibitor on contraction of the porcine urinary bladder," *Neurourology and Urodynamics*, vol. 28, no. 6, pp. 521–528, 2009.

[191] L. Boberg, M. Poljakovic, A. Rahman, R. Eccles, and A. Arner, "Role of Rho-kinase and protein kinase C during contraction of hypertrophic detrusor in mice with partial urinary bladder outlet obstruction," *BJU International*, vol. 109, no. 1, pp. 132–140, 2012.

[192] M. A. Claudino, C. F. Franco-Penteado, M. A. F. Corat et al., "Reduction of urinary bladder activity in transgenic sickle cell disease mice," *Blood*, vol. 114, abstract 2580, 2009, (ASH Annual Meeting Abstracts).

[193] W. F. Tarry, J. W. Duckett, and M. I. H. Snyder, "Urological complications of sickle cell disease in a pediatric population," *Journal of Urology*, vol. 138, no. 3, pp. 592–594, 1987.

[194] H. S. Zarkowsky, D. Gallagher, and F. M. Gill, "Bacteremia in sickle hemoglobinopathies," *Journal of Pediatrics*, vol. 109, no. 4, pp. 579–585, 1986.

[195] J. M. Miller Jr., "Sickle cell trait in pregnancy," *Southern Medical Journal*, vol. 76, no. 8, pp. 962–963, 1983.

[196] I. C. Baill and F. R. Witter, "Sickle trait and its association with birthweight and urinary tract infections in pregnancy," *International Journal of Gynecology and Obstetrics*, vol. 33, no. 1, pp. 19–21, 1990.

[197] L. M. Pasture, D. A. Savitz, and J. M. Thorp, "Predictors of urinary tract infection at the first prenatal visit," *Epidemiology*, vol. 10, no. 3, pp. 282–287, 1999.

[198] M. L. Portocarrero, M. L. Portocarrero, M. M. Sobral, I. Lyra, P. Lordêlo, and U. Barroso Jr., "Prevalence of enuresis and daytime urinary incontinence in children and adolescents with sickle cell disease," *Journal of Urology*, vol. 187, no. 3, pp. 1037–1040, 2012.

# 10

# Priapism in Sickle Cell Anemia: Emerging Mechanistic Understanding and Better Preventative Strategies

**Genevieve M. Crane and Nelson E. Bennett Jr.**

*Institute of Urology, Lahey Clinic, 41 Mall Road, Burlington, MA 01805, USA*

Correspondence should be addressed to Nelson E. Bennett Jr., nbennettjrmd@gmail.com

Academic Editor: Kanokwan Sanchaisuriya

Sickle cell anemia is a common and disabling disorder profoundly affecting mortality as well as quality of life. Up to 35% of men with sickle cell disease are affected by painful, prolonged erections termed ischemic priapism. A priapic episode may result in fibrosis and permanent erectile dysfunction. The severity of sickle cell disease manifestations is variable dependent on a number of contributing genetic factors; however, priapism tends to cluster with other severe vascular complications including pulmonary hypertension, leg ulceration, and overall risk of death. The mechanisms underlying priapism in sickle cell disease have begun to be elucidated including hemolysis-mediated dysregulation of the nitric oxide signaling pathway and dysregulation of adenosine-mediated vasodilation. A better understanding of these mechanisms is leading toward novel preventative strategies. This paper will focus on the mechanisms underlying development of ischemic priapism in sickle cell disease, current acute and preventative treatment strategies, and future directions for improved management of this disorder.

## 1. Introduction

Sickle cell disease (SCD) is a common disorder with 8% of African Americans heterozygous for the hemoglobin S point mutation (HbS) in the $\beta$-globin gene and approximately 50,000 Americans homozygous for this mutation [1, 2]. Hemoglobin is a tetrameric protein composed of two $\alpha$-chains and two $\beta$-globin chains. Deoxygenation results in aggregation and polymerization of HbS tetramers, formation of needle-like hemoglobin fibers, and distortion of red cells into the characteristic sickle shape.

Sickling is dependent on multiple variables including hemoglobin concentration and hydration status, pH and degree of deoxygenation. Sickling is more common in vascular beds with low-flow states including the splenic sinusoids, the bone marrow, the penile corpora during an erection, or any inflamed tissue. The combined influence of these factors can result in a vicious cycle of inflammation, hypoxia, and acidosis resulting in increased sickling, vessel occlusion, and ischemia [3].

Manifestations of SCD are widespread and generally secondary to ischemia from vessel occlusion and hemolysis from direct rupture of sickle cells that have lost normal red cell deformability. The type and severity of complications vary significantly between individuals. Common manifestations include vaso-occlusive crises, the result of hypoxic injury or infarction, which may affect the brain, pulmonary vessels, spleen, bone marrow, kidney, retina, penis or other tissues resulting in sequelae such acute chest syndrome with pulmonary infarction, stroke or splenic infarction. Splenic infarction and subsequent fibrosis ultimately contribute to increased susceptibility to infections from encapsulated bacteria leading to increased risk of septicemia and meningitis, the most common causes of death in children with SCD. Leg ulcers are another common manifestation of vaso-occlusion. A comprehensive discussion of the manifestations of SCD is beyond the scope of this paper.

This paper will focus on one common manifestation that can significantly affect quality of life of men with SCD, which is the development of prolonged, painful erections known as low-flow or ischemic priapism that result in tissue ischemia and attenuated or absent return of functional erections. Reports of the lifetime prevalence of ischemic priapism in SCD range from 2–35% [4, 5]. High flow priapism, which results from increased arterial flow generally caused by trauma, does not result in tissue ischemia and has not been associated with increased risk in SCD patients. The mechanisms underlying high and low-flow priapism completely differ, as do their treatments; therefore, this paper will focus only on ischemic priapism, which is substantially increased in SCD patients.

## 2. Pathophysiology of Priapism

In the flaccid state, the erectile tissue smooth muscle is tonically contracted as are the arterial and arteriolar vessels, allowing only a small amount of flow to meet nutritional needs. When neurotransmitters are released to signal an erection, there is smooth muscle relaxation resulting in filling of the sinusoids and ultimate compression of venous outflow resulting in trapping of blood. This results in an erection with pressure greater than that of systolic blood pressure. The corpora cavernosa are covered in a tunica albuginea, a bilayered structure with an inner layer that supports the cavernous tissue and an outer layer that runs longitudinally from the glans to insert onto the pubic rami. Emissary veins run between the inner and outer layers. During an erection, these are compressed along with the subtunical venous plexus to prevent venous outflow. The corpora spongiosum lacks the tunica, and therefore, serves as an arteriovenous fistula with less rigidity than the corpora cavernosa [6]. The principal neurotransmitter for erection is nitric oxide (NO), which is released by both nerve terminals and endothelial cells. The NO then diffuses into both trabecular cells and arterial smooth muscle cells. This activates guanylate cyclase, which catalyzes the formation of cGMP from GTP, and results in a cascade that decreases intracellular calcium and opens potassium channels to cause smooth muscle relaxation. Alternative pathways generate cAMP, which enhances this effect. Detumescence follows degradation of cGMP and cAMP. cGMP is degraded by phosphodiesterase-5 (PDE5), the target of sildenafil, vardenafil and tadalafil.

Stasis and low blood flow rates within the sinusoids of the erectile tissue make the penis a site at high risk for developing a veno-occlusive crisis in SCD. Ischemic priapism is characterized by a prolonged erection that is usually painful and not associated with sexual excitement or desire. Typically, the corpora cavernosa are tense, congested and tender to palpation while the glans and corpus spongiosum are usually soft and uninvolved. Classically, the primary mechanism is thought to be obstruction of venous drainage resulting in viscous, hypoxic blood [7] leading to interstitial edema and fibrosis of the cavernosa, ultimately resulting in impotence. The length of time of ischemia directly correlates with the likelihood of return of erectile function, and therefore, ischemic priapism is considered a urologic emergency. For example, in one study, all patients with ischemic priapism episodes of greater than 12 hours duration had reduction in erectile rigidity. No patients with priapism greater than 36 hours had return of spontaneous functional erections [4].

## 3. Mechanisms Underlying Sickle Cell-Induced Priapism

While anatomic factors and a low-flow state contribute to making erectile tissue prone to sickle cell-induced pain and ischemia, abnormal regulation of the nitric oxide (NO) pathway and its downstream signaling may be particularly key in the development of priapism and other vascular complications in SCD.

NO is a potent vasodilator and key to tumescence as described above, but free NO is readily scavenged in the blood by hemoglobin. It is converted to nitrate plus methemoglobin following reaction with oxyhemoglobin and to iron-nitrosylhemoglobin following reaction with deoxyhemoglobin [8]. The ability of hemoglobin to scavenge NO is normally dramatically reduced by its compartmentalization within red blood cells, which creates a cell-free and therefore hemoglobin-free zone adjacent to the vessel endothelium due to laminar flow (Figure 1(a)). In addition, the presence of the cell membrane, cytoskeleton and other factors increase the diffusion distance between NO and hemoglobin. As a result, hemoglobin contained in red cells has less than 0.2% of the scavenging capacity of free hemoglobin [9]. The chronic intravascular hemolysis in SCD changes this tight regulation of NO. SCD patients have elevated free hemoglobin concentrations compared to normal volunteers [8], and these concentrations were frequently sufficient to blunt vasodilation in response to nitroprusside administration. Pain crises may be exacerbated by further hemolysis, NO scavenging and prevention of vasodilation in the presence of ischemia.

Other studies have also associated risk for priapism with markers of hemolysis. Lactate dehydrogenase (LDH), bilirubin and reticulocyte count were all elevated in men with SCD who experienced priapism compared with men with SCD who had never experienced an episode of priapism [10]. In another study, LDH level closely correlated with the free-hemoglobin level in plasma, accelerated NO consumption and impaired vasodilation [11]. In addition, LDH levels in this study could be used to identify a subset of SCD patients at higher risk for vascular complications including pulmonary hypertension, priapism, and leg ulcers.

Chronic scavenging of NO results in a decreased expression of downstream regulatory molecules including PDE5 that normally degrades cGMP, the second messenger in NO signaling. Genetically modified mice homozygous for the sickle cell mutation ($SS^{-/-}$) have been shown to express decreased levels of PDE5 in penile tissue, and similar effects were seen in mice deficient for endothelial nitric oxide synthase ($eNOS^{-/-}$), which also develop priapism [12]. Nonetheless, following cavernosal nerve stimulation, these mice express high levels of cavernosal cGMP, likely secondary to the fact that NO released from nerve terminals is not as readily scavenged. The combination of chronically decreased PDE5 and normal cGMP generation following nerve stimulation may result in an unregulated, prolonged erection.

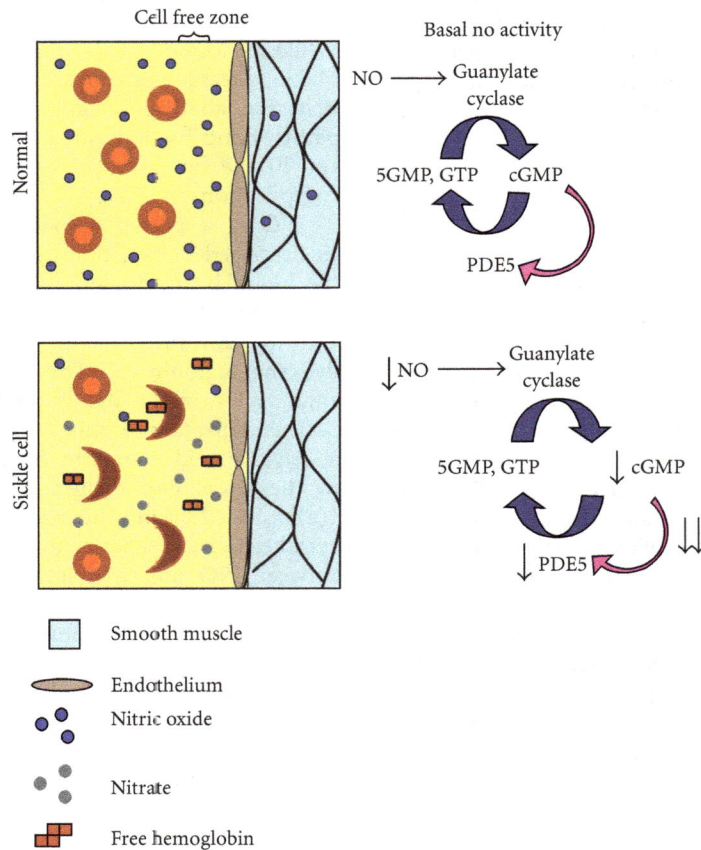

(a)

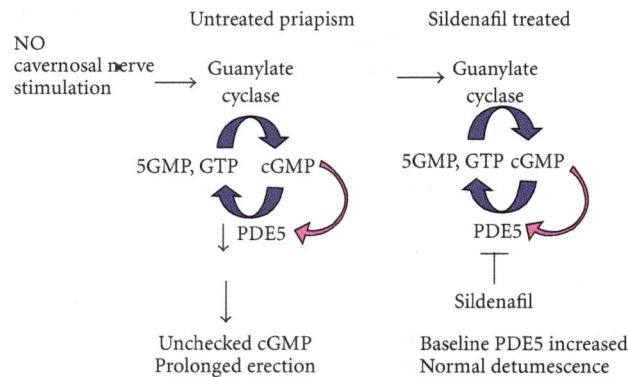

(b)

FIGURE 1: Abnormal nitric oxide signaling leads to priapism in SCD. NO can be readily scavenged by free hemoglobin and deactivated by conversion to nitrate. This is normally prevented by compartmentalization of hemoglobin in red cells and a cell free zone adjacent to the endothelium ((a), first panel adapted from Liao [9] and Rother et al. [23]). In SCD, chronic hemolysis leads to higher levels of free hemoglobin and decreased NO availability. This results in decreased basal levels of its downstream effector, cGMP, and decreased PDE5, which degrades cGMP. Following cavernosal nerve stimulation in SCD (b), normal levels of cGMP are achieved as NO is released from nerve terminals. However, PDE5 levels remain low, leading to prolonged cGMP activity and prolonged erection. This can be prevented by long-term treatment with sildenafil ((b), second panel). Inhibition of PDE5 by sildenafil results in increased cGMP, which then increases basal PDE5 levels through normal feedback mechanisms [13, 14].

There is complex regulation of PDE5 by cGMP and its effector, cGMP-dependent protein kinase (PKG) [13]. cGMP is the substrate for PDE5, but it can also bind at an additional allosteric site to alter the conformation of PDE5, exposing a phosphorylation site. This site can be phosphorylated by PKG, which then increases the activity of PDE5. Also, as a normal feedback mechanism, the promoters which regulate the expression PDE5 isoforms found in penile tissue are responsive to increasing concentrations of cGMP [14]. That is, cGMP stimulates PDE5 expression to regulate its own degradation, suggesting that PDE expression could be enhanced by agents that increase cGMP levels. This phenomenon has now been demonstrated both in vitro and in vivo. Culture of cavernous smooth muscle cells treated with sildenafil increased PDE5 expression, and young but not old rats treated with sildenafil for 3 weeks demonstrated an elevation of PDE5 expression in penile tissue following treatment [15].

The ability of elevated cGMP to stimulate increased expression of PDE5 has raised the possibility of a novel preventative strategy for priapism in SCD. While initially somewhat paradoxical, these results suggest that treatment of sickle cell patients with PDE5 inhibitors may actually help prevent priapism by correcting the chronically low levels of PDE5 in their cavernosal tissue (Figure 1(b)). Indeed, Burnett and colleagues who posed this hypothesis have found that long-term, low-dose PDE5 inhibitor treatment may help reduce priapism in a series of cases [13].

Additional pathways may also affect the development of priapism in SCD. One that has recently gained interest is the regulation of adenosine signaling. Similar to NO, adenosine is a potent vasodilator and neurotransmitter. Adenosine signals through G-protein coupled receptors to increase cAMP to result in smooth muscle relaxation, and intracavernosal injection of adenosine can be used to induce erection. Studies in adenosine deaminase deficient mice, which develop prolonged erections, have demonstrated that excessive adenosine accumulation and adenosine receptor signaling contribute to priapism through smooth muscle relaxation [16]. Adenosine signaling was similarly elevated in the sickle cell $SS^{-/-}$ mouse model. Elevated levels of adenosine appear to contribute to fibrosis, as adenosine deaminase enzyme therapy attenuated fibrosis in both mouse models [17]. These results suggest that the adenosine signaling pathway may be an excellent target for the development of new treatment strategies to prevent priapism or to limit fibrosis following a priapic episode.

In addition to pathways that regulate vasodilation, appropriate regulation of vasoconstriction is also necessary for normal erectile function. RhoA and its downstream effectors, Rho-kinases (ROCK1 and 2), help maintain the penis in a flaccid state and have been shown to have abnormal activation in erectile dysfunction [18] including in old age and diabetes. There is reduced activity of components of this pathway in both $eNOS^{-/-}$ and $SS^{-/-}$ mice with priapism [19, 20]. Additional work will be required to further clarify the role of this pathway in priapism as well as appropriate targets for therapy.

## 4. Treatment Strategies

Acute treatment for ischemic priapism should be instituted within hours given the increasing likelihood of cavernosal fibrosis and permanent erectile dysfunction. Standard treatment involves penile blood gas studies, corporeal aspiration, and phenylephrine injection to induce smooth muscle contraction and detumescence. SCD patients may benefit from early high-dose intracavernosal phenylephrine given that the acidic pH of the ischemic cavernosa may decrease the affinity of adrenergic receptors for their ligands [21]. If conservative measures fail, penile shunt surgery should be performed. This may involve anastamosing corpus spongiosum and corpora cavernosa to create an internal fistula. SCD patients may also benefit from hydration, blood transfusions, exchange transfusions, or hyperbaric oxygen.

Ideally, patients at high risk for the development of such episodes would be identified early to increase education of the risks of prolonged priapism and to institute potential prophylactic strategies. Increased awareness of the signs of priapism and education on the need for early treatment may be the best way to prevent longterm sequelae. Despite the risks of ischemic priapism and its association with SCD being well known in the medical community, few men receive education on the need to seek urgent medical attention for this issue [4]. In addition, it may be possible to identify the subset of SCD patients at highest risk for severe priapic episodes for education and prophylatic strategies before permanent damage has taken place. This is because prolonged episodes of priapism that result in intracavernosal fibrosis are often preceded by periods of "stuttering priapism" (72% of cases in one report [5]) or acute transient attacks as originally described by Hinman [7]. Treatment of individuals with stuttering priapism with PDE5 inhibitors has been reported to reduce the frequency of these episodes [13]. Use of PDE5 inhibitors to abort acute attacks has also been reported [22], but positive results would be less likely to be attributable to short-term changes in PDE5 levels and, in fact, such use could potentially worsen a priapic event [13]. However, it has been hypothesized that use of PDE5 inhibitors in acute attacks may result in vasodilatation of cavernosal tissue allowing egress of sickle cells.

There has been evidence to suggest that nocturnal oxygen desaturation, particularly in children, may contribute to the onset of painful crises [24, 25]. This could be particularly relevant to priapism given the normal physiology of nocturnal tumescence, and patients may benefit from prophylatic treatment including nocturnal oxygen or the use of continuous positive airway pressure machines.

Hormonal therapy has also been used to decrease the incidence of priapism [26] including GnRH analogs, stilbestrol [27] and antiandrogens which are associated with significant side effects including hot flashes and gynecomastia. More recently, one group has investigated the use of finasteride, a 5 $\alpha$-reductase inhibitor, to decrease the frequency of priapism in a population with SCD and recurrent priapism with a significant decrease in the number of episodes per month [28]. Unfortunately, these hormonal therapies may have significant or unknown effects on fertility and libido, posing a significant disadvantage for use in the typically young SCD patient population.

Long-term use of oral [29, 30] or intracavernous delivery [31] of $\alpha$-adrenergic agonists has also been investigated with some success as first described by Virag and colleagues. Digoxin has been used and is believed to exert its effect by inhibition of the Na/K ATPase pump to prevent relaxation of cavernosal smooth muscle. Neuromodulatory agents have also been used, particularly in spinal cord patients, to moderate the autonomic and somatic reflex pathways involved in erection. These include gabapentin, a synthetic analogue of GABA, an inhibitory neurotransmitter, and baclofen, a GABA receptor agonist. A detailed paper of these and other agents in the chronic treatment of ischemic priapism can be found in a recent paper by Chow and Payne [26].

If irreversible damage has been done, long-term management of erectile dysfunction may be treated with placement of a penile prosthesis to restore function depending on the preference of the patient, likelihood of success and a detailed discussion of the risks of the procedure. A severe and prolonged episode of priapism will result in cavernous smooth muscle necrosis, fibrosis, and ultimately penile shortening. If erectile function is unlikely to recover, immediate implantation of a penile prosthesis may, therefore, be considered to avoid the complications of penile fibrosis and shortening [32].

The type and severity of the complications of SCD are variable depending on a variety of modulating genetic factors including the presence of other types of hemoglobin, particularly persistent fetal hemoglobin (HbF). Normally after birth, a switch occurs in the $\beta$-globin locus from production of predominantly $\gamma$-globin to $\beta$-globin. Hydroxyurea, which blocks DNA synthesis, has been used to help induce HbF in the adult, thus helping to reduce the frequency of sickle cell crises; however, it results in significant side effects including anemia, neutropenia, and renal and liver dysfunction.

## 5. Conclusions

While the complications associated with the painful crises associated with sickle cell disease including ischemic priapism remain common and debilitating in the SCD population, a better understanding of the underlying biology is emerging. There is hope for new preventative treatments including long-term low-dose PDE5 inhibitors to normalize NO downstream signaling and potential inhibition of adenosine signaling to minimize fibrosis following an episode of priapism.

## References

[1] A. G. Motulsky, "Frequency of sickling disorders in U.S. blacks," *New England Journal of Medicine*, vol. 288, no. 1, pp. 31–33, 1973.

[2] S. H. Orkin and D. R. Higgs, "Sickle cell disease at 100 years," *Science*, vol. 329, no. 5989, pp. 291–292, 2010.

[3] V. Kumar, A. K. Abbas, N. Fausto, and J. Aster, *Robbins and Cotran Pathologic Basis of Disease*, Saunders, Philadelphia, Pa, USA, 2004.

[4] N. Bennett and J. Mulhall, "Sickle cell disease status and outcomes of African-American men presenting with priapism," *Journal of Sexual Medicine*, vol. 5, no. 5, pp. 1244–1250, 2008.

[5] A. B. Adeyoju, A. B. K. Olujohungbe, J. Morris et al., "Priapism in sickle-cell disease; incidence, risk factors and complications—an international multicentre study," *British Journal of Urology International*, vol. 90, no. 9, pp. 898–902, 2002.

[6] E. A. Tanagho and J. W. McAninch, *Smith's General Urology*, McGraw Hill Medical, New York, NY, USA, 2008.

[7] F. Hinman, "Priapism: report Of cases and a clinical study of the literature with reference to its pathogenesis and surgical treatment," *Annals of Surgery*, vol. 60, pp. 689–716, 1914.

[8] C. D. Reiter, X. Wang, J. E. Tanus-Santos et al., "Cell-free hemoglobin limits nitric oxide bioavailability in sickle-cell disease," *Nature Medicine*, vol. 8, no. 12, pp. 1383–1389, 2002.

[9] J. C. Liao, "Blood feud: keeping hemoglobin from nixing NO," *Nature Medicine*, vol. 8, no. 12, pp. 1350–1351, 2002.

[10] V. G. Nolan, D. F. Wyszynski, L. A. Farrer, and M. H. Steinberg, "Hemolysis-associated priapism in sickle cell disease," *Blood*, vol. 106, no. 9, pp. 3264–3267, 2005.

[11] G. J. Kato, V. McGowan, R. F. Machado et al., "Lactate dehydrogenase as a biomarker of hemolysis-associated nitric oxide resistance, priapism, leg ulceration, pulmonary hypertension, and death in patients with sickle cell disease," *Blood*, vol. 107, no. 6, pp. 2279–2285, 2006.

[12] H. C. Champion, T. J. Bivalacqua, E. Takimoto, D. A. Kass, and A. L. Burnett, "Phosphodiesterase-5A dysregulation in penile erectile tissue is a mechanism of priapism," *Proceedings of the National Academy of Sciences of the United States of America*, vol. 102, no. 5, pp. 1661–1666, 2005.

[13] A. L. Burnett, T. J. Bivalacqua, H. C. Champion, and B. Musicki, "Long-term oral phosphodiesterase 5 inhibitor therapy alleviates recurrent priapism," *Urology*, vol. 67, no. 5, pp. 1043–1048, 2006.

[14] C.-S. Lin, S. Chow, A. Lau, R. Tu, and T. F. Lue, "Human PDE5A gene encodes three PDE5 isoforms from two alternate promoters," *International Journal of Impotence Research*, vol. 14, no. 1, pp. 15–24, 2002.

[15] B. Musicki, H. C. Champion, R. E. Becker, T. Liu, M. F. Kramer, and A. L. Burnett, "Erection capability is potentiated by long-term sildenafil treatment: role of blood flow-induced endothelial nitric-oxide synthase phosphorylation," *Molecular Pharmacology*, vol. 68, no. 1, pp. 226–232, 2005.

[16] T. Mi, S. Abbasi, H. Zhang et al., "Excess adenosine in murine penile erectile tissues contributes to priapism via A2B adenosine receptor signaling," *Journal of Clinical Investigation*, vol. 118, no. 4, pp. 1491–1501, 2008.

[17] J. Wen, X. Jiang, Y. Dai et al., "Increased adenosine contributes to penile fibrosis, a dangerous feature of priapism, via A2B adenosine receptor signaling," *FASEB Journal*, vol. 24, no. 3, pp. 740–749, 2010.

[18] H. Wang, M. Eto, W. D. Steers, A. P. Somlyo, and A. V. Somlyo, "RhoA-mediated $Ca^{2+}$ sensitization in erectile function," *Journal of Biological Chemistry*, vol. 277, no. 34, pp. 30614–30621, 2002.

[19] T. J. Bivalacqua, T. Liu, B. Musicki, H. C. Champion, and A. L. Burnett, "Endothelial nitric oxide synthase keeps erection regulatory function balance in the penis," *European Urology*, vol. 51, no. 6, pp. 1732–1740, 2007.

[20] T. J. Bivalacqua, A. E. Ross, T. D. Strong et al., "Attenuated rhoA/rho-kinase signaling in penis of transgenic sickle cell mice," *Urology*, vol. 76, no. 2, pp. 510.e7–510.e12, 2010.

[21] C. Wen, R. Munarriz, I. Mcauley, I. Goldstein, A. Traish, and N. Kim, "Management of ischemic priapism with high-dose intracavernosal phenylephrine: from bench to bedside," *Journal of Sexual Medicine*, vol. 3, no. 5, pp. 918–922, 2006.

[22] E. S. Bialecki and K. R. Bridges, "Sildenafil relieves priapism in patients with sickle cell disease," *American Journal of Medicine*, vol. 113, no. 3, p. 252, 2002.

[23] R. P. Rother, L. Bell, P. Hillmen, and M. T. Gladwin, "The clinical sequelae of intravascular hemolysis and extracellular plasma hemoglobin: a novel mechanism of human disease," *Journal of the American Medical Association*, vol. 293, no. 13, pp. 1653–1662, 2005.

[24] M. B. Scharf, J. S. Lobel, and E. Caldwell, "Nocturnal oxygen desaturation in patients with sickle cell anemia," *Journal of the American Medical Association*, vol. 249, no. 13, pp. 1753–1755, 1983.

[25] B. N. Y. Setty, M. J. Stuart, C. Dampier, D. Brodecki, and J. L. Allen, "Hypoxaemia in sickle cell disease: biomarker modulation and relevance to pathophysiology," *Lancet*, vol. 362, no. 9394, pp. 1450–1455, 2003.

[26] K. Chow and S. Payne, "The pharmacological management of intermittent priapismic states," *British Journal of Urology International*, vol. 102, no. 11, pp. 1515–1521, 2008.

[27] G. R. Serjeant, K. De Ceulaer, and G. H. Maude, "Stilboestrol and stuttering priapism in homozygous sickle-cell disease," *Lancet*, vol. 2, no. 8467, pp. 1274–1276, 1985.

[28] D. Rachid-Filho, A. G. Cavalcanti, L. A. Favorito, W. S. Costa, and F. J. B. Sampaio, "Treatment of recurrent priapism in sickle cell anemia with finasteride: a new approach," *Urology*, vol. 74, no. 5, pp. 1054–1057, 2009.

[29] R. Virag, D. Bachir, K. Lee, and F. Galacteros, "Preventive treatment of priapism in sickle cell disease with oral and self-administered intracavernous injection of etilefrine," *Urology*, vol. 47, no. 5, pp. 777–781, 1996.

[30] I. Okpala, N. Westerdale, T. Jegede, and B. Cheung, "Etilefrine for the prevention of priapism in adult sickle cell disease," *British Journal of Haematology*, vol. 118, no. 3, pp. 918–921, 2002.

[31] D. J. Ralph, E. S. Pescatori, G. S. Brindley, and J. P. Pryor, "Intracavernosal phenylephrine for recurrent priapism: self-administration by drug delivery implant," *Journal of Urology*, vol. 165, no. 5, p. 1632, 2001.

[32] E. A. Salem and O. El Aasser, "Management of ischemic priapism by penile prosthesis insertion: prevention of distal erosion," *Journal of Urology*, vol. 183, no. 6, pp. 2300–2303, 2010.

# 11

# Elevated Circulating Angiogenic Progenitors and White Blood Cells Are Associated with Hypoxia-Inducible Angiogenic Growth Factors in Children with Sickle Cell Disease

**Solomon F. Ofori-Acquah,**[1] **Iris D. Buchanan,**[2] **Ifeyinwa Osunkwo,**[1]
**Jerry Manlove-Simmons,**[3] **Feyisayo Lawal,**[4] **Alexander Quarshie,**[5] **Arshed A. Quyyumi,**[6]
**Gary H. Gibbons,**[3] **and Beatrice E. Gee**[2]

[1] Department of Pediatrics, Division of Hematology/Oncology, Emory University School of Medicine, 2015 Uppergate Dr. NE,
 Atlanta, GA 30322, USA
[2] Department of Pediatrics, Morehouse School of Medicine, 720 Westview Drive, SW Atlanta, GA 30310-1495, USA
[3] Cardiovascular Research Institute, Morehouse School of Medicine, 720 Westview Drive, SW Atlanta, GA 30310-1495, USA
[4] Morehouse College, 830 Westview Dr SW, Atlanta, GA 30314, USA
[5] Biostatistics Core, Morehouse School of Medicine, 720 Westview Drive, SW Atlanta, GA 30310-1495, USA
[6] Department of Medicine, Division of Cardiology, 1462 Clifton Road N.E. Suite 507, Atlanta, GA 30322, USA

Correspondence should be addressed to Beatrice E. Gee, bgee@msm.edu

Academic Editor: Kenneth R. Peterson

We studied the number and function of angiogenic progenitor cells and growth factors in children aged 5–18 years without acute illness, 43 with Hemoglobin SS and 68 with normal hemoglobin. Hemoglobin SS subjects had at least twice as many mononuclear cell colonies and more circulating progenitor cell than Control subjects. Plasma concentrations of erythropoietin, angiopoietin-2, and stromal-derived growth factor (SDF)-1$\alpha$ were significantly higher in children with Hemoglobin SS compared to Control subjects. In a multivariate analysis model, SDF-1$\alpha$ concentration was found to be associated with both CPC number and total white blood cell count in the Hemoglobin SS group, suggesting that SDF-1$\alpha$ produced by ischemic tissues plays a role in mobilizing these cells in children with Hemoglobin SS. Despite having a higher number of angiogenic progenitor cells, children with Hemoglobin SS had slower migration of cultured mononuclear cells.

## 1. Introduction

Sickle cell anemia (Hemoglobin SS) is characterized by hemoglobin polymerization and the formation of inflexible sickled erythrocytes. Accumulation of sickled erythrocytes in the microcirculation causes acute vaso-occlusive events that lead to pain and acute organ injury. Chronic arterial vasculopathy, with intimal proliferation and arterial stenosis, can lead to complications such as stroke and pulmonary hypertension. The etiology of arterial stenosis in sickle cell anemia is poorly understood. We hypothesize that intimal proliferation in sickle cell anemia is due to abnormal reparative responses to ongoing vessel injury. Hemolytic anemia,

vaso-occlusion, and abnormal flow dynamics in sickle cell anemia may contribute to vessel injury. Chronic intravascular hemolysis releases free heme, which binds avidly to nitric oxide (NO), causing NO depletion, and subsequent vasoconstriction and inflammation [1]. Erythrocyte-derived reactive iron and oxygen species are also directly injurious to endothelium [2]. Repetitive episodes of acute vaso-occlusion cause tissue ischemia and reperfusion, which also lead to inflammation and increased oxidative stress [3]. Evidence of ongoing inflammation and vascular injury is present in people with sickle cell anemia even when asymptomatic, with elevated levels of high sensitivity C-reactive protein (hsCRP) [4] and circulating endothelial cells [5].

Reendothelization after vascular injury is a critically important process to restoring and maintaining vascular homeostasis. Endothelial progenitor cells (EPCs) are recruited from the bone marrow and home to sites of vascular injury. Recruitment and homing of EPCs are intimately regulated by cytokines and growth factors released at the sites of vascular insult. Reduced numbers of endothelial progenitor colonies have been found in adults with cardiovascular risk factors [6], diabetes [7], and those with established cerebrovascular disease [8]. Cardiovascular disorders are also associated with functional impairments in EPC migration or angiogenesis [9]. Endothelial progenitor cells are elevated during acute myocardial infarction [10], stimulated by hematopoietic growth factors such as erythropoietin [11], granulocyte colony-stimulating factor (G-CSF), or granulocyte-macrophage colony stimulating factor (GM-CSF), and by treatment with HMG-CoA reductase inhibitors (statins) [12] or angiotensin-2 receptor antagonists [13].

To date, there is limited information about the number and function of EPCs or the growth factors involved in EPC recruitment and homing in people who have sickle cell disease. Van Beem reported elevated numbers of circulating EPCs (expressing CD34 and VEGFR2) in adults with Hemoglobin SS or $S\beta^0$-thalassemia during painful crisis, but there was no difference between asymptomatic adults with sickle cell disease and healthy controls [14]. The higher number of circulating EPCs during painful crisis was associated with increased serum levels of erythropoietin, soluble VCAM-1 (sVCAM-1), and vascular endothelial growth factor (VEGF).

Several angiogenic growth factors have been found to be elevated in Hemoglobin SS. Angiopoietin (Ang)-2 and erythropoietin were higher in adults with Hemgoglobin SS compared to healthy controls and further elevated during acute painful crisis [15]. Higher levels of vascular endothelial growth factor (VEGF) were found in subjects with Hemoglobin SS compared to controls in some studies [16, 17], but not in others [15]. When present, higher VEGF levels were found to be associated with reduced odds of elevated tricuspid valve regurgitant velocity by echocardiography in children with sickle cell disease, a noninvasive measure suggesting pulmonary artery hypertension [16]. Conversely, children with sickle cell disease with elevated tricuspid regurgitant velocity had higher concentrations of platelet-derived growth factor (PDGF)-BB. Higher levels of SDF-1 have been found in adults with Hemoglobin SS than controls, particularly in those who had pulmonary hypertension [18].

There is ongoing debate about the *in vitro* phenotype of endothelial progenitor cells. Circulating cells expressing hematopoietic stem cell marker CD34, vascular endothelial growth factor receptor (VEGFR)-2, and early progenitor marker CD133 have been considered to represent EPCs, though recent studies show that these cells were immature hematopoietic cells that did not differentiate into EPCs or form vessels [19]. In a study of the effects of granulocyte-macrophage colony-stimulating factor (GM-CSF) on vascular function in adults with peripheral arterial disease, treatment-induced increase in the number of circulating CD34-expressing cells correlated with clinical improvements in flow-mediated dilation and pain-free walking time [20],

suggesting that undifferentiated hematopoietic cells have angiogenic potential or are a surrogate marker of vascular repair cells. In this paper, we refer to the cultured cells as mononuclear cells and the cells measured from the peripheral blood as circulating progenitors cells (CPCs) with angiogenic potential.

Taken together, there is evidence that people with sickle cell disease have vessel injury and proangiogenic growth factor responses, but limited information about vascular reparative function in sickle cell disease. We hypothesize that vascular complications in people with sickle cell disease arise from altered repair mechanisms, most likely due to abnormal angiogenic cell functions. We expect CPC numbers to be normal or elevated, stimulated by high levels of erythropoietin that is seen with chronic anemia. We report here our findings of cultured mononuclear colony and CPC number in children with Hemoglobin SS versus healthy Controls, their relationship to plasma levels of angiogenic growth factors, and the migration of cultured mononuclear cells.

## 2. Materials and Methods

*2.1. Blood Sample Collection.* The study protocol was approved by the Institutional Review Boards of Morehouse School of Medicine and Children's Healthcare of Atlanta, and the Grady Hospital Research Oversight Committee. Written informed consent was obtained from each participant's parent or guardian and verbal assent from the volunteer before sample collection. Venous blood was collected from African American children aged 5–18 years old without symptoms of acute illness. *Controls* had Hemoglobin AA or AC, and sickle cell anemia subjects had *Hemoglobin SS* or Hb $S$-$\beta^0$ thalassemia. Children treated with hydroxyurea, recent red blood cell transfusion within the previous 90 days, or who had cardiovascular risk factors, such as overweight or obesity, cigarette smoking, diabetes, or hypertension, were excluded. Complete blood counts were performed by standard methods by the clinical laboratories used by the clinic sites.

*2.2. Circulating Progenitor Cell Quantitation.* Whole blood samples were labeled with monoclonal antibodies for FITC-conjugated anti-human CD34 (clone 8G12, 0.6 $\mu$g/mL final concentration, Becton Dickinson, Franklin Lakes, NJ), PE-conjugated anti-human VEGFR2 (clone 89106, 1.2 $\mu$g/mL, R&D Systems, Minneapolis, MN), PERCP-conjugated anti-human CD45 (clone 2D1, 0.6 $\mu$g/mL, Becton Dickinson), APC-conjugated anti-human CD133/1 (clone AC133, 0.85 $\mu$g/mL, Miltenyi Biotec Inc., Auburn, CA), and PE-Cy7 conjugated anti-human CXCR4 (clone 12G5, 0.5 $\mu$g/mL, eBioscience Inc., San Diego, CA), or their isotype controls at the same concentrations, and analyzed by FACS. Thirty microliters of antibody cocktail was added to 300 $\mu$L of whole blood, or 15 $\mu$L of the isotype control cocktail was added to 150 $\mu$L of blood. Samples were incubated in the dark for 15 minutes. Red blood cells were lysed by adding 1.5 mL of lysing solution ($NH_4Cl$ 0.15 M, $KHCO_3$ 10 mM, EDTA 0.1 mM) into each tube. Lysis was stopped by adding 1.5 mL of staining media (phosphate-buffered saline [PBS] without $Mg^{++}$ or $Ca^{++}$, heat-inactivated fetal calf serum 3%, and $NaN_3$ 0.1%) and mixing gently. Immediately before acquisition on a flow cytometer, $100\,\mu L$ of Accucheck Counting Beads (PCB100, Invitrogen) were added and mixed gently. Cells were washed twice and resuspended in $500\,\mu L$ of staining media. Samples were kept in the dark until run on the flow cytometer, within 4 hours of initial processing. Data are reported for cells with low (dim) CD45 expression (which excludes mature leukocytes).

*2.3. Mononuclear Cell Colony Assay.* Mononuclear cell culture was performed according to a modification of the protocol of Hill et al. [6]. Peripheral blood mononuclear cells (PBMCs) were isolated from whole blood by density fractionation and cultured on fibronectin-coated plates (Becton Dickinson) in M199 medium (Invitrogen, Carlsbad, CA) with fetal calf serum 20% (Invitrogen) and penicillin 100 U/mL and streptomycin $100\,\mu g/mL$ (Invitrogen), at $37^\circ C$ in 5% $CO_2$. The same lot of fetal calf serum was used throughout the study for all samples. After 48 hours, nonadherent cells were replated at a concentration of $10^6$ per well in fibronectin-coated plates. Media were replenished every two days. Colony-forming units (>200 micron diameter) in each well were counted 7 days after replating. The reported number of colonies per well is the average of 3 wells per subject.

*2.4. Immunofluorescent Staining.* Mononuclear cells were seeded onto fibronectin-coated four-chamber slides (Becton Dickinson) at a concentration of $2 \times 10^6$ cells per chamber. Cells were grown to confluence over 14 days with media replenished every two days. Confluent monolayers were fixed with 4% paraformaldehyde in PBS. Cells were permeabilized with ice cold methanol for five minutes and blocked with goat serum 10% (Dako, Carpinteria, CA) for one hour. Cells were incubated overnight with murine primary antibodies directed against human CD31 (clone JC70A, $10\,\mu g/mL$ final concentration, Dako), human endothelial nitric oxide synthase (-eNOS, clone 3, $1.25\,\mu g/mL$, Becton Dickinson), human CD14 (clone TUK4, $0.5\,\mu g/mL$, Dako) or isotype controls at the same concentrations (mouse $IgG_1$ or mouse $IgG_{2a}$, Dako), in PBS with goat serum 2%. Cells were washed with PBS and incubated for one hour with secondary antibodies (Alexafluor (AF)-488 goat anti-mouse $IgG_1$ or AF-594 goat anti-mouse $IgG_{2a}$, Invitrogen) at $1:500$ dilution in PBS with goat serum 2%. Slides were counterstained with DAPI nuclear stain (Invitrogen).

*2.5. Wound Migration Assay.* Mononuclear cells were grown until confluent on fibronectin-coated plates for 14 days, as described above. An aseptic linear wound was made across the mononuclear cell monolayer using sterile $20\,\mu L$ pipette tip. Digital photographs were taken at 0 and 24 hours after the wound was made. The wound area was measured for each time point using image analysis software (Image-Pro Plus v. 6.2 for Windows, Bethesda, MD). The difference in wound area between hours 0 and 24 was expressed as

$$\%\text{Area migrated} = \frac{\text{Area}_{Hr0} - \text{Area}_{Hr24}}{\text{Area}_{Hr0}} \times 100. \quad (1)$$

The average wound area of 3 wells was reported for each subject.

*2.6. Angiogenic Growth Factor Assays.* Quantitative enzyme-linked immuno-sorbent assay (ELISA) for human erythropoietin, angiopoietin-2, and SDF-$1\alpha$ (R&D Systems, Minneapolis, MN), and a Human Angiogenesis Assay Panel (BioRad, Hercules, CA) were used to measure plasma concentrations of growth factors. Results for erythropoietin were expressed as mIU/mL or pg/mL of plasma for the other growth factors. Each ELISA sample was run in duplicate.

*2.7. Oxidative Stress Markers.* Plasma concentrations of the redox pairs cysteine and cystine (Cys, CySS) and reduced and oxidized glutathione (GSH, GSSG) were measured by high pressure liquid chromatography (HPLC), and the redox potentials for the Cys/CySS and GSH/GSSG couples ($E_h$CySS, $E_h$GSSG, resp.) were calculated using the method of Jones [21]. This method includes sample preparation and storage procedures to reduce artifacts that can be caused by hemolysis or GSH thiol-disulfide exchange. Urinary 8-isoprostanes (8-iso-Prostaglandin-$F_{2\alpha}$) were measured by ELISA (Enzo LifeLife Sciences, Plymouth Meeting, PA).

*2.8. Classification of Variables and Data*

*2.8.1. Outcome Variables.* The main outcome variables were blood-derived mononuclear cell colonies and CPC populations. Total white blood cell (WBC) count was analyzed as an intermediate outcome variable.

*2.8.2. Exposure Variables.* The main exposure variable was Hemoglobin Group, defined as a categorical variable with two levels, Hemoglobin SS and Control. The other exposure variables were the clinical characteristics (age, weight, sex), peripheral blood counts, angiogenic growth factors, and oxidative stress markers.

*2.9. Statistical Analysis.* Data were summarized using frequencies and percentages for categorical variables and means (and standard deviation) for continuous variables. Data that were not normally distributed were transformed using natural logarithm transformation. The antilogarithms of the means of the transformed data are reported as geometric means.

*2.9.1. Univariate Analyses.* Simple linear regression models were fitted to determine the relationships between the number of each CPC type (outcome variables) and individual clinical variables or biomarkers (exposure variables).

*2.9.2. Multivariate Analyses.* Bivariate linear regression models were fitted to examine the relationship between hemoglobin group SS and number of CPCs, as well as the confounding effects of the other exposure variables. Confounders were defined as those variables causing at least 25% reduction in the $\beta$-coefficient compared to the main exposure variable alone. Multiple linear regression analyses were then performed to examine the relationship between

TABLE 1: Subject characteristics and hematologic parameters. There was no difference in age and sex of the participants in each group. Hemoglobin SS subjects had significantly lower hemoglobin concentration and higher WBC and platelet counts (indicated by asterisks (*)).

| | | Control | | | Hemoglobin SS | | P value |
|---|---|---|---|---|---|---|---|
| | $n$ | Arithmetic mean (95th% CI) | Geometric mean (95th% CI) | $n$ | Arithmetic mean (95th% CI) | Geometric mean (95th% CI) | |
| Age (yrs) | 68 | 12.8 (12–13.8) | 12.3 (11.4–13.3) | 43 | 12 (11–13) | 11.5 (10.4–12.6) | 0.26 |
| Sex (males) | 68 | 30 (44%) | | 43 | 20 (47%) | | |
| Hemoglobin (gm/dL) | 39 | 13.6 (12.1–15.2) | 13.2 (12.4–14.1) | 19 | 8.4 (7.8–9) | 8.3* (7.7–8.9) | <0.001 |
| WBC ($\times 10^3$/mL) | 39 | 5.4 (4.9–6) | 5.2 (4.7–5.7) | 18 | 12.1 (9.6–14.4) | 11.4* (9.7–13.4) | <0.001 |
| Platelets ($\times 10^3$/mL) | 39 | 280 (261–298) | 274 (257–293) | 18 | 413 (373–454) | 406* (368–448) | <0.001 |

TABLE 2: Number of mononuclear cell colonies and CPCs for each Hemoglobin Group. Children with Hemoglobin SS had more mononuclear cell colonies and circulating progenitor cells than Controls. Mononuclear cell colonies are reported per well, and CPCs in cells/$\mu$L. Significant differences in geometric means between Control and Hemoglobin SS groups are indicated by asterisks (*).

| | Main exposure variables (Hemoglobin Group) | | | | | | | |
|---|---|---|---|---|---|---|---|---|
| Outcome variables | | Control | | | Hemoglobin SS | | Fold difference | P value |
| | $n$ | Arithmetic mean (95th% CI) | Geometric mean (95th% CI) | $n$ | Arithmetic mean (95th% CI) | Geometric mean (95th% CI) | | |
| Colonies | 63 | 13.5 (8.5–18.5) | 8.1 (5.8–11.5) | 39 | 28.8 (16.1–41.6) | 16.5* (11–24.6) | 2 | 0.01 |
| CD34 | 43 | 1.7 (1.3–2.1) | 1.4 (1.2–1.7) | 17 | 5.4 (2.3–8.5) | 3.6* (2.3–5.6) | 2.6 | <0.001 |
| CD34/CD133 | 43 | 1.0 (0.7–1.2) | 0.8 (0.7–1.0) | 17 | 2.0 (1.0–2.9) | 1.3 (0.8–2.2) | | 0.1 |
| CD34/CXCR4 | 43 | 0.6 (0.5–0.7) | 0.48 (0.4–0.6) | 17 | 3.2 (1.2–5.2) | 1.66* (0.9–3.2) | 3.5 | <0.001 |
| CD34/VEGFR2 | 43 | 0.12 (0.09–0.15) | 0.08 (0.06–0.1) | 17 | 0.68 (0.2–1.1) | 0.36* (0.2–0.6) | 2.6 | <0.001 |
| CD34/CXCR4/VEGFR2 | 43 | 0.2 (0.1–0.3) | 0.1 (0.07–01) | 17 | 0.6 (0.2–1) | 0.29* (0.15–0.5) | 2.9 | 0.002 |

hemoglobin group and number of CPCs, controlling for all confounding variables.

Similar univariate and multivariate analyses were performed using WBC as an intermediate outcome. All analyses were performed using STATA Data Analysis and Statistical software (College Station, TX), and level of statistical significance was set at 0.05.

## 3. Results

A total of 111 children were studied, 68 Controls and 43 with Hemoglobin SS. Clinical features are shown in Table 1. As expected, children with Hemoglobin SS had significantly lower hemoglobin concentration, and higher white blood cell and platelet counts than Controls. There were no significant differences in age or sex between the two groups.

*3.1. Angiogenic Progenitor Cells.* On average, twice as many mononuclear cell colonies were grown from the blood of children with Hemoglobin SS than healthy Control children (geometric mean 16.5 versus 8.1 colonies/well, $P < 0.05$) (Table 2). A subset of the cultured cells expressed platelet endothelial cell adhesion molecule (PECAM or CD31) and endothelial nitric oxide synthase (eNOS), two markers of mature endothelial cells (Figure 1). There was no significant difference in percentage of cultured cell expressing CD31 or eNOS between Hemoglobin SS and Control groups, and the cells did not express the monocytic marker, CD14 (data not shown).

Similarly, there were at least twice as many CPCs expressing CD34, CD34/VEGFR2, CD34/CXCR4, or CD34/CXCR4/VEGFR2 in the children with Hemoglobin SS compared to Controls (Table 2), but no difference in the number of cells expressing CD34/CD133. Circulating progenitor cells expressing CD34/CD133/VEGFR2 are not reported due to very low numbers. The differences between Hemoglobin SS and Controls were highest in CPC expressing CXCR4 (SDF-$1\alpha$ receptor). Thus, using two different assay methods, we found that asymptomatic children with Hemoglobin SS have a higher number of circulating angiogenic progenitor cells.

*3.2. Angiogenic Growth Factors.* Plasma concentrations of three angiogenic growth factors were significantly higher in children with Hemoglobin SS compared to Control subjects: erythropoietin (13.5-fold), angiopoietin-2 (4-fold), and stromal derived growth factor (1.7-fold) (Table 3). In the angiogenesis multiplex assay, there were no significant differences between Hemoglobin SS and Control subjects in plasma concentrations of vascular endothelial growth factor (VEGF), hepatic growth factor (HGF), interleukin (IL)-8, follistatin, platelet endothelial cell adhesion molecule (PECAM)-1, or platelet-derived growth factor (PDGF-BB) (20 subjects tested in each group) (data not shown). The concentrations of the three elevated angiogenic growth factors were found to be collinear, which is consistent with their common regulation by hypoxia inducible factor (HIF) (data not shown).

CD31          eNOS

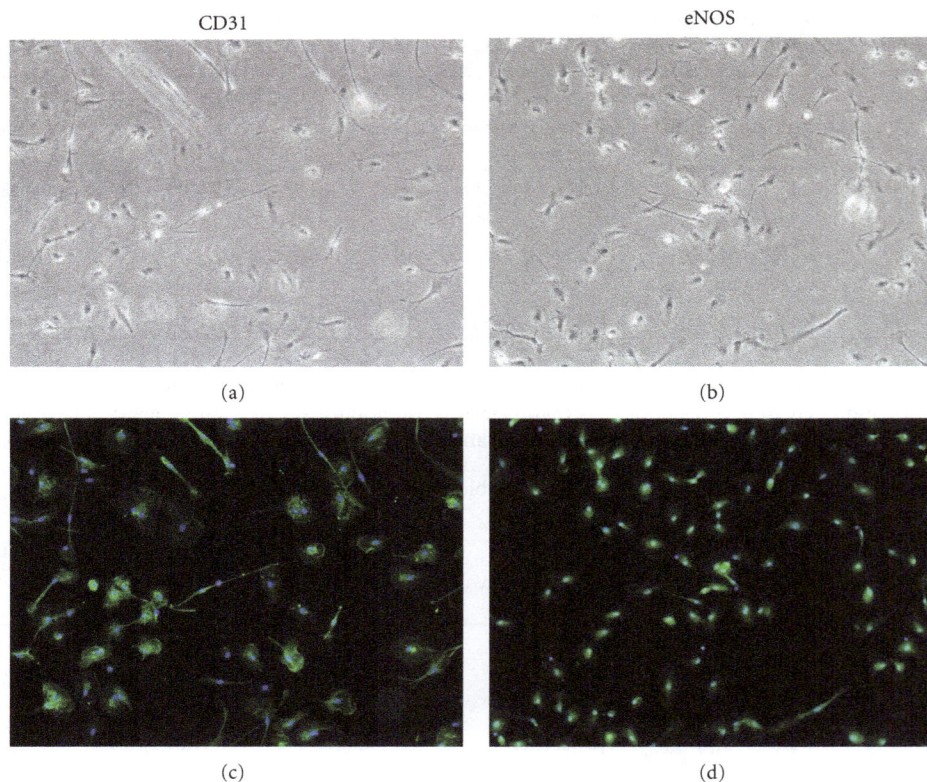

(a)          (b)

(c)          (d)

FIGURE 1: Immunofluorescent staining of cultured mononuclear cells for endothelial antigens CD31 and endothelial nitric oxide synthase (eNOS). CD31 and eNOS staining was observed in a subset of cells. A representative sample from a subject with Hemoglobin SS is shown. (a) shows phase contrast image and (c) shows CD31 staining (green) with nuclei stained with DAPI (blue) in the same field. (b) Shows phase contrast and (d) shows eNOS staining (green) for the same sample.

*3.3. Oxidative Markers.* Both cysteine and cystine were significantly higher (1.5-fold) in the children with Hemoglobin SS compared to Controls. There was no difference in levels of reduced glutathione (GSH) between groups, whereas the oxidized form of glutathione (GSSG) was 2-fold lower in the children with Hemoglobin SS (Table 3). The calculated redox potential for CyS/CySS ($E_h$CySS) was significantly lower (more reduced) in the Hemoglobin SS group than Controls, but there was no difference in $E_h$GSSG between groups. Urinary isoprostane levels were also not different between groups.

*3.4. Wound Migration.* Migration across a linear wound was measured in a subset of mononuclear cell samples. Mononuclear cells from Hemoglobin SS subjects ($n = 5$) migrated over a significantly smaller percentage of the original wound area in 24 hours than cells from healthy Controls ($n = 8$) (28 versus 59%, respectively, $P < 0.01$) (Figure 2). The assay was not performed if samples had not grown to confluence within the 14–16-day culture period.

*3.5. Multivariate Analyses.* Supplementary Table 1 (available online at doi:10.1155/2012/156598) shows the results of univariate analyses. Circulating progenitor cell number was significantly associated with erythropoietin, angiopoietin, SDF-$1\alpha$, hemoglobin concentration, WBC and platelet counts,

and CySS and CySH levels. The strongest associations were found with total WBC, SDF-$1\alpha$, or erythropoietin.

A multivariate model was then used to test the role of the exposure variables as possible determinants of the elevated number of CPCs in children with Hemoglobin SS. Total white blood cell count was strongly associated with all CPC types (Table 4). When CPC number was corrected per 100 WBC, CD34/VEGFR2-expressing cells remained significantly higher in the Hemoglobin SS group than Controls (mean 0.61 versus 0.25 per 100 WBC/$\mu$L, $P = 0.04$), but there were no differences for the other CPC types. To test for the effects of the angiogenic growth factors alone, WBC was excluded from the initial model.

Erythropoietin was associated with CD34 and CD34/CXCR4 numbers, and angiopoietin-2 was associated with CD34/CXCR4/VEGFR2 number. However, SDF-$1\alpha$ was consistently associated with the number of all CPC types in the Hemoglobin SS group (Table 5). SDF-$1\alpha$ in combination with either erythropoietin or angiopoietin-2 had slightly stronger associative effects. None of the other exposure variables or biomarkers, including total hemoglobin, reticulocytes, or platelet count were found to be associated with CPC number in the Hemoglobin SS group.

White blood cells were then analyzed as a possible intermediate outcome. In univariate analysis, total WBC was

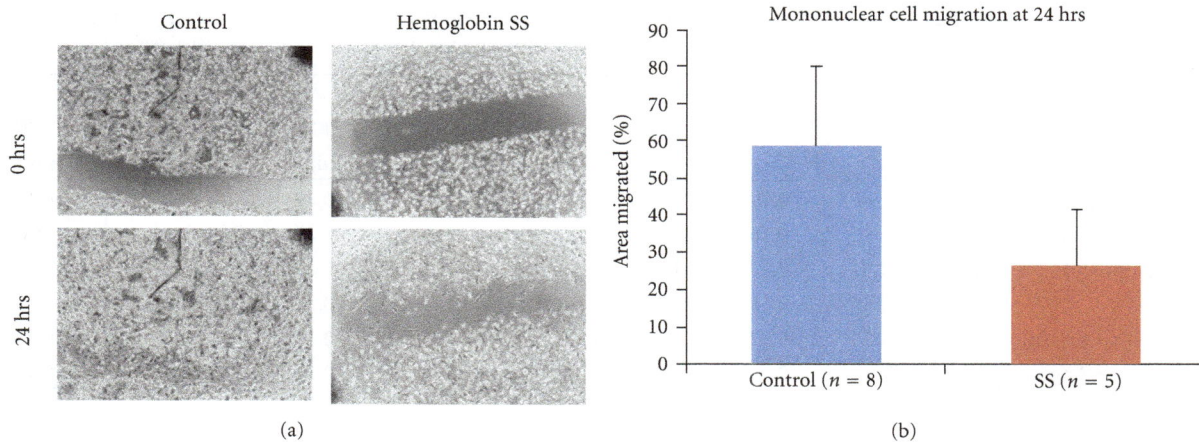

(a)

(b)

FIGURE 2: Mononuclear cell migration. Migration across a wound over 24 hours *was significantly less* in children with Hemoglobin SS than Controls. (a) shows a representative pair of Control and Hemoglobin SS wound migration assays. The freshly made wound was photographed at 0 (zero) hours, and the area migrated is measured after 24 hours. (b) shows the cumulative data for 8 Control and 5 Hemoglobin SS samples. The mean area migrated was less in children with Hemoglobin SS (28% versus 59% of the original wound area, $P < 0.01$).

TABLE 3: Angiogenic growth factors and oxidant stress markers for each Hemoglobin Group. Children with Hemoglobin SS had higher levels of three angiogenic growth factors, higher cysteine and cystine, and lower oxidized glutathione than Controls. Significant differences in the geometric means between Control and Hemoglobin SS groups are indicated by asterisks (*).

| Other exposure variables | Main exposure variables (Hemoglobin Group) | | | | | | Fold difference | P value |
|---|---|---|---|---|---|---|---|---|
| | Control | | | Hemoglobin SS | | | | |
| | $n$ | Arithmetic mean (95th% CI) | Geometric mean (95th% CI) | $n$ | Arithmetic mean (95th% CI) | Geometric mean (95th% CI) | | |
| Erythropoietin (IU/mL) | 68 | 6.6 (4.8, 8.4) | 4.2 (3.2, 5.5) | 42 | 72.4 (55.6, 89) | 56.6* (43.9, 73) | 13.5 | <0.001 |
| Angiopoietin-2 (pg/mL) | 45 | 1922 (1343, 2501) | 1144 (809, 1616) | 27 | 5946 (4661, 7231) | 4968* (3820, 6461) | 4.3 | <0.001 |
| SDF-1$\alpha$ (pg/mL) | 64 | 2376 (2192, 2561) | 2270 (2104, 2449) | 38 | 4065 (3660, 4471) | 3877* (3491, 4305) | 1.7 | <0.001 |
| CyS ($\mu$M) | 44 | 8.0 (7, 9) | 7.4 (6.5, 8.4) | 19 | 11.5 (9.5, 13.5) | 10.8* (9, 13) | 1.5 | 0.001 |
| CySS ($\mu$M) | 44 | 23.9 (22.3, 25.5) | 23.4 (21.9, 24.9) | 19 | 34.6 (30.4, 38.8) | 33.7* (30, 37.8) | 1.5 | <0.001 |
| $E_h$CySS (mV) | 44 | −81.1 (−84, −78) | | 18 | −87.1* (−92, −83) | | | 0.026 |
| GSH ($\mu$M) | 44 | 1.1 (1, 1.2) | 1.0 (0.9, 1.2) | 19 | 1.1 (0.7, 1.5) | 0.89 (0.7, 1.2) | | 0.38 |
| GSSG ($\mu$M) | 44 | 0.1 (0.08, 0.1) | 0.08 (0.07, 0.1) | 19 | 0.08 (0, 0.17) | 0.04* (0.02, 0.07) | 0.5 | 0.002 |
| $E_h$GSSG (mV) | 44 | −117.2 (−121, −113) | | 18 | 124.1 (−132, −117) | | | 0.11 |
| Urinary 8-isoprostanes (ng/mL) | 40 | 15 (9.7, 20.2) | 8.88 (6.2, 12.7) | 16 | 8.9 (7.2, 10.5) | 8.4 (7, 10.1) | | 0.83 |

TABLE 4: Bivariate linear regression showing relationship between Hemoglobin SS group, WBC, and CPC types. WBC was found to be a strongly associated with CPC number in the Hemoglobin SS group. Significant reductions in the beta-coefficient (>25%) compared to the main exposure variable are marked with an asterisk (*).

| Exposure variables | Outcome variables | | | | | | | |
|---|---|---|---|---|---|---|---|---|
| | CD34 | | CD34/CXCR4 | | CD34/VEGFR2 | | CD34/CXCR4/VEGFR2 | |
| | $\beta$ | Adj $r^2$ | $\beta$ | Adj $r^2$ | $\beta$ | Adj $r^2$ | $\beta$ | Adj $r^2$ |
| Group = Hb SS | 0.94 | 0.19 | 1.24 | 0.28 | 1.45 | 0.29 | 1.06 | 0.14 |
| Hb SS + WBC | −0.11* | 0.36 | 0.22* | 0.39 | 1.06* | 0.29 | 0.32* | 0.17 |

TABLE 5: Multivariate linear regression showing relationship between Hemoglobin SS group, angiogenic growth factors, and CPC populations. SDF-1$\alpha$ was consistently associated with the relationship between Hemoglobin SS status and all CPC types (highlighted). Significant reductions in the beta-coefficient ($>25\%$) compared to the main exposure variable are marked with an asterisk ($*$).

| | Outcome variables | | | | | | | |
|---|---|---|---|---|---|---|---|---|
| Exposure variables | CD34 | | CD34/CXCR4 | | CD34/VEGFR2 | | CD34/CXCR4/VEGFR2 | |
| | $\beta$ | Adj $r^2$ | $\beta$ | Adj $r^2$ | $\beta$ | Adj $r^2$ | $\beta$ | Adj $r^2$ |
| Group = Hb SS | 0.94 | 0.19 | 1.24 | 0.28 | 1.45 | 0.29 | 1.06 | 0.14 |
| Hb SS + Erythropoietin | 0.57* | 0.16 | 0.51* | 0.29 | 1.44 | 0.25 | 1.02 | 0.1 |
| Hb SS + Angiopoietin-2 | 1.0 | 0.17 | 1.12 | 0.26 | 1.24 | 0.25 | 0.76* | 0.11 |
| Hb SS + SDF-1$\alpha$ | 0.54* | 0.18 | 0.68* | 0.3 | 1.0* | 0.27 | 0.37* | 0.15 |
| Hb SS + SDF-1$\alpha$ + Erythropoietin | 0.42* | 0.17 | 0.3* | 0.31 | 1.24 | 0.26 | 0.54* | 0.14 |
| Hb SS + SDF-1$\alpha$ + Angiopoietin-2 | 0.71 | 0.19 | 0.73* | 0.29 | 0.98* | 0.26 | 0.3* | 0.14 |

TABLE 6: Multivariate linear regression showing relationship between Hemoglobin SS group, angiogenic growth factors, and WBC. Each angiogenic growth factor was strongly associated with the relationship between Hemoglobin SS and WBC. Significant reductions in the beta-coefficient ($>25\%$) compared to the main exposure are marked with an asterisk ($*$).

| | Intermediate outcome variable | |
|---|---|---|
| Exposure variables | WBC | |
| | $\beta$ | Adj $r^2$ |
| Group = Hb SS | 0.79 | 0.73 |
| Hb SS + Erythropoietin | 0.007 | 0.26 |
| Hb SS + Angiopoietin-2 | <0.001 | 0.17 |
| Hb SS + SDF-1$\alpha$ | 0.004 | 0.32 |

found to have a similar pattern of relationships to the exposure variables as the CPCs (Supplementary Table 2). Multivariate analysis showed that each of the hypoxia-inducible angiogenic growth factors was strongly associated with the relationship between Hemoglobin SS group and elevated WBC (Table 6).

## 4. Discussion

Vascular complications of sickle cell anemia, such as stroke and pulmonary hypertension, begin in childhood and are characterized by early development of intimal proliferation in cerebral and pulmonary arteries in the absence of cardiovascular risk factors, such as hypertension or hyperlipidemia. The mechanisms linking the primary genetic mutation in $\beta$-globin structure to the development of intimal proliferation and arterial stenosis are unknown. We hypothesize that sickle cell anemia is associated with abnormal vascular repair.

We have found that children with sickle cell anemia have a pro-angiogenic phenotype, with a higher numbers of cultured mononuclear cells that express mature endothelial markers, and CPCs with angiogenic potential, and higher angiogenic growth factor levels. The higher number of CPCs in Hemoglobin SS was associated with hypoxia-inducible angiogenic growth factors, either individually or in combination. Stromal derived factor-1$\alpha$ was found to be

associated with the number of all CPC types in children with Hemoglobin SS. In contrast, the severity of anemia (hemoglobin level) was not associated with CPC number. White blood cell count was found to be an intermediate outcome, responding in a similar way to the hypoxia-inducible angiogenic growth factors. When corrected for WBC, the number of CD34/VEGFR2 cells was higher in the Hemoglobin SS group, while there were no differences in the other CPC populations. This implies that the elevation in most of the CPC populations in Hemoglobin SS was a secondary effect of WBC mobilization, but that the number of circulating CD34/VEGFR2 cells was independent of elevated WBC.

Despite a higher number of CPCs in children with Hemoglobin SS, cultured mononuclear cells in this group migrated over a smaller area in a 24-hour period, suggesting abnormal reparative function. The wound migration assay is a well-established functional assay for endothelial progenitor cells. A limitation of our study is the small number of subjects whose cells were tested in the wound migration assay. The wound assay was not performed when the cells did not form a confluent monolayer within the two-week culture period. If the cells were tested after becoming confluent over a longer culture period, we were concerned that cell senescence would contribute to variability in the results. Therefore, our results represent only those samples with better *in vitro* cell growth.

Our findings suggest that bone marrow-derived CD34/VEGFR2 cells in asymptomatic children with Hemoglobin SS are mobilized by hypoxia-inducible angiogenic growth factors from ongoing tissue ischemia, probably due to subclinical sickle cell vaso-occlusion. We predict that numbers will be elevated during acute sickle cell complications, that there will be progressive decline in both CPC number and function with increasing age, and that those individuals with the most severe vascular complications may have impaired function. If validated as a consistent finding, impaired mononuclear cell migration may be due to alterations in SDF-1$\alpha$-mediated CXCR4 signaling. Endothelial progenitor cells from people with coronary artery disease were found to have slower migration, reduced vascular tube formation, and less effect in restoring circulation in a rodent ischemic limb model, in association with lower SDF-1$\alpha$-induced phosphorylation of JAK-2, a downstream target of CXCR4 [22].

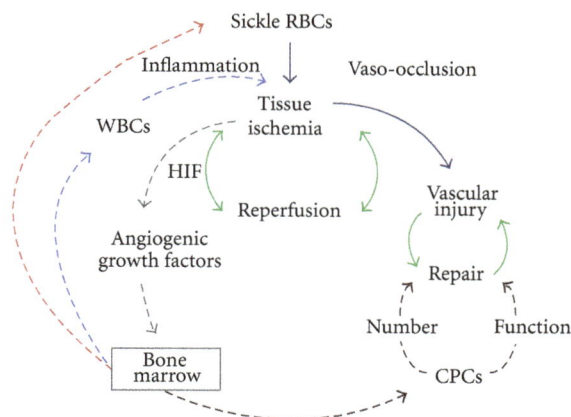

FIGURE 3: Diagram of CPC and WBC mobilization by vaso-occlusion induced tissue ischemia. Vaso-occlusion by sickled red blood cells (RBCs, red) results in tissue ischemia and reperfusion (navy blue). Repeated episodes of vascular ischemia are likely to promote vessel injury (black). Green arrows depict balanced physiologic processes that aim to restore equilibrium. Hypoxia-inducible factor (HIF, gray) produced by ischemic tissues stimulates angiogenic growth factors and bone marrow mobilization of angiogenic progenitor cells (CPCs, brown) that participate in vascular repair, white blood cells (light blue) that promote inflammation, and more sickle red blood cells.

If functional abnormalities in EPCs can be identified and corrected, EPCs in people with sickle cell disease can possibly be harnessed as cellular therapy to prevent or treat vasculopathy.

In addition, our data suggest that elevated WBC count in children with Hemoglobin SS is also due to mobilization by hypoxia-inducible angiogenic growth factors produced by tissue ischemia. This finding provides a mechanistic link between vaso-occlusion and the well-described elevations of white blood cells and inflammatory mediators in sickle cell disease (Figure 3). This relationship is consistent with findings from the Cooperative Study of Sickle Cell Disease (CSSCD) and a more recent cohort study, which describe elevated baseline leukocytosis as a risk factor for adverse sickle cell disease complications [23, 24]. Total WBC in the asymptomatic state, when not modified by transfusion or hydroxyurea therapy, may be a biomarker for tissue ischemia in sickle cell disease.

## 5. Conclusions

We found angiogenic CPC number to be elevated in this group of asymptomatic children with Hemoglobin SS, while mononuclear cell migration was slower than in healthy Control children. Stromal-derived factor-1$\alpha$, a hypoxia-inducible angiogenic growth factor, is strongly associated with the elevated numbers of CPCs and total WBC in children with Hemoglobin SS. Tissue ischemia resulting from vaso-occlusion may promote both proangiogenic and proinflammatory states in sickle cell disease.

## Acknowledgments

This paper was supported by Grants NIH NCRR 5U54RR022814, NHLBI HL088026, HL07776, Morehouse School of Medicine RCMI 5P20RR11104, NIH S21 MD000101-05, and Atlanta-CTSI UL1 RR025008. The authors thank the research volunteers, the clinical staff of Morehouse Medical Associates Pediatric Clinic and Children's Healthcare of Atlanta Sickle Cell Programs at Hughes Spalding and Egleston campuses, Allyson Belton for subject enrollment and sample collection, Natalia Silvestrov of the Clinical Chemistry Core Lab at Morehouse School of Medicine for measuring oxidative markers, Yao Huang for immunofluorescence staining, and Qunna Li of the Cardiovascular Clinical Research Institute at Emory University for running 5-color FACS analyses.

## References

[1] G. J. Kato, M. T. Gladwin, and M. H. Steinberg, "Deconstructing sickle cell disease: reappraisal of the role of hemolysis in the development of clinical subphenotypes," *Blood Reviews*, vol. 21, no. 1, pp. 37–47, 2007.

[2] K. J. Woollard, S. Sturgeon, J. P. F. Chin-Dusting, H. H. Salem, and S. P. Jackson, "Erythrocyte hemolysis and hemoglobin oxidation promote ferric chloride-induced vascular injury," *The Journal of Biological Chemistry*, vol. 284, no. 19, pp. 13110–13118, 2009.

[3] K. C. Wood and D. N. Granger, "Sickle cell disease: role of reactive oxygen and nitrogen metabolites," *Clinical and Experimental Pharmacology and Physiology*, vol. 34, no. 9, pp. 926–932, 2007.

[4] S. Krishnan, Y. Setty, S. G. Betal et al., "Increased levels of the inflammatory biomarker C-reactive protein at baseline are associated with childhood sickle cell vasocclusive crises," *British Journal of Haematology*, vol. 148, no. 5, pp. 797–804, 2010.

[5] A. Solovey, Y. Lin, P. Browne, S. Choong, E. Wayner, and R. P. Hebbel, "Circulating activated endothelial cells in sickle cell anemia," *The New England Journal of Medicine*, vol. 337, no. 22, pp. 1584–1590, 1997.

[6] J. M. Hill, G. Zalos, J. P. J. Halcox et al., "Circulating endothelial progenitor cells, vascular function, and cardiovascular risk," *The New England Journal of Medicine*, vol. 348, no. 7, pp. 593–600, 2003.

[7] C. J. M. Loomans, E. J. P. de Koning, F. J. T. Staal et al., "Endothelial progenitor cell dysfunction: a novel concept in the pathogenesis of vascular complications of type 1 diabetes," *Diabetes*, vol. 53, no. 1, pp. 195–199, 2004.

[8] U. Ghani, A. Shuaib, A. Salam et al., "Endothelial progenitor cells during cerebrovascular disease," *Stroke*, vol. 36, no. 1, pp. 151–153, 2005.

[9] O. M. Tepper, R. D. Galiano, J. M. Capla et al., "Human endothelial progenitor cells from type II diabetics exhibit impaired proliferation, adhesion, and incorporation into vascular structures," *Circulation*, vol. 106, no. 22, pp. 2781–2786, 2002.

[10] M. Massa, V. Rosti, M. Ferrario et al., "Increased circulating hematopoietic and endothelial progenitor cells in the early phase of acute myocardial infarction," *Blood*, vol. 105, no. 1, pp. 199–206, 2005.

[11] F. H. Bahlmann, K. DeGroot, T. Duckert et al., "Endothelial progenitor cell proliferation and differentiation is regulated by

erythropoietin," *Kidney International*, vol. 64, no. 5, pp. 1648–1652, 2003.

[12] U. Landmesser, N. Engberding, F. H. Bahlmann et al., "Statin-induced improvement of endothelial progenitor cell mobilization, myocardial neovascularization, left ventricular function, and survival after experimental myocardial infarction requires endothelial nitric oxide synthase," *Circulation*, vol. 110, no. 14, pp. 1933–1939, 2004.

[13] F. H. Bahlmann, K. de Groot, O. Mueller, B. Hertel, H. Haller, and D. Fliser, "Stimulation of endothelial progenitor cells: a new putative therapeutic effect of angiotensin II receptor antagonists," *Hypertension*, vol. 45, no. 4, pp. 526–529, 2005.

[14] R. T. van Beem, E. Nur, J. J. Zwaginga et al., "Elevated endothelial progenitor cells during painful sickle cell crisis," *Experimental Hematology*, vol. 37, no. 9, pp. 1054–1059, 2009.

[15] A. J. Duits, T. Rodriguez, and J. J. B. Schnog, "Serum levels of angiogenic factors indicate a pro-angiogenic state in adults with sickle cell disease," *British Journal of Haematology*, vol. 134, no. 1, pp. 116–119, 2006.

[16] X. Niu, M. Nouraie, A. Campbell et al., "Angiogenic and inflammatory markers of cardiopulmonary changes in children and adolescents with sickle cell disease," *PLoS One*, vol. 4, no. 11, Article ID e7956, 2009.

[17] A. Solovey, L. Gui, S. Ramakrishnan, M. H. Steinberg, and R. P. Hebbel, "Sickle cell anemia as a possible state of enhanced anti-apoptotic tone: survival effect of vascular endothelial growth factor on circulating and unanchored endothelial cells," *Blood*, vol. 93, no. 11, pp. 3824–3830, 1999.

[18] P. P. Landburg, E. Nur, N. Maria et al., "Elevated circulating stromal-derived factor-1 levels in sickle cell disease," *Acta Haematologica*, vol. 122, no. 1, pp. 64–69, 2009.

[19] J. Case, L. E. Mead, W. K. Bessler et al., "Human CD34+AC133+VEGFR-2+ cells are not endothelial progenitor cells but distinct, primitive hematopoietic progenitors," *Experimental Hematology*, vol. 35, no. 7, pp. 1109–1118, 2007.

[20] V. Subramaniyam, E. K. Waller, J. R. Murrow et al., "Bone marrow mobilization with granulocyte macrophage colony-stimulating factor improves endothelial dysfunction and exercise capacity in patients with peripheral arterial disease," *American Heart Journal*, vol. 158, no. 1, pp. 53–60, 2009.

[21] D. P. Jones and Y. Liang, "Measuring the poise of thiol/disulfide couples in vivo," *Free Radical Biology and Medicine*, vol. 47, no. 10, pp. 1329–1338, 2009.

[22] D. H. Walter, J. Haendeler, J. Reinhold et al., "Impaired CXCR4 signaling contributes to the reduced neovascularization capacity of endothelial progenitor cells from patients with coronary artery disease," *Circulation Research*, vol. 97, no. 11, pp. 1142–1151, 2005.

[23] S. T. Miller, L. A. Sleeper, C. H. Pegelow et al., "Prediction of adverse outcomes in children with sickle cell disease," *The New England Journal of Medicine*, vol. 342, no. 2, pp. 83–89, 2000.

[24] C. T. Quinn, N. J. Lee, E. P. Shull, N. Ahmad, Z. R. Rogers, and G. R. Buchanan, "Prediction of adverse outcomes in children with sickle cell anemia: a study of the Dallas Newborn Cohort," *Blood*, vol. 111, no. 2, pp. 544–548, 2008.

# 12

# Asthma in Sickle Cell Disease: Implications for Treatment

**Kathryn Blake and John Lima**

*Biomedical Research Department, Center for Clinical Pharmacogenomics and Translational Research, Nemours Children's Clinic, 807 Children's Way, Jacksonville, FL 32207, USA*

Correspondence should be addressed to Kathryn Blake, kblake@nemours.org

Academic Editor: Maurizio Longinotti

*Objective.* To review issues related to asthma in sickle cell disease and management strategies. *Data Source.* A systematic review of pertinent original research publications, reviews, and editorials was undertaken using MEDLINE, the Cochrane Library databases, and CINAHL from 1947 to November 2010. Search terms were [asthma] and [sickle cell disease]. Additional publications considered relevant to the sickle cell disease population of patients were identified; search terms included [sickle cell disease] combined with [acetaminophen], [pain medications], [vitamin D], [beta agonists], [exhaled nitric oxide], and [corticosteroids]. *Results.* The reported prevalence of asthma in children with sickle cell disease varies from 2% to approximately 50%. Having asthma increases the risk for developing acute chest syndrome , death, or painful episodes compared to having sickle cell disease without asthma. Asthma and sickle cell may be linked by impaired nitric oxide regulation, excessive production of leukotrienes, insufficient levels of Vitamin D, and exposure to acetaminophen in early life. Treatment of sickle cell patients includes using commonly prescribed asthma medications; specific considerations are suggested to ensure safety in the sickle cell population. *Conclusion.* Prospective controlled trials of drug treatment for asthma in patients who have both sickle cell disease and asthma are urgently needed.

## 1. Introduction

Asthma and sickle cell disease are interrelated, and the presence of asthma increases morbidity and mortality in sickle cell patients. This paper discusses the relationships between asthma and sickle cell disease and suspected pathophysiological commonalities. A review of guideline appropriate treatment in patients with asthma without sickle cell disease and specific recommendations for sickle cell patients in the treatment of persistent asthma and acute asthma exacerbation is provided. Specific cautions for use of $\beta_2$ agonists, leukotriene modifiers, and systemic corticosteroid therapies in patients with sickle cell disease are provided.

## 2. Search Strategy

The PubMed search engine of the National Library of Medicine was used to identify English-language and non-English language articles published from 1947 to November 2010 pertinent to asthma in sickle cell disease. Keywords and topics included: asthma, sickle cell disease, acute chest syndrome, drug classes and specific drug names used in the treatment of asthma, vitamin D, acetaminophen, exhaled nitric oxide, QTc, and pharmacogenetics. The same strategy was used for the Cochrane Library Database and CINAHL. Reference types included randomized controlled trials, reviews, and editorials. All publications were reviewed by the authors and those most relevant were used to support the topics covered in this paper.

## 3. Epidemiology and the Comorbidities: Asthma and Sickle Cell Disease

Sickle cell disease is a common genetic disorder believed to affect up to 100,000 persons in the United States though the actual prevalence is unknown [1, 2]. It occurs in approximately 1 in 350 African Americans,1 in every 32,000 Hispanic Americans (western states), and 1 in 1,000 Hispanic Americans (eastern states) [1, 3].

Asthma affects 23 million persons in the US (8 in every 100 persons) [4]. The prevalence rate of people ever told that they had asthma was 115/1000 persons in 2007 [4]. African-American children ages 0 to 17 years old are disproportionately affected having a 62% greater prevalence rate for asthma than European Caucasians (12.8% versus 7.9%, resp.), a 250% higher hospitalization rate, and a 500% higher death rate [5].

There is now ample evidence that asthma is a commonly occurring comorbidity in children with sickle cell disease. The diagnosis of asthma often includes evidence of airway bronchodilator response to inhaled $\beta_2$ agonists or bronchoconstriction in response to methacholine, cold air, or exercise in addition to medical history. The published reported prevalence of asthma in children with sickle cell disease has varied from 2% to approximately 50% [6–12]. Even more children appear to have airway dysfunction as the prevalence of airways hyperresponsiveness, measured by bronchodilator response to inhaled $\beta_2$ agonists or bronchoconstrictive response to cold air or exercise, ranges from 40% to 77% of sickle cell disease patients [7–11, 13]. While airways hyperresponsiveness can occur in the absence of asthma, the large disparity between the prevalence of airways hyperresponsiveness and asthma suggests that asthma could be underdiagnosed in the sickle cell disease population. However, a recent study found no relationship between asthma diagnosis and other asthma indices and airway hyperresponsiveness measured by methacholine sensitivity [14].

It is not yet known if asthma in sickle cell disease is a disease resulting from sickle cell disease pathophysiology or caused by similar genetic and environmental factors found in typical asthma. A recent study determined that even after controlling for a personal history of asthma in the child with sickle cell disease, simply having a sibling with asthma increased sickle cell disease morbidity (pain: 1.91 episodes/year, 95% confidence interval (CI) = 1.18–3.09; acute chest syndrome (ACS): 1.48 episodes/year, 95% CI 0.97–2.26) [15]. While these data do not distinguish between a genetic versus environmental effect on asthma, results from a segregation analysis study of the familial pattern of inheritance of asthma found that a major gene effect was present and followed Mendelian expectations [16]. These findings suggest that asthma in sickle cell disease patients is likely a comorbid condition rather than a disease due to sickle cell disease induced airway inflammation/bronchoconstriction.

## 4. Risks of Acute Chest Syndrome and Death in Children with Sickle Cell Disease and Asthma

The presence of asthma in sickle cell disease patients carries significant risks of morbidity and mortality in excess of that found in children with sickle cell disease without asthma [5, 17]. Acute chest syndrome is characterized by a new pulmonary infiltrate with fever and/or signs and symptoms of respiratory distress. A strong relationship is present between having asthma and risk for developing acute chest syndrome [18]. Children with sickle cell disease and asthma

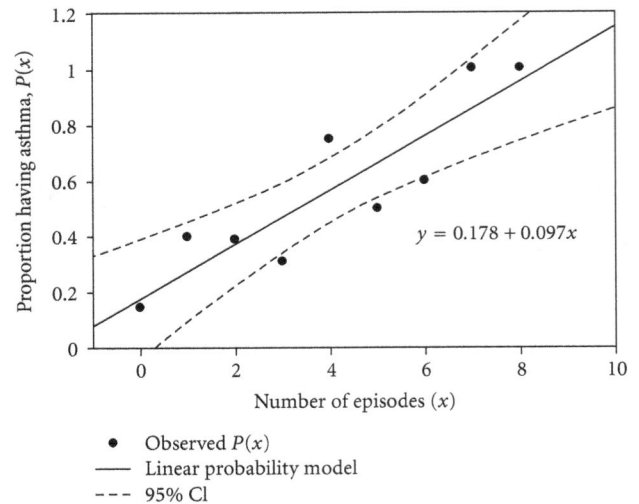

FIGURE 1: Prevalence of physician-diagnosed asthma and ACS episodes. The proportion of SCD patients having physician diagnosed asthma was plotted against the number of episodes of ACS in children with SCD. SCD: sickle cell disease, ACS: acute chest syndrome, reproduced with permission from [18].

have a greater than 5-fold risk of developing acute chest syndrome compared to children with sickle cell disease but without asthma (Figure 1) [8, 17–19]. The median time to an acute chest syndrome event in children with asthma has been observed to be shorter by nearly half compared to children without asthma [20]. The diagnosis of asthma tends to precede the first episode of acute chest syndrome by 0.5 to 7 years suggesting that the presence of asthma may predispose children to developing acute chest syndrome [21]. In one study, asthma increased the risk of acute chest syndrome the greatest in children aged 2 to 4 years, and continues to confer a greater risk of ACS until at least 12 years of age [20].

It is likely that the increased rate of acute chest syndrome in children with asthma contributes to greater mortality in this group. Children who experience acute chest syndrome early in life are at risk of acute chest syndrome episodes throughout childhood [22] and acute chest syndrome contributes to the cause of death in over 60% of patients with sickle cell disease [23, 24]. One study reported that children with sickle cell disease with asthma have a 2.36 (hazard ratio) greater risk of death compared to children with sickle cell disease without asthma [17]. Despite the strong association between asthma and acute chest syndrome, it is not clear if asthma triggers more frequent episodes of acute chest syndrome or if children with frequent episodes of acute chest syndrome are more likely to have asthma [18, 20].

## 5. Acute Chest Syndrome, Asthma, and the Nitric Oxide Pathway

Perturbations of the nitric oxide pathway contribute to the pathophysiology of both asthma and sickle cell disease. Under homeostatic conditions, arginine is a substrate for the arginase I and II, and nitric oxide synthase (NOS; isoforms 1, 2, and 3) enzymes and these enzymes coregulate the function of each other [25]. In asthma, arginine metabolized by arginase forms ornithine and subsequently forms polyamines and proline leading to smooth muscle contraction, collagen formation, and cell proliferation [26]; whereas arginine metabolized by NOS produces nitric oxide (NO) which also produces epithelial damage and airway hyperreactivity [25]. Upregulation of NOS2, and contributions from NOS1 and NOS3, results in greater production of NO which can be measured in expired air. Exhaled NO is increasingly used as clinical biomarker of airway inflammation and response to anti-inflammatory treatment [27–30]. In sickle cell disease, erythrocyte hemolysis increases availability of plasma arginase, which increases production of ornithine, polyamines, and proline from arginine [31, 32]. Less arginine is available as a substrate for NOS and production of NO is decreased in this population [31–33]. However, there are currently no data directly linking disruptions in NO pathway homeostasis in the vasculature to that occurring in the lung. The signaling mechanisms regulating enzyme activity and metabolism of L-arginine are exceedingly complex and the effect of polymorphisms in the arginase and NOS genes on nitric oxide and ornithine production are only beginning to be evaluated.

Despite the known alterations in the arginine pathway in sickle cell disease resulting in reduced NO formation, the association between fraction of expired NO ($FE_{NO}$) levels and frequency of ACS events is not consistent [33–36]. It is possible that polymorphisms in the nitric oxide pathway may modify this relationship as the greater the number of nitric oxide synthase gene 1 (*NOS1*) AAT repeats, the lower the $FE_{NO}$ levels in children with sickle cell disease [33]. Furthermore, in sickle cell patients without asthma but not in those with asthma, the number of AAT repeats associates with the risk of acute chest syndrome ($r^2 = 0.76$) (Figure 2) [18]. If future studies confirm that this *NOS1* polymorphism could be used to identify those children whose acute chest syndrome episodes are unrelated to asthma versus those whose acute chest syndrome episodes are related to asthma, one could speculate that treatment strategies may differ for the management of acute chest syndrome events (see Section 16). Currently however, there are no data describing the relationship between exhaled nitric oxide levels and acute chest syndrome in children with sickle cell disease and asthma.

## 6. Painful Episodes and Respiratory Symptoms

Painful episodes, defined as body pain complaints (excluding head pain) which require administration of opioids, are the most common cause of morbidity in sickle cell disease and are associated with an increased risk of early death [37]. Children with >3 episodes of pain per year have higher reports of breathing difficulty and chest pain [38]. Pain occurs at least 2 times more frequently in children with asthma and sickle cell disease compared to those without asthma [20]. Monthly episodes of mild-to-moderate pain

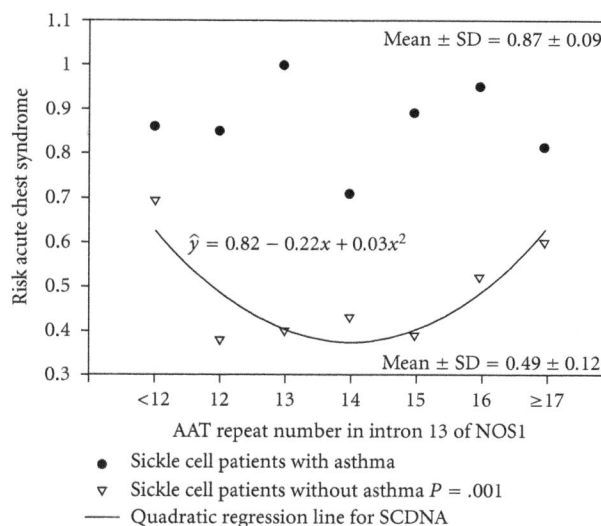

FIGURE 2: Risk of ACS and NOS1 AAT repeats in intron 13. The risk of ACS (1-[controls/(cases+controls)]) is plotted against the number of NOS1 AAT repeats in patients with SCD with physician-diagnosed asthma (closed circles) and without physician- diagnosed asthma (SCDNA). ACS: acute chest syndrome, NOS1: nitric oxide synthase 1 gene, SCDNA: sickle cell disease physician diagnosed asthma, reproduced with permission from [18].

managed at home occur in up to 40% of children with sickle cell disease and pain can occur on 30% of days [39, 40]. In children with asthma, respiratory symptoms are 3 times more likely to precede, or 5 times more like to occur concurrently with, painful episodes than in patients without asthma [41].

## 7. Leukotrienes and Asthma and Pain in Sickle Cell Disease

Inflammatory mediators are increased in both asthma and sickle cell disease. Leukotrienes, interleukins, soluble vascular adhesion molecules, tumor necrosis factor, and C-reactive protein are elevated in, and are believed to contribute to the chronicity of, both asthma and sickle cell disease [42, 43]. Cysteinyl leukotrienes (LT) are potent mediators of inflammation and are synthesized from arachidonic acid located in membrane-phospholipids by cytosolic phospholipase A2 in response to stimulation [44, 45]. Arachidonic acid is converted to 5-hydroperoxyeicosatetraenoic acid and LTA4 by membrane-bound 5-lipoxygenase (ALOX5) and 5-lipoxygenase activating protein (FLAP) [46]. In human mast cells, basophils, eosinophils, and macrophages, LTA4 is converted to LTB4 by LTA4 hydrolase (LTA4H), or is conjugated with reduced glutathione by LTC4 synthase to form LTC4 [45]. LTC4 is transported to the extracellular space mainly by the multidrug resistance protein 1 (MRP1) [47]. LTC4 is converted to LTD4 and LTE4 by γ-glutamyltransferase and dipeptidase; LTE4 is excreted in the urine and is a measure of whole body leukotriene production [48–50]. Leukotrienes can also be produced by transcellular biosynthesis [51].

Experimentally induced asthma in a transgenic murine model of sickle cell disease caused greater mortality due to increased allergic lung inflammation (elevations in eosinophils, eosinophil peroxidase, and IgE levels) compared with control sickle cell disease mice without induced asthma [52]. Eosinophils are a major source of leukotrienes in asthma and elevations of LTB4 and LTC4 in blood and LTE4 in urine occur of patients with sickle cell disease [53–57].

A recent study found that urinary LTE4 levels were elevated at baseline in children with sickle cell disease and that higher levels were associated with a greater than 2-fold increased rate of hospitalization for pain episodes compared with lower levels in children without sickle cell disease [57]. Other data show that urinary LTE4 levels are directly associated with increased rate of pain and acute chest syndrome episodes in sickle cell disease patients [55, 56].

## 8. Leukotriene Pathway Genes in Asthma and Sickle Cell Disease

Typical symptoms of asthma caused by cysteinyl leukotrienes (LTC4, LTD4, and LTE4) are mediated by the cysteinyl leukotriene-1 and cysteinyl leukotriene-2 receptors [44, 58, 59]. The ALOX5 gene located on 10q11.21 encodes ALOX5, a key enzyme in the synthesis of cysteinyl leukotrienes [45]. Early studies identified addition and deletion variants (wildtype $n = 5$; variant $n \neq 5$) in the core promoter of the ALOX5 gene that were associated with diminished promoter-reporter activity in tissue culture [60] which has been confirmed in both healthy African Americans and patients with asthma [61, 62]. Recently, expression of 5-lipoxygenase and 5-lipoxygenase activating protein were shown to be elevated in peripheral blood mononuclear cells from patients with sickle cell disease [63]. Increased expression was mediated by placenta growth factor, an angiogenic growth factor, and increased levels correlated with sickle cell disease severity [63, 64]. Thus, the leukotriene pathway, and in particular the ALOX5 gene, are implicated in both asthma and sickle cell disease severity and morbidity.

## 9. Potential Relevance of Vitamin D and Childhood Use of Acetaminophen on Asthma in Sickle Cell Disease

Several epidemiological and association studies support a link between hypovitaminosis D (either insufficiency or deficiency) and asthma. The prevalence of hypovitaminosis D among African American youths has been found to be greater in individuals with asthma (86%) compared to controls without asthma (19%) [65]. Epidemiological studies also report an inverse association between maternal intake of vitamin D and the risk of childhood wheezing and asthma in offspring [66, 67].

Among individuals with asthma, hypovitaminosis D has been associated with asthma, asthma severity and reduced steroid response. Brehm et al reported vitamin D insufficiency in 28% of children with asthma living in Costa Rica [68], which is near the equator. Additionally, vitamin D levels were inversely associated with airway responsiveness (methacholine challenge), total IgE and eosinophils count. Increasing vitamin D levels were also associated with reduced odds of hospitalization and with reduced odds of inhaled corticosteroid use. In a recent study of adults with asthma, higher vitamin D levels were associated with greater lung function, while hypovitaminosis D was associated with increased airway hyperresponsiveness and reduced glucocorticoid response [69]. These studies, though small in number, suggest an important link between hypovitaminosis D and asthma.

Vitamin D deficiency in sickle cell disease patients has become well recognized in the past decade. Between 33% and 76% of children and adults are classified as Vitamin D deficient (<10 to12 ng/mL) and 65% to 98% are Vitamin D insufficient (<20 to 30 ng/mL) [70–75]. There are no reports of Vitamin D levels in patients with both sickle cell disease and asthma. It is possible that the low Vitamin D levels observed in patients with sickle cell disease and patients with asthma contributes to the significantly increased morbidity and mortality that is observed in patients with both sickle cell disease and asthma compared to those without asthma.

Painful vaso-occlusive crises may occur as early as 6 to 12 months of age and monthly episodes of mild-to-moderate pain managed at home occur in up to 40% of children with sickle cell disease and pain can occur on 30% of days [39, 40, 76]. Acetaminophen is the most commonly used analgesic for the management of mild-to-moderate pain [76] and is a component of up to 47% of pain medications in children with sickle cell disease [77]. Thus, patients with sickle cell disease have significant exposure to acetaminophen during their lifetime.

Over the past decade, several publications have reported an association with acetaminophen use prenatally and during childhood and an increased risk of developing asthma [78]. In a worldwide assessment of asthma, acetaminophen use was associated with an increased risk of asthma in young children and adolescents (odds ratio 1.43–3.23) [79, 80]. Several putative mechanisms have been suggested. The formation of $N$-acetyle-$\rho$I-benzoquinoneimine, a highly reactive metabolite of acetaminophen, may result in decreased glutathione. Glutathione serves as an antioxidant and oxygen radicals are known to produce tissue injury, bronchoconstriction and hyperreactivity, and stimulation of inflammatory mediators [78, 81]. Glutathione levels in alveolar fluid in patients with asthma are associated with levels of bronchial hyperresponsiveness [78]. Reduced glutathione may also shift cytokine production from Th1 to Th2 responses. A functional genetic polymorphism in the glutathione $S$-transferase P1 gene (GSTP1) is most common in Hispanics and African Americans and has been associated with susceptibility to asthma development and most recently in the relationship between acetaminophen use and the subsequent development of asthma [78, 82]. Research is needed to determine if there is an association between acetaminophen use in early life for the management of pain in children with sickle cell disease and the increased prevalence of asthma or airway hyperreactivity.

## 10. Management of Chronic Asthma in Patients with Sickle Cell Disease

Medications for the treatment of asthma are classified as long-term control or quick-relief medications [83]. Quick-relief medications include bronchochodilators such as short-acting $\beta_2$ agonists, short-acting anticholinergics, and systemic corticosteroids; long-term control medications include inhaled corticosteroids with or without long-acting $\beta_2$ agonists, leukotriene modifiers, omalizumab, and less commonly these days, theophylline and cromolyn. The National Heart, Lung, and Blood Institute revised the Guidelines for the Diagnosis and Management of Asthma in 2007 for different age groups (Figures 3 and 4) [83].

For quick relief of symptoms in patients of all ages and asthma severity, short-acting $\beta_2$ agonists are the preferred therapy because of the rapid onset of effect and overall effectiveness in relieving symptoms. They are also the primary treatment for patients who have intermittent asthma (Step 1) which is defined as mild impairment (symptoms less than twice per week, no interference with normal activity, no nocturnal awakenings, normal forced expiratory volume in the first second ($FEV_1$), and one or fewer exacerbations requiring oral steroids per year). For patients with mild-to-severe persistent asthma, long-term control medications are recommended and inhaled corticosteroids are the preferred first-line drugs with leukotriene modifiers, cromolyn, or theophylline as alternative drugs in children over 5-year-old and adults. In patients insufficiently controlled with low or medium doses of inhaled corticosteroids, a long-acting $\beta_2$-agonist, leukotriene modifier, or theophylline may be added though controversy surrounds the use of adding a long-acting $\beta_2$-agonist (see Section 14). Patients with severe persistent asthma with allergic disease may require additional add-on treatment with omalizumab or oral corticosteroid.

Initial severity classification and treatment recommendations and changes are guided by assessments of a patient's level of current impairment (symptoms, nighttime awakenings, short-acting $\beta_2$-agonist use, pulmonary function, and asthma control questionnaire assessments) and future risk (exacerbations requiring oral corticosteroid treatment loss of lung function over time, adverse effects of treatment).

There are currently no published data from prospective controlled trials of drug treatment for asthma symptoms in patients who have both sickle cell disease and asthma [32, 84]. At Nemours Children's Clinic in Florida and Delaware only 27%, 35%, and 49% of patients with sickle cell disease and physician diagnosed asthma are treated with a corticosteroid+long acting $\beta_2$-agonist inhaler, leukotriene modifier, or corticosteroid inhaler, respectively, suggesting undertreatment of asthma (personal data). One abstract of a retrospective analysis observed a reduced rate of pain crises and acute chest syndrome in children with sickle cell disease

and asthma treated with inhaled corticosteroids ± a long-acting $\beta_2$-agonist [85].

## 11. Inhaled Short-Acting $\beta_2$-Agonists

There are two potential concerns with the use of inhaled short-acting $\beta_2$ agonists in patients with sickle cell disease: genotype at the $\beta_2$-adrenergic receptor gene (ADRB2) and inherent cardiovascular effects of $\beta_2$-adrenergic stimulation.

Historically, use of inhaled $\beta_2$ agonists for the management of asthma has been fraught with controversy relating to epidemics of increased asthma mortality associated with their initial introduction in the late1950s [86–89] and more recently with analysis of drug prescription records associating use with an increased risk of death or near death from asthma [90]. However, a controlled trial of regularly scheduled albuterol use in patients with asthma with mild disease to examine potential adverse effects demonstrated no deterioration in asthma control with albuterol use [91]. However, in current practice, regular scheduled use of short acting inhaled $\beta_2$ agonists is discouraged and as-needed use is promoted as a way to minimize exposure and to monitor changes in asthma control. Whether these adverse effects on asthma control are due to genetic polymorphisms in ADRB2 or inherent pharmacological effects of $\beta_2$ agonists has been the recent focus of this controversy.

The ADRB2 is a small, intronless gene and two common nonsynonomous variants at amino acid positions 16 (Gly16Arg) and 27 (Gln27Glu) have functional relevance in vitro [92, 93], and clinical studies have focused on outcomes resulting from the Gly16Arg polymorphism. Several retrospective studies, though results have been inconsistent, have found that patients who are homozygous Arg16 have worse asthma control during regularly scheduled albuterol use compared to homozygous Gly16 patients [94–97]. However a carefully controlled prospective study found a better relative response by patients homozygous for Gly16 treated with regularly scheduled albuterol compared with patients who were homozygous Arg16; the authors suggest that a different class of bronchodilator (e.g., anticholinergics) may be appropriate for patients harboring the homozygous Arg16 genotype [98]. These findings are relevant to African Americans with sickle cell disease because African Americans are more likely to be homozygous Arg16 (23–30% of the population) compared to Whites (14–16%) [99, 100]. In addition, African Americans have a poorer bronchodilator response to acute use of albuterol compared to Whites [101, 102] which may place them at risk of overuse of their albuterol inhaler for relief of symptoms.

Though rare, $\beta_2$ agonists can have adverse cardiovascular effects including increased atrial or ventricular ectopy and prolongation of the QTc interval [103, 104]. In patients with prolonged QTc, the use of $\beta_2$ agonists doubles the risk of cardiac events (hazard ratio 2.0, 95% CI 1.26, to 3.15) with a greater risk in the first year of use [103]. Because of the increased frequency of prolonged QTc in patients with sickle cell disease, $\beta_2$-agonist use may pose a specific risk in this population [32, 105, 106].

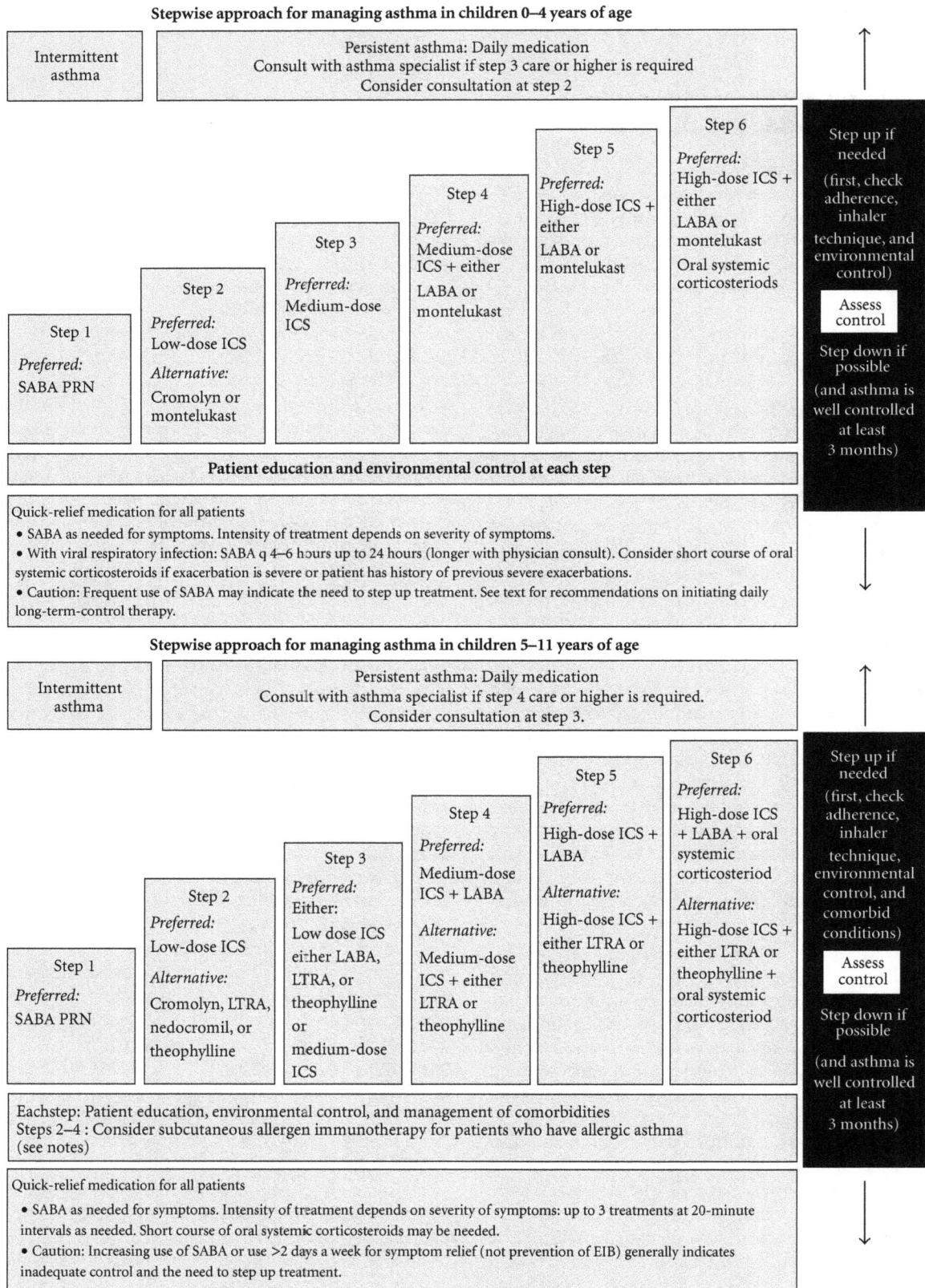

FIGURE 3: Guideline recommended stepwise approach to managing asthma in young children. ICS: inhaled corticosteroid, EIB: exercise induced bronchospasm, LABA: long-acting $\beta_2$-agonist, LTRA: leukotriene receptor antagonist, and SABA: short-acting $\beta_2$-agonist, reproduced from [83].

**Stepwise approach for managing asthma in youths 12 years of age and adult**

| Intermittent asthma | Persistent asthma: Daily medication<br>Consult with asthma specialist if step 4 care or higher is required<br>Consider consultation at step 3 |
|---|---|

**Step 1**
*Preferred:*
SABA PRN

**Step 2**
*Preferred:*
Low-dose ICS
*Alternative:*
Cromolyn, LTRA, nedocromil, or theophylline

**Step 3**
*Preferred:*
Low-dose ICS + LABA or medium-dose
*Alternative:*
low-dose ICS + either LTRA, theophylline, or zileuton

**Step 4**
*Preferred:*
Medium-dose ICS + LABA
*Alternative:*
Medium-dose ICS + either LTRA or theophylline, or zileuton

**Step 5**
*Preferred:*
High-dose ICS + LABA

AND

Consider omalizumab for patients who have allergies

**Step 6**
*Preferred:*
High-dose ICS + LABA + oral corticosteriod

AND

Consider omalizumab for patients who have allergies

Step up if needed
(first, check adherence, environmental control, and comorbid conditions)

**Assess control**

Step down if possible
(and asthma is well controlled at least 3 months)

Each step: patient education, environmental control, and management of comorbidities
Steps 2–4 :Consider subcutaneous allergen immunotherapy for patients who have allergic asthma (see notes)

Quick-relief medication for all patients
- SABA as needed for symptoms. Intensity of treatment depends on severity of symptoms: up to 3 treatments at 20-minute intervals as needed. Short course of oral systemic corticosteroids may be needed
- Use of SABA >2 days a week for symptom relief (not prevention of EIB) generally indicates inadequate control and the need to step up treatment

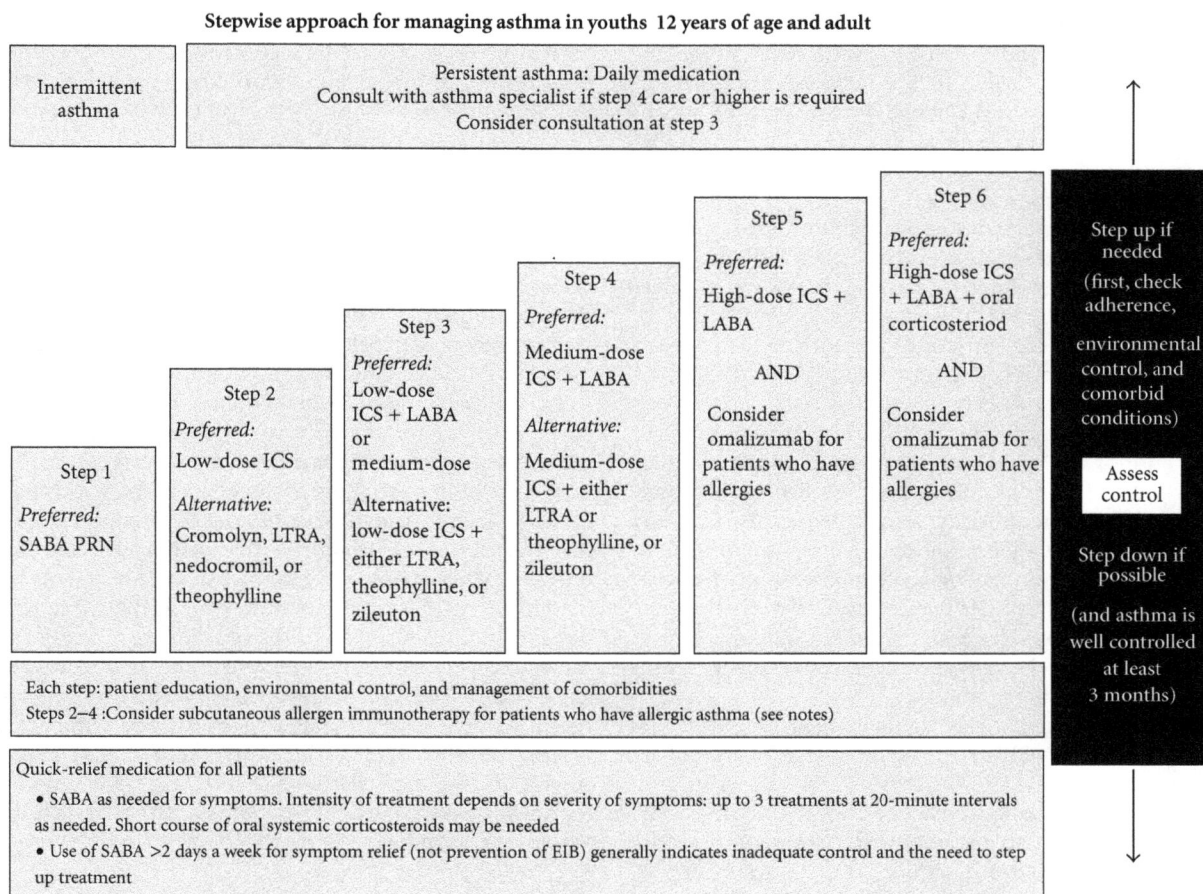

FIGURE 4: Guideline recommended stepwise approach to managing asthma in adolescents and adults. ICS: inhaled corticosteroid, EIB: exercise induced bronchospasm, LABA: long-acting $\beta_2$-agonist, LTRA: leukotriene receptor antagonist, and SABA: short-acting $\beta_2$-agonist, reproduced from [83].

Despite these issues, inhaled short-acting $\beta_2$ agonists should remain as first-line therapy for prevention and treatment of acute bronchospasm. Inhaled short-acting anticholinergic drugs (see Section 16) are an alternative and can be used if there are concerns for a specific patient and the use of short-acting $\beta_2$ agonists.

## 12. Inhaled Corticosteroids

Inhaled corticosteroids are the preferred treatment for long-term control of persistent asthma symptoms [83]. There are no concerns unique to patients with sickle cell disease and asthma which would preclude use in this population. Issues related to systemic corticosteroid use are discussed in Section 16.

## 13. Leukotriene Modifiers

Leukotrienes are a known component of airway inflammation in asthma and in sickle cell disease though the added contribution of asthma on leukotriene level production in patients with sickle cell disease has not been specifically

studied. However, it is reasonable to suspect that blockade of leukotriene receptor activity by a leukotriene modifier could be effective in patients who have both sickle cell disease and asthma.

Leukotriene modifiers include a 5-lipoxygenase inhibitor (zileuton) and three leukotriene receptor antagonists (montelukast, zafirlukast, and pranlukast, the latter is available only in Japan). Leukotriene receptor antagonists exert their beneficial effects in asthma by binding to the cys-leukotriene 1 receptor and antagonizing the detrimental effects of the cysteinyl leukotrienes in airways. Despite leukotriene synthesis blockade through inhibition of 5-lipoxygenase, there is no evidence for clinical differences between 5-lipoxygenase inhibitors and leukotriene receptor antagonists in asthma [107]. Several *in vitro* trials have documented zileuton, a hydroxyurea derivative, may have potential beneficial effects in sickle cell disease pathology including effects on nitric oxide, sickle red blood cell retention and adhesion in the pulmonary circulation, and decreased interleukin-13 secretion [108–112].

Montelukast, however, would be the preferred leukotriene modifier in patients with sickle cell disease and asthma because it has well-established effects on the improvements of asthma symptoms and it can be given once daily [107, 113, 114]. The safety profile of montelukast is similar to placebo and its safety record extends over 10 years of use in millions of patients. The other available LTD4 inhibitor at the CysLT1 receptor, zafirlukast, must be given twice daily and may require liver function testing.

Zileuton, a leukotriene synthesis inhibitor, must be given twice daily and treatment has been associated with increased hepatic enzymes most often appearing in the first three months of treatment with the extended release product. These abnormalities can progress, remain unchanged, or may resolve with continued treatment. Use of the immediate release product has been associated with severe liver injury including symptomatic jaundice, hyperbilirubinemia, aspartate aminotransferase elevations greater than 8 times the upper limit of normal, life-threatening liver injury, and death. Liver function monitoring should be performed prior to the start of therapy, then monthly for three months, then every two-to-three months for the remainder of the first year, and then periodically. If liver dysfunction develops or transaminase elevations are more than 5 times the upper limits of normal, then the drug should be discontinued (from Zileuton prescribing information).

Response to montelukast is highly variable and limits its usefulness in asthma [115–117]; heterogeneity in response is due in large part to genetic variability [115, 118–120]. The pharmacogenetics of leukotriene pathway and transporter genes may be relevant to patients with asthma and sickle cell disease. In a six-month clinical trial of montelukast therapy in patients with asthma, in which 80% of European Caucasians and 47% of African Americans, carried five tandem repeats of the ALOX5 promoter sp1 tandem repeat polymorphism, European Caucasian participants carrying a variant number (either 2, 3, 4, 6, or 7) repeats of the ALOX5 promoter on one allele had a 73% reduction in the risk of having one or more asthma exacerbations compared with homozygotes for the five repeat alleles [115]. In contrast, there were no differences in exacerbation risk by genotype in placebo treated patients. African Americans were not studied for the association analysis due to too few numbers of African American participants. However, African Americans were nearly 3 times more likely than Whites to carry a variant number of repeats (53% versus 20%) suggesting that African Americans with asthma and sickle cell disease may have significant improvements in asthma control with montelukast therapy [115].

Montelukast is an orally administered drug in which response is directly related to blood concentration and wide ranges of response to the same doses has been observed [115, 117, 121]. Montelukast is a substrate for OATP2B1, a member of the SLCO family of organic anion membrane transport proteins encoded by SLCO2B1 [119]. A nonsynonomous polymorphism, rs1242149 (c935G > A), in SLCO2B1 has been found to associate with significantly reduced plasma concentrations of montelukast and Asthma Symptom Utility Index (ASUI) in patients with asthma treated with montelukast for 6 months [119, 122]. The ASUI is a validated tool that assesses patient preferences for combinations of asthma-

related symptoms and drug effects and correlates with patient perception of asthma control [123]. If these findings are confirmed, future studies would be needed to examine dose-response relationships by genotype to determine if specific genotype-driven doses are required for effectiveness.

Montelukast use has been associated with behavior changes which recently prompted labeling changes to include information that agitation, aggressive behavior or hostility, anxiousness, depression, dream abnormalities, hallucinations, insomnia, irritability, restlessness, somnambulism, suicidal thinking and behavior (including suicide), and tremor may occur with montelukast use. Analyses from two recent publications (authored by employees of Merck and Co, Inc.) involving over 20,000 patients treated with montelukast found no evidence of "possibly suicidality related adverse events" nor "behavior-related adverse events" [124, 125]. In addition, analysis of three recent large asthma trials in 569 patients treated with montelukast conducted by the American Lung Association Asthma Clinical Research Centers network have uncovered no behavioral problems [126].

However, these adverse events could be of concern in patients with sickle cell disease who are already at risk for suicide ideation and attempted suicide and depression [127, 128]. The Duke University Psychiatry Department recently published data that 29% of patients with sickle cell disease reported suicide ideation and 8% had attempted suicide during their lifetime [127]. Therefore, monitoring for these adverse effects in patients with sickle cell disease would be reasonable.

## 14. Inhaled Long-Acting $\beta_2$-Agonists

Long-acting $\beta_2$ agonists (salmeterol and formoterol) may be associated with particular risks in African Americans. Several clinical studies and meta-analyses have documented an increased risk of asthma exacerbations or death due to asthma in patients using long-acting $\beta_2$ agonists with and without inhaled corticosteroid therapy [129–132]. These risks were identified in clinical trials prior to the marketing of salmeterol, the first long-acting $\beta_2$-agonist available in this country [129]. A large postmarketing study, demonstrated a 2-fold increase in respiratory-related deaths and over 4-fold increase in asthma-related deaths in patients treated with salmeterol versus placebo over 6 months and these increases were driven largely by the increases in African American subpopulation (4- and 7-fold increases, resp.) [130]. Similar effects on exacerbation rates have been found for formoterol [133]. Long-acting $\beta_2$ agonists are not to be used as monotherapy and are to only be used with an anti-inflammatory drug (preferably inhaled corticosteroids). These risks appear to be even greater in children and adolescents compared to adults based upon results presented at an FDA Advisory Committee meeting in 2008 [134]. Guidelines for the Diagnosis and Management of Asthma state that long-acting $\beta_2$ agonists are to be used only in patients who are not controlled on low- to medium-doses of inhaled corticosteroids or whose disease is considered severe enough to warrant initial treatment with two maintenance therapies [83, 83].

Results from retrospective pharmacogenetic association studies of long-acting $\beta_2$ agonists (salmeterol and formoterol) on asthma control in patients with and without concomitant inhaled corticosteroid treatment have largely failed to find any association between the Gly16Arg genotype and asthma control even in studies specifically evaluating effects in African Americans [100, 135–138]. Two prospective genotype driven, randomized, double-blind trials examining the effects of salmeterol plus inhaled corticosteroid therapy have failed to find any significant effects on adverse asthma outcomes by the Gly16Arg genotype [139, 140].

However, given the adverse consequences found for African Americans in the large post marketing study with salmeterol and FDA analysis [130, 134] it would be prudent to carefully evaluate the risk to benefit of adding either salmeterol or formoterol to treatment in patients with sickle cell disease and asthma.

## 15. Other Treatments for Long-Term Control in Persistent Asthma

Theophylline, cromolyn, and omalizumab are additional treatment options for the patient with asthma and sickle cell disease. Theophylline is not a particularly attractive choice because of its cardiostimulatory effects and adverse gastrointestinal effects (nausea, dyspepsia) [141]. Inhaled cromolyn is exceedingly safe but is rarely used because it requires four times daily dosing and use has been supplanted by montelukast in the pediatric asthma population. Omalizumab is an add-on option for a select set of patients 12 years and older with moderate to severe persistent asthma who have a positive skin test or *in vitro* reactivity to a perennial aeroallergen and symptoms that are inadequately controlled with inhaled corticosteroids plus a long-acting $\beta_2$-agonist [83]. Omalizumab is an anti-IgE monoclonal antibody which binds to the C$\varepsilon$3 domain of free IgE in the serum and not to IgE already bound to mast cells. The omalizumab-IgE complex prevents IgE from binding to the Fc$\varepsilon$-R1 on mast cells and basophils; cross-linking IgE bound to mast cells and basophils causes mast cell and basophil degranulation with release of histamine, tryptase, bradykinin, prostaglandin E2, prostaglandin F2, and leukotrienes. Omalizumab must be given by subcutaneous injection (1 to 3 injections) every 2 or 4 weeks and patients must be observed for a period of time after dosing for the development of an anaphylactic reaction. Thus, omalizumab treatment requires considerable motivation on behalf of the patient in order to be effective.

## 16. Management of Acute Asthma in Patients with Sickle Cell Disease

Risks of pharmacologic treatment during acute exacerbations of asthma in patients with sickle cell disease may require specific considerations to ensure effectiveness with minimization of adverse effects. Emergency department and hospital-based pharmacologic care of asthma in the absence of sickle cell disease includes the use of frequent inhaled short-acting $\beta_2$-agonist treatment with oral (or intravenous, if hospitalized) corticosteroids [83]. Inhaled ipratropium (an anticholinergic drug) can be added to short-acting $\beta_2$-agonist treatment in severe exacerbations. Corticosteroid treatment should be continued until lung function is at least 70% of predicted normal function or the patient's personal best value, and symptoms have resolved [83]. Corticosteroid treatment may require up to 10 days of therapy or longer but dose tapering is not needed for treatments less than 14 days [83].

The potential risks associated with high doses of inhaled short-acting $\beta_2$ agonists in the acute management of patients with asthma and sickle cell disease are no different than those previously described for as-needed use in persistent asthma. However, because African Americans may be less responsive to acute use of short-acting $\beta_2$ agonists, higher doses may be required compared to White patients [101, 102]. The risks of therapy associated with prolongation of the QTc should be considered when administering multiple inhaled treatments or continuous nebulization of short-acting $\beta_2$ agonists [32]. There are no reasons to expect anticholinergic efficacy or toxicity would be any different for patients with asthma and sickle cell disease compared to those without sickle cell disease.

Systemic corticosteroid use in the management of acute chest syndrome in sickle cell patients has been associated with rebound pain and increased early (within 2 weeks) readmission rates in many but not all studies [142–146]. Readmission rates after treatment with corticosteroids for acute chest syndrome in patients with asthma is no different than rates for all patients (including those without asthma). While the time to readmission is longer after corticosteroid with a taper versus without a taper, patients with a taper are more likely to be readmitted than those without [145]. It is not clear however if the increased risk of readmission in patients with a corticosteroid taper is actually due to underdosing of corticosteroid during the taper period resulting in inadequate resolution of symptoms prior to discontinuation of corticosteroid treatment. This same study showed that in patients with asthma, readmission rates are greater in those who are treated with corticosteroids alone compared with corticosteroids plus transfusions or no therapy [145]. In a large study examining over 5,000 admissions for acute chest syndrome in over 3,000 individuals, 48% of patients with asthma received corticosteroid treatment [143]. The relative risk of readmission of patients with asthma (compared to those without asthma) was 3.2 which was slightly reduced (relative risk 2.9) in those who also received bronchodilators [143]. It is not clear if the increase in relative risk is due to the undertreatment with corticosteroid therapy (only 48% of patients with asthma receiving corticosteroid treatment) or a reflection of more severe acute chest syndrome events in patients with asthma. A smaller study of 53 children found no adverse effect of a short course of prednisone on readmission rate after acute chest syndrome, though a Type II error may have precluded observing an effect [142]. Another study found a shorter length of stay in patients with asthma treated for acute chest syndrome compared to those without asthma (6.4 days versus 8.6 days, resp.) which may have been due to the use of bronchodilators and corticosteroids for acute chest syndrome (not currently standard treatment for acute chest syndrome) and favored a response in those with asthma; readmission rate was not evaluated [12]. Thus, available evidence suggests that even in patients with asthma, systemic corticosteroid treatment is not without risk. Whether management of asthma exacerbations occurring in the absence of acute chest syndrome would identify a satisfactory risk to benefit ratio is unknown but deserves study in a controlled trial. Also unclear is whether a sufficiently long corticosteroid taper would lessen the risk of readmission in patients with asthma. However, unraveling these issues is complicated due to the overlap between the diagnosis of acute chest syndrome events and asthma exacerbations in patients with asthma. With the presently available data, patients with asthma should receive standard guideline appropriate care [83] which would include aggressive use of bronchodilators with systemic corticosteroid treatment with consideration for a sufficiently long taper after discharge until symptoms are completely resolved as recommended in the current asthma guidelines [83]. In addition, all patients with asthma should be discharged with prescribed inhaled corticosteroid treatment for the long-term management of asthma.

## 17. Conclusions

Patients with sickle cell disease and asthma have unique characteristics that suggest they are a subpopulation of patients with asthma that require special considerations for management of persistent and acute asthma symptoms. Until further evidence is available from controlled clinical trials, the management of asthma in the patient with sickle cell disease should be consistent with the published Guidelines for the Diagnosis and Management of Asthma. The pharmacogenomics of asthma therapy is of interest but there is little firm evidence that research findings can be translated to the clinic setting at present. Given the overall preference for, and better adherence with, oral versus inhaled medications, even in low-income African Americans with asthma [147–149], and the evidence indicating a predominate contribution of leukotrienes in both diseases, montelukast may be an attractive choice for the treatment of persistent asthma. Systemic corticosteroid use in acute asthma exacerbations presents a conundrum that is not resolved. In the typical patient with asthma without sickle cell disease, systemic corticosteroids are standard of care but in those with sickle cell disease may worsen sickle cell disease outcomes after discontinuation of treatment. At present, guideline appropriate care may be warranted. Clearly, this population of patients with asthma requires large controlled trials to clearly define the most appropriate care.

## Conflicts of Interests

The authors have no conflicts of interests to report.

## References

[1] K. L. Hassell, "Population estimates of sickle cell disease in the U.S.," *American Journal of Preventive Medicine*, vol. 38, no. 4, pp. S512–S521, 2010.

[2] A. Ashley-Koch, Q. Yang and R. S. Olney, "Sickle hemoglobin (Hb S) allele and sickle cell disease: a HuGE review," *American Journal of Epidemiology*, vol. 151, no. 9, pp. 839–845, 2000.

[3] R. S. Olney, "Newborn screening for sickle cell disease: public health impact and evaluation," in *Part IV. Developing, Implementing, and Evaluating Population Interventions*, chapter 22, Oxford University Press, Oxford, UK, 2000, http://www.cdc.gov/genomics/resources/books/21stcent/chap22.htm.

[4] "Trends in Asthma morbidity and mortality-January 2009," American Lung Association Epidemiology & Statistics Unit Research Epidemiology & Statistics Unit, January 2009.

[5] L. Akinbami, "The state of childhood asthma, United States, 1980–2005," *Advance data*, no. 381, pp. 1–24, 2006.

[6] E. P. Vichinsky, L. D. Neumay, A. N. Earles et al., "Causes and outcomes of the acute chest syndrome in sickle cell disease," *New England Journal of Medicine*, vol. 342, no. 25, pp. 1855–1865, 2000.

[7] M. A. Leong, C. Dampier, L. Varlotta, and J. L. Allen, "Airway hyperreactivity in children with sickle cell disease," *Journal of Pediatrics*, vol. 131, no. 2, pp. 278–285, 1997.

[8] J. M. Knight-Madden, T. S. Forrester, N. A. Lewis, and A. Greenough, "Asthma in children with sickle cell disease and its association with acute chest syndrome," *Thorax*, vol. 60, no. 3, pp. 206–210, 2005.

[9] A. C. Koumbourlis, H. J. Zar, A. Hurlet-Jensen, and M. R. Goldberg, "Prevalence and reversibility of lower airway obstruction in children with sickle cell disease," *Journal of Pediatrics*, vol. 138, no. 2, pp. 188–192, 2001.

[10] K. P. Sylvester, R. A. Patey, G. F. Rafferty, D. Rees, S. L. Thein, and A. Greenough, "Airway hyperresponsiveness and acute chest syndrome in children with sickle cell anemia," *Pediatric Pulmonology*, vol. 42, no. 3, pp. 272–276, 2007.

[11] O. Y. Ozbek, B. Malbora, N. Sen, A. C. Yazici, E. Ozyurek, and N. Ozbek, "Airway hyperreactivity detected by methacholine challenge in children with sickle cell disease," *Pediatric Pulmonology*, vol. 42, no. 12, pp. 1187–1192, 2007.

[12] R. Bryant, "Asthma in the pediatric sickle cell patient with acute chest syndrome," *Journal of Pediatric Health Care*, vol. 19, no. 3, pp. 157–162, 2005.

[13] R. C. Strunk, M. S. Brown, J. H. Boyd, P. Bates, J. J. Field, and M. R. DeBaun, "Methacholine challenge in children with sickle cell disease: a case series," *Pediatric Pulmonology*, vol. 43, no. 9, pp. 924–929, 2008.

[14] J. J. Field, J. Stocks, F. J. Kirkham et al., "Airway hyperresponsiveness in children with sickle cell anemia," *Chest*. In press.

[15] J. J. Field, E. A. Macklin, Y. Yan, R. C. Strunk, and M. R. DeBaun, "Sibling history of asthma is a risk factor for pain in children with sickle cell anemia," *American Journal of Hematology*, vol. 83, no. 11, pp. 855–857, 2008.

[16] K. L. Phillips, P. An, J. H. Boyd et al., "Major gene effect and additive familial pattern of inheritance of asthma exist among families of probands with sickle cell anemia and asthma," *American Journal of Human Biology*, vol. 20, no. 2, pp. 149–153, 2008.

[17] J. H. Boyd, E. A. Macklin, R. C. Strunk, and M. R. DeBaun, "Asthma is associated with increased mortality in individuals with sickle cell anemia," *Haematologica*, vol. 92, no. 8, pp. 1115–1118, 2007.

[18] L. Duckworth, L. Hsu, H. Feng et al., "Physician-diagnosed asthma and acute chest syndrome: associations with NOS polymorphisms," *Pediatric Pulmonology*, vol. 42, no. 4, pp. 332–338, 2007.

[19] F. Bernaudin, R. C. Strunk, A. Kamdem et al., "Asthma is associated with acute chest syndrome, but not with an increased rate of hospitalization for pain among children in France with sickle cell anemia: a retrospective cohort study," *Haematologica*, vol. 93, no. 12, pp. 1917–1918, 2008.

[20] J. H. Boyd, E. A. Macklin, R. C. Strunk, and M. R. DeBaun, "Asthma is associated with acute chest syndrome and pain in children with sickle cell anemia," *Blood*, vol. 108, no. 9, pp. 2923–2927, 2006.

[21] K. P. Sylvester, R. A. Patey, S. Broughton et al., "Temporal relationship of asthma to acute chest syndrome in sickle cell disease," *Pediatric Pulmonology*, vol. 42, no. 2, pp. 103–106, 2007.

[22] C. T. Quinn, E. P. Shull, N. Ahmad, N. J. Lee, Z. R. Rogers, and G. R. Buchanan, "Prognostic significance of early vaso-occlusive complications in children with sickle cell anemia," *Blood*, vol. 109, no. 1, pp. 40–45, 2007.

[23] D. S. Darbari, P. Kple-Faget, J. Kwagyan, S. Rana, V. R. Gordeuk, and O. Castro, "Circumstances of death in adult sickle cell disease patients," *American Journal of Hematology*, vol. 81, no. 11, pp. 858–863, 2006.

[24] C. D. Fitzhugh, N. Lauder, J. C. Jonassaint et al., "Cardiopulmonary complications leading to premature deaths in adult patients with sickle cell disease," *American Journal of Hematology*, vol. 85, no. 1, pp. 36–40, 2010.

[25] N. Zimmermann and M. E. Rothenberg, "The arginine-arginase balance in asthma and lung inflammation," *European Journal of Pharmacology*, vol. 533, no. 1–3, pp. 253–262, 2006.

[26] D. Vercelli, "Arginase: marker, effector, or candidate gene for asthma?" *Journal of Clinical Investigation*, vol. 111, no. 12, pp. 1815–1817, 2003.

[27] "ATS/ERS recommendations for standardized procedures for the online and offline measurement of exhaled lower respiratory nitric oxide and nasal nitric oxide, 2005," *American Journal of Respiratory and Critical Care Medicine*, vol. 171, no. 8, pp. 912–930, 2005.

[28] A. D. Smith, J. O. Cowan, K. P. Brassett, G. P. Herbison, and D. R. Taylor, "Use of exhaled nitric oxide measurements to guide treatment in chronic asthma," *New England Journal of Medicine*, vol. 352, no. 21, pp. 2163–2173, 2005.

[29] S. A. Kharitonov, D. Yates, R. A. Robbins, R. Logan-Sinclair, E. A. Shinebourne, and P. J. Barnes, "Increased nitric oxide in exhaled air of asthmatic patients," *Lancet*, vol. 343, no. 8890, pp. 133–135, 1994.

[30] S. A. Kharitonov, D. H. Yates, and P. J. Barnes, "Inhaled glucocorticoids decrease nitric oxide in exhaled air of asthmatic patients," *American Journal of Respiratory and Critical Care Medicine*, vol. 153, no. 1, pp. 454–457, 1996.

[31] C. R. Morris, M. T. Gladwin, and G. J. Kato, "Nitric oxide and arginine dysregulation: a novel pathway to pulmonary hypertension in hemolytic disorders," *Current Molecular Medicine*, vol. 8, no. 7, pp. 620–632, 2008.

[32] C. R. Morris, "Asthma management: reinventing the wheel in sickle cell disease," *American Journal of Hematology*, vol. 84, no. 4, pp. 234–241, 2009.

[33] K. J. Sullivan, N. Kissoon, L. J. Duckworth et al., "Low exhaled nitric oxide and a polymorphism in the NOS I gene is associated with acute chest syndrome," *American Journal of Respiratory and Critical Care Medicine*, vol. 164, no. 12, pp. 2186–2190, 2002.

[34] K. J. Sullivan, N. Kissoon, E. Sandler et al., "Effect of oral arginine supplementation on exhaled nitric oxide concentration in sickle cell anemia and acute chest syndrome," *Journal of Pediatric Hematology/Oncology*, vol. 32, no. 7, pp. e249–e258, 2010.

[35] R. E. Girgis, M. A. Qureshi, J. Abrams, and P. Swerdlow, "Decreased exhaled nitric oxide in sickle cell disease: relationship with chronic lung involvement," *American Journal of Hematology*, vol. 72, no. 3, pp. 177–184, 2003.

[36] S. S. Pawar, J. A. Panepinto, and D. C. Brousseau, "The effect of acute pain crisis on exhaled nitric oxide levels in children with sickle cell disease," *Pediatric Blood and Cancer*, vol. 50, no. 1, pp. 111–113, 2008.

[37] P. Niscola, F. Sorrentino, L. Scaramucci, P. de Fabritiis, and P. Cianciulli, "Pain syndromes in sickle cell disease: an update," *Pain Medicine*, vol. 10, no. 3, pp. 470–480, 2009.

[38] E. Jacob, M. M. Sockrider, M. Dinu, M. Acosta, and B. U. Mueller, "Respiratory symptoms and acute painful episodes in sickle cell disease," *Journal of Pediatric Oncology Nursing*, vol. 27, no. 1, pp. 33–39, 2010.

[39] B. S. Shapiro, D. F. Dinges, E. C. Orne et al., "Home management of sickle cell-related pain in children and adolescents: natural history and impact on school attendance," *Pain*, vol. 61, no. 1, pp. 139–144, 1995.

[40] C. Dampier, B. N. Y. Setty, B. Eggleston, D. Brodecki, P. O'Neal, and M. Stuart, "Vaso-occlusion in children with sickle cell disease: clinical characteristics and biologic correlates," *Journal of Pediatric Hematology/Oncology*, vol. 26, no. 12, pp. 785–790, 2004.

[41] J. Glassberg, J. F. Spivey, R. Strunk, S. Boslaugh, and M. R. DeBaun, "Painful episodes in children with sickle cell disease and asthma are temporally associated with respiratory symptoms," *Journal of Pediatric Hematology/Oncology*, vol. 28, no. 8, pp. 481–485, 2006.

[42] S. T. Holgate, "Pathogenesis of asthma," *Clinical and Experimental Allergy*, vol. 38, no. 6, pp. 872–897, 2008.

[43] O. S. Platt, "Sickle cell anemia as an inflammatory disease," *Journal of Clinical Investigation*, vol. 106, no. 3, pp. 337–338, 2000.

[44] J. M. Drazen, E. Israel, and P. M. O'Byrne, "Treatment of asthma with drugs modifying the leukotriene pathway," *New England Journal of Medicine*, vol. 340, no. 3, pp. 197–206, 1999.

[45] Y. Kanaoka and J. A. Boyce, "Cysteinyl leukotrienes and their receptors: cellular distribution and function in immune and inflammatory responses," *Journal of Immunology*, vol. 173, no. 3, pp. 1503–1510, 2004.

[46] J. W. Woods, J. F. Evans, D. Ethier et al., "5-lipoxygenase and 5-lipoxygenase-activating protein are localized in the nuclear envelope of activated human leukocytes," *Journal of Experimental Medicine*, vol. 178, no. 6, pp. 1935–1946, 1993.

[47] B. K. Lam, W. F. Owen, K. F. Austen, and R. J. Soberman, "The identification of a distinct export step following the biosynthesis of leukotriene C by human eosinophils," *Journal of Biological Chemistry*, vol. 264, no. 22, pp. 12885–12889, 1989.

[48] M. E. Anderson, R. D. Allison, and A. Meister, "Interconversion of leukotrienes catalyzed by purified γ-glutamyl transpeptidase: concomitant formation of leukotriene D4 and γ-glutamyl amino acids," *Proceedings of the National Academy of Sciences of the United States of America*, vol. 79, no. 4, pp. 1088–1091, 1982.

[49] C. W. Lee, R. A. Lewis, E. J. Corey, and K. F. Austen, "Conversion of leukotriene D to leukotriene E by a dipeptidase released from the specific granule of human polymorphonuclear leukocytes," *Immunology*, vol. 48, no. 1, pp. 27–35, 1983.

[50] N. Rabinovitch, "Urinary leukotriene E," *Immunology and Allergy Clinics of North America*, vol. 27, no. 4, pp. 651–664, 2007.

[51] G. Folco and R. C. Murphy, "Eicosanoid transcellular biosynthesis: from cell-cell interactions to in vivo tissue responses," *Pharmacological Reviews*, vol. 58, no. 3, pp. 375–388, 2006.

[52] S. D. Nandedkar, T. R. Feroah, W. Hutchins et al., "Histopathology of experimentally induced asthma in a murine model of sickle cell disease," *Blood*, vol. 112, no. 6, pp. 2529–2538, 2008.

[53] B. N. Y. Setty and M. J. Stuart, "Eicosanoids in sickle cell disease: potential relevance of neutrophil leukotriene B to disease pathophysiology," *Journal of Laboratory and Clinical Medicine*, vol. 139, no. 2, pp. 80–89, 2002.

[54] B. O. Ibe, J. Kurantsin-Mills, J. U. Raj, and L. S. Lessin, "Plasma and urinary leukotrienes in sickle cell disease: possible role in the inflammatory process," *European Journal of Clinical Investigation*, vol. 24, no. 1, pp. 57–64, 1994.

[55] J. J. Field, R. C. Strunk, J. E. Knight-Perry, M. A. Blinder, R. R. Townsend, and M. R. DeBaun, "Urinary cysteinyl leukotriene E significantly increases during pain in children and adults with sickle cell disease," *American Journal of Hematology*, vol. 84, no. 4, pp. 231–233, 2009.

[56] J. J. Field, J. Krings, N. L. White et al., "Urinary cysteinyl leukotriene e is associated with increased risk for pain and acute chest syndrome in adults with sickle cell disease," *American Journal of Hematology*, vol. 84, no. 3, pp. 158–160, 2009.

[57] J. E. Jennings, T. Ramkumar, J. Mao et al., "Elevated urinary leukotriene E levels are associated with hospitalization for pain in children with sickle cell disease," *American Journal of Hematology*, vol. 83, no. 8, pp. 640–643, 2008.

[58] J. M. Drazen and K. F. Austen, "Leukotrienes and airway responses," *American Review of Respiratory Disease*, vol. 136, no. 4, pp. 985–998, 1987.

[59] M. D. Thompson, J. Takasaki, V. Capra et al., "G-protein-coupled receptors and asthma endophenotypes: the cysteinyl leukotriene system in perspective," *Molecular Diagnosis and Therapy*, vol. 10, no. 6, pp. 353–366, 2006.

[60] K. H. In, K. Asano, D. Beier et al., "Naturally occurring mutations in the human 5-lipoxygenase gene promoter that modify transcription factor binding and reporter gene transcription," *Journal of Clinical Investigation*, vol. 99, no. 5, pp. 1130–1137, 1997.

[61] S. Vikman, R. M. Brena, P. Armstrong, J. Hartiala, C. B. Stephensen, and H. Allayee, "Functional analysis of 5-lipoxygenase promoter repeat variants," *Human Molecular Genetics*, vol. 18, no. 23, pp. 4521–4529, 2009.

[62] O. Kalayci, E. Birben, C. Sackesen et al., "ALOX5 promoter genotype, asthma severity and LTC production by eosinophils," *Allergy*, vol. 61, no. 1, pp. 97–103, 2006.

[63] N. Patel, C. S. Gonsalves, M. Yang, P. Malik, and V. K. Kalra, "Placenta growth factor induces 5-lipoxygenase-activating protein to increase leukotriene formation in sickle cell disease," *Blood*, vol. 113, no. 5, pp. 1129–1138, 2009.

[64] N. Perelman, S. K. Selvaraj, S. Batra et al., "Placenta growth factor activates monocytes and correlates with sickle cell disease severity," *Blood*, vol. 102, no. 4, pp. 1506–1514, 2003.

[65] R. J. Freishtat, S. F. Iqbal, D. K. Pillai et al., "High prevalence of vitamin D deficiency among inner-city African American youth with asthma in Washington, DC," *Journal of Pediatrics*, vol. 156, no. 6, pp. 948–952, 2010.

[66] R. Beasley, "The burden of asthma with specific reference to the United States," *Journal of Allergy and Clinical Immunology*, vol. 109, no. 5, pp. S482–S489, 2002.

[67] C. A. Camargo Jr., S. L. Rifas-Shiman, A. A. Litonjua et al., "Maternal intake of vitamin D during pregnancy and risk of recurrent wheeze in children at 3 y of age," *American Journal of Clinical Nutrition*, vol. 85, no. 3, pp. 788–795, 2007.

[68] J. M. Brehm, J. C. Celedón, M. E. Soto-Quiros et al., "Serum vitamin D levels and markers of severity of childhood asthma in Costa Rica," *American Journal of Respiratory and Critical Care Medicine*, vol. 179, no. 9, pp. 765–771, 2009.

[69] E. R. Sutherland, E. Goleva, L. P. Jackson, A. D. Stevens, and D. Y. M. Leung, "Vitamin D levels, lung function, and steroid response in adult asthma," *American Journal of Respiratory and Critical Care Medicine*, vol. 181, no. 7, pp. 699–704, 2010.

[70] B. M. Goodman III, N. Artz, B. Radford, and I. A. Chen, "Prevalence of vitamin D deficiency in adults with sickle cell disease," *Journal of the National Medical Association*, vol. 102, no. 4, pp. 332–335, 2010.

[71] E. Chapelon, M. Garabedian, V. Brousse, J. C. Souberbielle, J. L. Bresson, and M. de Montalembert, "Osteopenia and vitamin D deficiency in children with sickle cell disease," *European Journal of Haematology*, vol. 83, no. 6, pp. 572–578, 2009.

[72] A. J. Rovner, V. A. Stallings, D. A. Kawchak, J. I. Schall, K. Ohene-Frempong, and B. S. Zemel, "High risk of vitamin D deficiency in children with sickle cell disease," *Journal of the American Dietetic Association*, vol. 108, no. 9, pp. 1512–1516, 2008.

[73] A. H. Adewoye, T. C. Chen, Q. Ma et al., "Sickle cell bone disease: response to vitamin D and calcium," *American Journal of Hematology*, vol. 83, no. 4, pp. 271–274, 2008.

[74] A. Lal, E. B. Fung, Z. Pakbaz, E. Hackney-Stephens, and E. P. Vichinsky, "Bone mineral density in children with sickle cell anemia," *Pediatric Blood and Cancer*, vol. 47, no. 7, pp. 901–906, 2006.

[75] A. M. Buison, D. A. Kawchak, J. Schall, K. Ohene-Frempong, V. A. Stallings, and B. S. Zemel, "Low vitamin D status in children with sickle cell disease," *Journal of Pediatrics*, vol. 145, no. 5, pp. 622–627, 2004.

[76] J. Stinson and B. Naser, "Pain management in children with sickle cell disease," *Pediatric Drugs*, vol. 5, no. 4, pp. 229–241, 2003.

[77] S. L. Yoon and S. Black, "Comprehensive, integrative management of pain for patients with sickle-cell disease," *Journal of Alternative and Complementary Medicine*, vol. 12, no. 10, pp. 995–1001, 2006.

[78] H. Farquhar, A. Stewart, E. Mitchell et al., "The role of paracetamol in the pathogenesis of asthma," *Clinical and Experimental Allergy*, vol. 40, no. 1, pp. 32–41, 2010.

[79] R. W. Beasley, T. O. Clayton, J. Crane et al., "Acetaminophen use and risk of asthma, rhinoconjunctivitis and eczema in adolescents: ISAAC phase three," *American Journal of Respiratory and Critical Care Medicine*. In press.

[80] R. Beasley, T. Clayton, J. Crane et al., "Association between paracetamol use in infancy and childhood, and risk of asthma, rhinoconjunctivitis, and eczema in children aged 6-7 years: analysis from Phase Three of the ISAAC programme," *The Lancet*, vol. 372, no. 9643, pp. 1039–1048, 2008.

[81] V. W. Persky, "Acetaminophen and Asthma," *Thorax*, vol. 65, no. 2, pp. 99–100, 2010.

[82] M. S. Perzanowski, R. L. Miller, D. Tang et al., "Prenatal acetaminophen exposure and risk of wheeze at age 5 years in an urban low-income cohort," *Thorax*, vol. 65, no. 2, pp. 118–123, 2010.

[83] EPR 3. National Asthma Education and Prevention Program, *Expert Panel Report 3: Guidelines for the diagnosis and management of asthma*, U.S. Department of Health and Human Services, Public Health Service, National Institutes of Health, National Heart, Lung, and Blood Institute, Bethesda, Md, USA, August 2007, no. 08-4051.

[84] J. J. Field and M. R. DeBaun, "Asthma and sickle cell disease: two distinct diseases or part of the same process?" *Hematology/American Society of Hematology. Education Program*, pp. 45–53, 2009.

[85] S. A. Schroeder and A. G. Nepo, "Treatment of asthma in children with sickle cell disease can prevent recurrences of acute chest syndrome," *American Journal of Respiratory and Critical Care Medicine*, vol. 177, article A262, 2008.

[86] C. G. Giuntini and P. L. Paggiaro, "Present state of the controversy about regular inhaled β-agonists in asthma," *European Respiratory Journal*, vol. 8, no. 5, pp. 673–678, 1995.

[87] M. R. Sears, R. M. Sly, and R. O'Donnell, "Relationships between asthma mortality and treatment," *Annals of Allergy*, vol. 70, no. 5, pp. 425–426, 1993.

[88] W. H. Inman and A. M. Adelstein, "Rise and fall of asthma mortality in England and Wales in relation to use of pressurised aerosols," *Lancet*, vol. 2, no. 7615, pp. 279–285, 1969.

[89] N. Pearce, R. Beasley, J. Crane, C. Burgess, and R. Jackson, "End of the New Zealand asthma mortality epidemic," *Lancet*, vol. 345, no. 8941, pp. 41–44, 1995.

[90] W. O. Spitzer, S. Suissa, P. Ernst et al., "The use of β-agonists and the risk of death and near death from asthma," *New England Journal of Medicine*, vol. 326, no. 8, pp. 501–506, 1992.

[91] J. M. Drazen, E. Israel, H. A. Boushey et al., "Comparison of regularly scheduled with as-needed use of albuterol in mild asthma," *New England Journal of Medicine*, vol. 335, no. 12, pp. 841–847, 1996.

[92] S. A. Green, J. Turki, M. Innis, and S. B. Liggett, "Amino-terminal polymorphisms of the human β₂-adrenergic receptor impart distinct agonist-promoted regulatory properties," *Biochemistry*, vol. 33, no. 32, pp. 9414–9419, 1994.

[93] S. A. Green, J. Turki, P. Bejarano, I. P. Hall, and S. B. Liggett, "Influence of beta 2-adrenergic receptor genotypes on signal transduction in human airway smooth muscle cells," *American Journal of Respiratory Cell and Molecular Biology*, vol. 13, no. 1, pp. 25–33, 1995.

[94] E. Israel, J. M. Drazen, S. B. Liggett et al., "The effect of polymorphisms of the β₂-adrenergic receptor on the response to regular use of albuterol in asthma," *American Journal of Respiratory and Critical Care Medicine*, vol. 162, no. 1, pp. 75–80, 2000.

[95] D. R. Taylor, J. M. Drazen, G. P. Herbison, C. N. Yandava, R. J. Hancox, and G. I. Town, "Asthma exacerbations during long term β agonist use: influence of β₂ adrenoceptor polymorphism," *Thorax*, vol. 55, no. 9, pp. 762–767, 2000.

[96] D. K. C. Lee, C. E. Bates, and B. J. Lipworth, "Acute systemic effects of inhaled salbutamol in asthmatic subjects expressing common homozygous β₂-adrenoceptor haplotypes at positions 16 and 27," *British Journal of Clinical Pharmacology*, vol. 57, no. 1, pp. 100–104, 2004.

[97] R. J. Hancox, M. R. Sears, and D. R. Taylor, "Polymorphism of the β₂-adrenoceptor and the response to long-term β-agonist therapy in asthma," *European Respiratory Journal*, vol. 11, no. 3, pp. 589–593, 1998.

[98] E. Israel, V. M. Chinchilli, J. G. Ford et al., "Use of regularly scheduled albuterol treatment in asthma: genotype-stratified, randomised, placebo-controlled cross-over trial," *Lancet*, vol. 364, no. 9444, pp. 1505–1512, 2004.

[99] G. A. Hawkins, K. Tantisira, D. A. Meyers et al., "Sequence, haplotype, and association analysis of ADRβ2 in a multi-ethnic asthma case-control study," *American Journal of Respiratory and Critical Care Medicine*, vol. 174, no. 10, pp. 1101–1109, 2006.

[100] E. R. Bleecker, R. M. Lawrance, H. J. Ambrose, and M. Goldman, "Beta2-adrenergic receptor gene polymorphisms: is Arg/Arg genotype associated with serious adverse events during treatment with budesonide and formoterol in one pressurized metered-dose inhaler (BUD/FM pMDI) within racial groups?" *American Journal of Respiratory and Critical Care Medicine*, vol. 177, article A775, 2008.

[101] K. Blake, R. Madabushi, H. Derendorf, and J. Lima, "Population pharmacodynamic model of bronchodilator response to inhaled albuterol in children and adults with asthma," *Chest*, vol. 134, no. 5, pp. 981–989, 2008.

[102] G. E. Hardie, J. K. Brown, and W. M. Gold, "Adrenergic responsiveness: FEV1 and symptom differences in Whites and African Americans with mild asthma," *Journal of Asthma*, vol. 44, no. 8, pp. 621–628, 2007.

[103] P. Thottathil, J. Acharya, A. J. Moss et al., "Risk of cardiac events in patients with asthma and long-QT syndrome treated with beta₂ agonists," *American Journal of Cardiology*, vol. 102, no. 7, pp. 871–874, 2008.

[104] S. R. Salpeter, T. M. Ormiston, and E. E. Salpeter, "Cardiovascular effects of β-agonists in patients with asthma and COPD: a meta-analysis," *Chest*, vol. 125, no. 6, pp. 2309–2321, 2004.

[105] B. U. Mueller, K. J. Martin, W. Dreyer, L. I. Bezold, and D. H. Mahoney, "Prolonged QT interval in pediatric sickle cell disease," *Pediatric Blood and Cancer*, vol. 47, no. 6, pp. 831–833, 2006.

[106] F. Akgül, E. Seyfeli, I. Melek et al., "Increased QT dispersion in sickle cell disease: effect of pulmonary hypertension," *Acta Haematologica*, vol. 118, no. 1, pp. 1–6, 2007.

[107] H. W. Kelly, "Non-corticosteroid therapy for long-term control of asthma," *Expert Opinion on Pharmacotherapy*, vol. 8, no. 13, pp. 2077–2087, 2007.

[108] B. A. Rohrman and D. A. Mazziotti, "Quantum chemical design of hydroxyurea derivatives for the treatment of sickle-cell anemia," *Journal of Physical Chemistry B*, vol. 109, no. 27, pp. 13392–13396, 2005.

[109] J. Haynes Jr., B. Obiako, J. A. King, R. B. Hester, and S. Ofori-Acquah, "Activated neutrophil-mediated sickle red blood cell adhesion to lung vascular endothelium: role of phosphatidylserine-exposed sickle red blood cells," *American Journal of Physiology*, vol. 291, no. 4, pp. H1679–H1685, 2006.

[110] S. Kuvibidila, B. S. Baliga, R. Gardner et al., "Differential effects of hydroxyurea and zileuton on interleukin-13 secretion by activated murine spleen cells: implication on the expression of vascular cell adhesion molecule-1 and vasoocclusion in sickle cell anemia," *Cytokine*, vol. 30, no. 5, pp. 213–218, 2005.

[111] J. Haynes Jr., B. S. Baliga, B. Obiako, S. Ofori-Acquah, and B. Pace, "Zileuton induces hemoglobin F synthesis in erythroid progenitors: role of the L-arginine-nitric oxide signaling pathway," *Blood*, vol. 103, no. 10, pp. 3945–3950, 2004.

[112] J. Haynes Jr. and B. Obiako, "Activated polymorphonuclear cells increase sickle red blood cell retention in lung: role of phospholipids," *American Journal of Physiology*, vol. 282, no. 1, pp. H122–H130, 2002.

[113] K. V. Blake, "Montelukast: data from clinical trials in the management of asthma," *Annals of Pharmacotherapy*, vol. 33, no. 12, pp. 1299–1314, 1999.

[114] G. P. Currie and K. McLaughlin, "The expanding role of leukotriene receptor antagonists in chronic asthma," *Annals of Allergy, Asthma and Immunology*, vol. 97, no. 6, pp. 731–741, 2006.

[115] J. J. Lima, S. Zhang, A. Grant et al., "Influence of leukotriene pathway polymorphisms on response to montelukast in asthma," *American Journal of Respiratory and Critical Care Medicine*, vol. 173, no. 4, pp. 379–385, 2006.

[116] K. Malmstrom, G. Rodriguez-Gomez, J. Guerra et al., "Oral montelukast, inhaled beclomethasone, and placebo for chronic asthma: a randomized, controlled trial," *Annals of Internal Medicine*, vol. 130, no. 6, pp. 487–495, 1999.

[117] S. J. Szefler, B. R. Phillips, F. D. Martinez et al., "Characterization of within-subject responses to fluticasone and montelukast in childhood asthma," *Journal of Allergy and Clinical Immunology*, vol. 115, no. 2, pp. 233–242, 2005.

[118] M. Klotsman, T. P. York, S. G. Pillai et al., "Pharmacogenetics of the 5-lipoxygenase biosynthetic pathway and variable clinical response to montelukast," *Pharmacogenetics and Genomics*, vol. 17, no. 3, pp. 189–196, 2007.

[119] E. B. Mougey, H. Feng, M. Castro, C. G. Irvin, and J. J. Lima, "Absorption of montelukast is transporter mediated: a common variant of OATP2B1 is associated with reduced plasma concentrations and poor response," *Pharmacogenetics and Genomics*, vol. 19, no. 2, pp. 129–138, 2009.

[120] J. J. Telleria, A. Blanco-Quiros, D. Varillas et al., "ALOX5 promoter genotype and response to montelukast in moderate persistent asthma," *Respiratory Medicine*, vol. 102, no. 6, pp. 857–861, 2008.

[121] B. Knorr, S. Holland, J. D. Rogers, H. H. Nguyen, and T. F. Reiss, "Montelulkast adult (10-mg film-coated tablet) and pediatric (5-mg chewable tablet) dose selections," *Journal of Allergy and Clinical Immunology*, vol. 106, no. 3, pp. S171–S178, 2000.

[122] C. G. Irvin, D. A. Kaminsky, N. R. Anthonisen et al., "Clinical trial of low-dose theophylline and montelukast in patients with poorly controlled asthma," *American Journal of Respiratory and Critical Care Medicine*, vol. 175, no. 3, pp. 235–242, 2007.

[123] D. A. Revicki, N. K. Leidy, F. Brennan-Diemer, S. Sorensen, and A. Togias, "Integrating patient preferences into health outcomes assessment: the multiattribute asthma symptom utility index," *Chest*, vol. 114, no. 4, pp. 998–1007, 1998.

[124] G. Philip, C. Hustad, G. Noonan et al., "Reports of suicidality in clinical trials of montelukast," *Journal of Allergy and Clinical Immunology*, vol. 124, no. 4, pp. 691–696.e6, 2009.

[125] G. Philip, C. M. Hustad, M. P. Malice et al., "Analysis of behavior-related adverse experiences in clinical trials of montelukast," *Journal of Allergy and Clinical Immunology*, vol. 124, no. 4, pp. 699–706.e3, 2009.

[126] J. T. Holbrook and R. Harik-Khan, "Montelukast and emotional well-being as a marker for depression: results from 3 randomized, double-masked clinical trials," *Journal of Allergy and Clinical Immunology*, vol. 122, no. 4, pp. 828–829, 2008.

[127] C. L. Edwards, M. Green, C. C. Wellington et al., "Depression, suicidal ideation, and attempts in black patients with sickle cell disease," *Journal of the National Medical Association*, vol. 101, no. 11, pp. 1090–1095, 2009.

[128] J. U. Ohaeri, W. A. Shokunbi, K. S. Akinlade, and L. O. Dare, "The psychosocial problems of sickle cell disease sufferers and their methods of coping," *Social Science and Medicine*, vol. 40, no. 7, pp. 955–960, 1995.

[129] W. Castle, R. Fuller, J. Hall, and J. Palmer, "Serevent nationwide surveillance study: comparison of salmeterol with salbutamol in asthmatic patients who require regular bronchodilator treatment," *British Medical Journal*, vol. 306, no. 6884, pp. 1034–1037, 1993.

[130] H. S. Nelson, S. T. Weiss, E. E. Bleecker, S. W. Yancey, and P. M. Dorinsky, "The salmeterol multicenter asthma research trial: a comparison of usual pharmacotherapy for asthma or usual pharmacotherapy plus salmeterol," *Chest*, vol. 129, no. 1, pp. 15–26, 2006.

[131] S. R. Salpeter, N. S. Buckley, T. M. Ormiston, and E. E. Salpeter, "Meta-analysis: effect of long-acting $\beta$-agonists on severe asthma exacerbations and asthma-related deaths," *Annals of Internal Medicine*, vol. 144, no. 12, pp. 904–912, 2006.

[132] S. R. Salpeter, A. J. Wall, and N. S. Buckley, "Long-acting beta-agonists with and without inhaled corticosteroids and catastrophic asthma events," *American Journal of Medicine*, vol. 123, no. 4, pp. 322–328.e2, 2010.

[133] M. Mann, B. Chowdhury, E. Sullivan, R. Nicklas, R. Anthracite, and R. J. Meyer, "Serious asthma exacerbations in asthmatics treated with high-dose formoterol," *Chest*, vol. 124, no. 1, pp. 70–74, 2003.

[134] J. M. Kramer, "Balancing the benefits and risks of inhaled long-acting beta-agonists—the influence of values," *New England Journal of Medicine*, vol. 360, no. 16, pp. 1592–1595, 2009.

[135] E. R. Bleecker, S. W. Yancey, L. A. Baitinger et al., "Salmeterol response is not affected by $\beta_2$-adrenergic receptor genotype in subjects with persistent asthma," *Journal of Allergy and Clinical Immunology*, vol. 118, no. 4, pp. 809–816, 2006.

[136] E. R. Bleecker, D. S. Postma, R. M. Lawrance, D. A. Meyers, H. J. Ambrose, and M. Goldman, "Effect of ADRB2 polymorphisms on response to longacting $\beta_2$-agonist therapy: a pharmacogenetic analysis of two randomised studies," *Lancet*, vol. 370, no. 9605, pp. 2118–2125, 2007.

[137] E. R. Bleecker, R. Lawrance, H. Ambrose, and M. Goldman, "Beta2-adrenergic receptor Gly16Arg variation: effect on response to budesonide/formoterol (BUD/FM) or budesonide (BUD; post-formoterol) in children and adolescents with asthma," *American Journal of Respiratory and Critical Care Medicine*, vol. 177, article A776, 2008.

[138] W. Anderson, S. A. Bacanu, E. R. Bleecker et al., "A prospective haplotype analysis of beta2-adrenergic receptor polymorphisms and clinical response to salmeterol and salmeterol/fluticasone propionate," *American Journal of Respiratory and Critical Care Medicine*, vol. 177, article A775, 2008.

[139] M. E. Wechsler, S. J. Kunselman, V. M. Chinchilli et al., "Effect of $\beta_2$-adrenergic receptor polymorphism on response to longacting $\beta_2$ agonist in asthma (LARGE trial): a genotype-stratified, randomised, placebo-controlled, crossover trial," *The Lancet*, vol. 374, no. 9703, pp. 1754–1764, 2009.

[140] E. R. Bleecker, H. S. Nelson, M. Kraft et al., "$\beta_2$-receptor polymorphisms in patients receiving salmeterol with or without fluticasone propionate," *American Journal of Respiratory and Critical Care Medicine*, vol. 181, no. 7, pp. 676–687, 2010.

[141] K. Blake, "Theophylline," in *Pediatric Asthma*, S. Murphy and H. W. Kelly, Eds., pp. 363–431, Marcel Dekker, New York, 1999.

[142] R. Kumar, S. Qureshi, P. Mohanty, S. P. Rao, and S. T. Miller, "A short course of prednisone in the management of acute chest syndrome of sickle cell disease," *Journal of Pediatric Hematology/Oncology*, vol. 32, no. 3, pp. e91–e94, 2010.

[143] A. Sobota, D. A. Graham, M. M. Heeney, and E. J. Neufeld, "Corticosteroids for acute chest syndrome in children with sickle cell disease: variation in use and association with length of stay and readmission," *American Journal of Hematology*, vol. 85, no. 1, pp. 24–28, 2010.

[144] D. S. Darbari, O. Castro, J. G. Taylor et al., "Severe vasoocclusive episodes associated with use of systemic corticosteroids in patients with sickle cell disease," *Journal of the National Medical Association*, vol. 100, no. 8, pp. 948–951, 2008.

[145] J. J. Strouse, C. M. Takemoto, J. R. Keefer, G. J. Kato, and J. F. Casella, "Corticosteroids and increased risk of readmission after acute chest syndrome in children with sickle cell disease," *Pediatric Blood and Cancer*, vol. 50, no. 5, pp. 1006–1012, 2008.

[146] M. S. Isakoff, J. A. Lillo, and J. N. Hagstrom, "A single-institution experience with treatment of severe acute chest syndrome: lack of rebound pain with dexametha-sone plus transfusion therapy," *Journal of Pediatric Hematology/Oncology*, vol. 30, no. 4, pp. 322–325, 2008.

[147] M. P. Celano, J. F. Linzer, A. Demi et al., "Treatment adherence among low-income, african american children with persistent asthma," *Journal of Asthma*, vol. 47, no. 3, pp. 317–322, 2010.

[148] L. Hendeles, M. Asmus, and S. Chesrown, "What is the role of budesonide inhalation suspension for nebulization?" *The Journal of Pediatric Pharmacology and Therapeutics*, vol. 6, pp. 162–166, 2001.

[149] C. Rand, A. Bilderback, K. Schiller, J. M. Edelman, C. M. Hustad, and R. S. Zeiger, "Adherence with montelukast or fluticasone in a long-term clinical trial: results from the mild asthma montelukast versus inhaled corticosteroid trial," *Journal of Allergy and Clinical Immunology*, vol. 119, no. 4, pp. 916–923, 2007.

# 13

# Cormic Index Profile of Children with Sickle Cell Anaemia in Lagos, Nigeria

**Samuel Olufemi Akodu, Olisamedua Fidelis Njokanma, and Omolara Adeolu Kehinde**

*Department of Paediatrics, Lagos State University Teaching Hospital, P.O. Box 11950, Ikeja, Lagos 100001, Nigeria*

Correspondence should be addressed to Samuel Olufemi Akodu; femiakodu@hotmail.com

Academic Editor: Aurelio Maggio

*Background.* Sickle cell disorders are known to have a negative effect on linear growth. This could potentially affect proportional growth and, hence, Cormic Index. *Objective.* To determine the Cormic Index in the sickle cell anaemia population in Lagos. *Methodology.* A consecutive sample of 100 children with haemoglobin genotype SS, aged eight months to 15 years, and 100 age and sex matched controls (haemoglobin genotype AA) was studied. Sitting height (upper segment) and full length or height were measured. Sitting height was then expressed as a percentage of full length/height (Cormic Index). *Results.* The mean Cormic Index decreased with age among primary subjects (SS) and AA controls. The overall mean Cormic Index among primary subjects was comparable to that of controls ($55.0 \pm 4.6\%$ versus $54.5 \pm 5.2\%$; $54.8 \pm 4.5\%$ versus $53.6 \pm 4.9\%$) in boys and girls, respectively. In comparison with AA controls, female children with sickle cell anaemia who were older than 10 years had a significantly lower mean Cormic Index. *Conclusion.* There was a significant negative relationship between Cormic Index and height in subjects and controls irrespective of gender. Similarly, a significant negative correlation existed between age, sitting height, subischial leg length, weight, and Cormic Index in both subjects and controls.

## 1. Introduction

Sickle cell anaemia is a group of genetic disorders most commonly seen in man and it is found in people of African descent but it is also seen in people of other ethnic groups [1]. It has been shown that, as a group, children with sickle cell anaemia have poor growth [2, 3]. Anthropometry is the principal method of assessing growth and height/length-for-age is the most useful linear measurement that gives an indication of past nutrition [4].

The Cormic Index expresses sitting height as a proportion of full height. It is a measure of the relative length of trunk and lower limb and it varies between individuals and groups [5]. It is the most common bivariate index of shape [5]. The Cormic Index is most often used to correct for variability in body shape when Body Mass Index (BMI) is used to compare the nutritional status in or between different populations [6]. For example, individuals who are very tall may be wrongly classified as being underweight despite having normal body weight for their culture. Similarly, in muscular people BMI may be more likely to indicate overweight, as lean body mass

tissue is denser than fat tissue. The BMI can be modified using Cormic Index to help correct for this variability in body shape. Used as such, it adjusts for population differences in phenotype that may impact BMI. It is important to recognize that this type of adjustment mainly has been applied to adults and not to children or adolescents [7].

It has been evident that there is variability in the growth of spinal length compared with limb length during the prepubertal period and during adolescence. Previous studies have shown that increase in sitting height is relatively faster than leg length in later childhood [8, 9]. The negative effect of sickle cell anaemia on spinal growth and, hence, Cormic Index would therefore be expected to be more obvious in older children during the period of expected rapid growth. Shorter spinal length relative to the height increases the Cormic Index.

To the best of the authors' knowledge, there is no prior report of the Cormic Index among children with sickle cell anaemia in Nigeria or elsewhere. Studies have been conducted among African [10], Australian aborigines [11], and Asian [12] population without specific reference to haemoglobin genotype. However, the direct effect of sickle cell anaemia on linear growth may limit the application of findings in the general population to affected children.

The appraisal of the Cormic Index among children with sickle cell anaemia is therefore of clinical and scientific interest. Therefore, the main objective of the present report was to determine the Cormic Index among children with sickle cell anaemia.

## 2. Materials and Methods

The cross-sectional study was conducted between October and December 2009 among children with sickle cell anaemia attending the sickle cell disease clinic of the Department of Paediatrics of Lagos State University Teaching Hospital, Ikeja, in Southwest Nigeria. The hospital is an urban tertiary health centre in Lagos State, Western Nigeria. It is a major referral center serving the whole state, which is a major point of entry into Nigeria from different parts of the world and is the economic nerve centre of Nigeria.

Approval for the study was obtained from the Ethics Committee of Lagos State University Teaching Hospital and written informed consent was obtained from each parent. Consecutive patients with sickle cell anaemia who came for routine follow-up clinic that gave consent and met the study criteria were eligible for enrollment in the study. Healthy controls were children with haemoglobin genotype "AA" from the general outpatient and follow-up clinics and healthy children attending other specialist clinics like the Paediatric Dermatology Clinic. Controls were matched with primary subjects for age and sex. Two hundred children were studied—one hundred each with haemoglobin genotypes SS and AA. In order to have fairly equal representation of ages, the subjects stratified as follows: <2 years, >2 to 5 years, >5 to 10 years, and >10 to 15 years.

### 2.1. Inclusion Criteria

(1) Age six months to fifteen years.

(2) Confirmed HbSS by electrophoresis.

(3) Signed, informed consent of the caregiver.

(4) Subjects who were in steady state, that is, absence of any crisis in the preceding four weeks, no recent drop in the haemoglobin level, and absence of any symptoms or signs attributable to acute illness [13].

(5) Children who were not taking medications known to affect growth, for example, steroids.

### 2.2. Exclusion Criteria

(1) Children with congenital cardiac abnormality, chronic renal disease, or abnormal chest wall deformity or chronic respiratory disorder.

(2) Refusal of consent.

(3) Children with history of cerebrovascular accident.

(4) Sickle cell anaemia patients with history of long-term transfusion therapy.

The inclusion and exclusion criteria for the controls were the same as for subjects except that the haemoglobin genotype was AA.

### 2.3. Measurement of Height.
Children two years of age and older had their heights measured using a stadiometer while the length of those below two years was measured using an infantometer.

### 2.4. Measurement of Weight.
Subjects' weights were measured barefooted and wearing light clothing. Weight measurements were taken on a Seca 761 series mechanical floor scale to the nearest 0.1 Kg.

### 2.5. Measurement of Sitting Height.
Sitting height was measured using a sitting height table. Sitting height was measured from the vertex of the head to the seated buttocks. The subject's head was positioned in the Frankfort horizontal plane, the shoulders relaxed, the back straight, and the head plate was brought into firm contact with the vertex [14].

The various linear measurements were taken three times and the mean was recorded. Subjects were measured wearing light clothing and shoes were removed. The measurements were taken following the standard techniques. The measurements were carried out by the researchers.

### 2.6. Derivation of Subischial Leg Length.
It is expressed as the difference between height/length and sitting height.

### 2.7. Derivation of Body Mass Index.
The body mass index was expressed as weight in Kg/height in metre$^2$ (Kg/m$^2$).

### 2.8. Derivation of Cormic Index.
It is expressed as

$$\left( \frac{\text{Sitting height}}{\text{height}} \right) \times 100. \tag{1}$$

Social classification was done using the scheme proposed by Oyedeji [15] in which subjects are grouped into five classes (I–V) based on the occupation and educational attainments of both parents. Analysis was done using Statistical Package for Social Science (SPSS) version 17.0. Comparison of mean values was done using Student's $t$-test and $P < 0.05$ is considered significant. The Pearson correlation coefficient ($r$) was attempted for understanding the overall relationship of anthropometric variables and age with Cormic Index.

In order to standardize the calculated BMI, the model developed by Norgan [16] was modified and applied. In the original model, standardized BMI was obtained using the formula $BMI_{std} = BMI_{52.0} + (BMI_0 - BMI_1)$, where

$BMI_{std}$ is standardized BMI,

$BMI_{52.0}$ is estimated BMI at Cormic Index of 54.9% (the mean Cormic Index for the European population),

TABLE 1: Mean Cormic Index distribution of study subjects according to age and gender.

| Variable | SS Mean (SD) | AA Mean (SD) | $t$-value | $P$ value |
|---|---|---|---|---|
| Age group | | | | |
| ≤2 yrs | | | | |
| Males | 60.3 (2.6) | 60.1 (1.8) | −0.228 | 0.822 |
| Females | 59.5 (2.8) | 60.8 (2.6) | 1.192 | 0.245 |
| Males and females | 59.9 (2.7) | 60.5 (2.2) | 0.783 | 0.437 |
| >2 yrs–5 yrs | | | | |
| Males | 54.5 (2.3) | 56.6 (3.3) | 1.914 | 0.068 |
| Females | 55.0 (2.3) | 54.8 (1.5) | −0.267 | 0.792 |
| Males and females | 54.7 (2.2) | 55.7 (2.7) | 1.408 | 0.165 |
| >5 yrs–10 yrs | | | | |
| Males | 52.1 (5.6) | 51.5 (1.2) | −0.385 | 0.704 |
| Females | 51.4 (1.6) | 51.6 (2.2) | 0.337 | 0.739 |
| Males and females | 51.8 (4.0) | 51.6 (1.7) | −0.208 | 0.836 |
| >10 yrs–15 yrs | | | | |
| Males | 50.4 (3.6) | 51.1 (3.5) | 0.475 | 0.640 |
| Females | 48.1 (2.2) | 51.5 (2.9) | 3.181 | 0.004 |
| Males and females | 49.3 (3.1) | 51.3 (3.2) | 2.213 | 0.032 |
| Socioeconomic strata | | | | |
| Upper | 55.15 (5.15) | 55.02 (4.89) | 0.128 | 0.899 |
| Other | 53.10 (4.70) | 54.57 (4.18) | 1.612 | 0.110 |

SD: standard deviation.

$BMI_0$ is actual (observed) BMI,

$BMI_1$ is estimated BMI at actual (observed) Cormic Index.

Note: Cormic Index should be expressed as a percentage.

Modification to the Norgan model was done by substituting the mean Cormic Index of the European population with that for the haemoglobin AA population in the current study.

## 3. Results

*3.1. Cormic Index of Study Subjects.* The Cormic Index of the SS subjects ranged from 44.5% to 68.2% while that for AA controls ranged from 45.9% to 65.0%. The mean Cormic Index of the SS group of 54.1 (±5.1)% was not statistically different from 54.9 (±4.5)% in the AA-control group (t-value = 1.240, $P$ = 0.216). The overall mean Cormic Index was 54.5 (±4.8)%. The mean Cormic Index of the study subjects according to age, gender, and socioeconomic strata was shown in Table 1. Mean Cormic Index decreased with age irrespective of gender or haemoglobin genotype. In each age group, the value observed in males with genotype SS was comparable to that of their AA counterparts. This was also the pattern in females except in the oldest age group in which AA controls had a significantly higher index. Within the haemoglobin "SS" group, the mean Cormic Index values of males were comparable to those of females across all age groups. The same was true of "AA" subjects across all age groups.

The mean Cormic Index was significantly higher in sickle cell anaemia subjects of the upper socioeconomic class than in those of the other classes ($P$ = 0.047). On the other hand, the difference between mean values for upper class and lower class controls was not significant ($P$ = 0.63).

*3.2. Correlation between Cormic Index and Height.* Table 2 shows the results of correlation analysis between Cormic Index and height of study subjects with and without sickle cell anaemia. Overall, the Cormic Index had strong negative correlations with height ($r$ = −0.850, −0.860, in subjects and controls, resp.). The pattern of negative correlation was observed in both sexes and in all age groups but the coefficients were not consistently significant. Significant positive correlations were detected between sitting height and subischial leg length ($r$ = 0.895, 0.925: $P$ = 0.000 each) in subjects and controls, respectively.

*3.3. Correlation between Cormic Index and Other Anthropometrics and Age.* Anthropometric variables tested were weight, BMI, sitting height, and subischial leg length. The Pearson correlation coefficient ($r$) for understanding the overall relationship of anthropometric variables and age with Cormic Index is shown in Table 3. Examination on the Pearson correlation coefficient revealed a significant ($P$ < 0.05) negative correlation between age, sitting height, subischial leg length, weight, and Cormic Index in both subjects and controls. Also, a weak correlation was observed between BMI and Cormic Index among subjects with HbSS and controls. However, it was in subjects with sickle cell anaemia that the

TABLE 2: Correlation analysis between height and Cormic Index in study subjects.

| Age group | Correlation coefficient ($r$) | | $P$ value | |
|---|---|---|---|---|
| | AA | SS | AA | SS |
| ≤2 yrs | | | | |
| Males | −0.679 | −0.411 | 0.011 | 0.164 |
| Females | −0.786 | −0.604 | 0.001 | 0.029 |
| Males and females | −0.708 | −0.465 | 0.000 | 0.017 |
| >2 yrs–5 yrs | | | | |
| Males | −0.887 | −0.680 | 0.000 | 0.011 |
| Females | −0.571 | −0.861 | 0.042 | 0.000 |
| Males and females | −0.827 | −0.769 | 0.000 | 0.000 |
| >5 yrs–10 yrs | | | | |
| Males | −0.460 | −0.641 | 0.133 | 0.025 |
| Females | −0.594 | −0.235 | 0.042 | 0.462 |
| Males and females | −0.552 | −0.569 | 0.005 | 0.004 |
| >10 yrs–15 yrs | | | | |
| Males | −0.453 | −0.644 | 0.139 | 0.024 |
| Females | −0.299 | −0.047 | 0.345 | 0.885 |
| Males and females | −0.381 | −0.495 | 0.066 | 0.014 |

TABLE 3: The Pearson correlation of Cormic Index with other anthropometrics and age.

| Characteristics | Correlation coefficient ($r$) | | $P$ value | |
|---|---|---|---|---|
| | AA | SS | AA | SS |
| Age | −0.752 | −0.744 | 0.000 | 0.000 |
| BMI | 0.120 | 0.386 | 0.241 | 0.000 |
| Subischial leg length | −0.922 | −0.919 | 0.000 | 0.000 |
| Sitting height | −0.728 | −0.670 | 0.000 | 0.000 |
| Weight | −0.565 | −0.700 | 0.000 | 0.000 |

TABLE 4: Regression of BMI on Cormic Index of subjects and controls.

| Independent variables | Equation | $R^2$ | SEE (cm) |
|---|---|---|---|
| Sickle cell anaemia subjects | | | |
| Males | 3.73 + 0.21 CI | 0.162 | 2.448 |
| Females | 6.10 + 0.15 CI | 0.126 | 1.951 |
| Males and females | 4.60 + 0.18 CI | 0.149 | 2.215 |
| Controls | | | |
| Males | 6.52 + 0.16 CI | 0.063 | 2.901 |
| Females | 15.26 + 0.02 CI | 0.000 | 3.961 |
| Males and females | 10.84 + 0.09 CI | 0.014 | 3.459 |

CI: Cormic Index.
Note: Cormic Index should be expressed as a percentage.

correlation coefficient was significant ($P = 0.000$). Table 3 also shows that the correlation between Cormic Indices and subischial leg length is higher in both subjects with sickle cell anaemia and controls.

*3.4. Regression of BMI and Cormic Index.* A simple regression equation was derived from the relationship between BMI as dependent variable and Cormic Index as independent variable (Table 4). Separate regression equations for the sexes were derived for BMI on the Cormic Index. Testing by covariance analysis showed that the slopes and intercepts were not significantly different. Therefore, the sexes were combined and a single equation was used to calculate expected BMI values.

Standardized BMI using the modified Norgan model was obtained as follows:

$$BMI_{std} = BMI_{54.9} + (BMI_0 - BMI_1). \qquad (2)$$

Using 54.9 (the mean Cormic Index of haemoglobin AA controls) in the regression equation for estimating BMI yielded a value of 14.5.

Thus, the final model is

$$BMI_{std} = 14.5 + (BMI_0 - BMI_1). \qquad (3)$$

$z$-scores were generated for observed BMI as well as the standardized BMI. On the basis of the $z$-scores, study subjects were then categorized into "thin," "normal," or "overweight." Table 5 shows the prevalence of thinness and overweight using both the actual (observed) and the standardized BMI values. Table 5 shows that, altogether, sixty subjects were classified as thin on the basis of $z$-scores of observed BMI. Of these 60, six were identified as thin using $z$-scores of standardized BMI. Also, five subjects were adjudged overweight using observed BMI: four of these five subjects were identified as overweight using standardized BMI.

## 4. Discussion

Cormic Indices were comparable between male and female children with sickle cell anaemia. Unfortunately, there are no local or international figures for comparison. However, mean Cormic Index decreased progressively with age both in primary subjects and in controls. This is consistent with the expected physiologic trend in which the lower limbs grow relatively faster than the trunk in early childhood.

Specifically, comparison of mean Cormic Index between HbSS subjects and controls older than 10 years showed that controls have significantly higher mean Cormic Index values than sickle cell anaemia subjects irrespective of gender. Interestingly, the significant difference was not recorded in males following gender stratification. The explanation for the different pattern in males and females is not clear. This significantly lower mean value among females with sickle cell anaemia older than 10 years translates to relatively shorter trunks which may be explained by narrowing of intervertebral discs as a result of repeated vasoocclusion [17, 18]. Added to this explanation is the fact that increase in sitting height is relatively faster than leg length in later childhood [8, 19]. The negative effect of sickle cell anaemia on spinal growth would therefore be expected to be more obvious in older children during the period of expected rapid growth.

Thus, the finding of lower Cormic Index in older subjects might be expected but the limitation of the observation to girls is not readily explained. It is plausible that the observation represents a relatively minor trend that has

TABLE 5: The effect of adjusting the BMI of subjects with sickle cell anaemia for a mean Cormic Index of 54.9%.

| Age group | Thinness | | Overweight | |
| --- | --- | --- | --- | --- |
| | Actual | Adjusted | Actual | Adjusted |
| ≤2 yrs | | | | |
| Males | 8 (61.5) | 4 (30.8) | 1 (7.7) | 0 (0.0) |
| Females | 4 (30.8) | 1 (7.7) | 1 (7.7) | 1 (7.7) |
| Males and females | 12 (46.2) | 5 (19.2) | 2 (7.7) | 1 (7.7) |
| >2 yrs–5 yrs | | | | |
| Males | 7 (53.8) | 0 (0.0) | 1 (7.7) | 0 (0.0) |
| Females | 7 (53.8) | 0 (0.0) | 0 (0.0) | 0 (0.0) |
| Males and females | 14 (53.8) | 0 (0.0) | 1 (3.9) | 0 (0.0) |
| >5 yrs–10 yrs | | | | |
| Males | 5 (41.7) | 0 (0.0) | 1 (8.3) | 1 (8.3) |
| Females | 8 (66.7) | 1 (8.3) | 0 (0.0) | 0 (0.0) |
| Males and females | 13 (54.2) | 1 (4.2) | 1 (8.3) | 1 (8.3) |
| >10 yrs–15 yrs | | | | |
| Males | 9 (75.0) | 0 (0.0) | 1 (8.3) | 2 (16.7) |
| Females | 12 (100) | 0 (0.0) | 0 (0.0) | 0 (0.0) |
| Males and females | 21 (87.5) | 0 (0.0) | 1 (4.2) | 1 (4.2) |
| All | | | | |
| Males | 29 (58.0) | 4 (8.0) | 4 (8.0) | 3 (6.0) |
| Females | 31 (82.0) | 2 (4.0) | 1 (2.0) | 1 (2.0) |
| Males and females | 60 (60.0) | 6 (6.0) | 5 (5.0) | 4 (4.0) |

been exaggerated by peculiar circumstances of the female subjects in the current study. Only further studies, possibly with much larger subgroups, can elucidate the situation. A plausible explanation could be that there was a fortuitous concentration of female sickle cell anaemia with relatively less severe affection of height.

Significant negative correlations were detected between Cormic Index and height ($r$ = −0.868, −0.855) in boys and girls, respectively. This is purely an arithmetical relationship: height is the denominator in the Cormic Index. Therefore, the ratio should increase as the denominator reduces and vice versa.

It was also observed that strong negative correlations existed between Cormic Index and age (0.752, 0.744). Similar observations have been reported in a study of healthy Bengalee children aged six years to 12 years [5]. Both the sitting height and height are linear measurements which increase physiologically in the same direction with age. Arithmetically, this ratio could be reduced if the sitting height is relatively short. Several previous studies have shown that increase in sitting height is faster than leg length in later childhood [20, 21]. A disease like sickle cell anaemia that affects growth is therefore more likely to adversely affect sitting height in later childhood.

From the result of this study there is significant positive correlation when sitting height was compared to subischial height. This study has also demonstrated that Cormic Index has a direct relationship with sitting height and subischial leg length. That is to say, it is the size of the trunk that mainly determines the body Cormic Index and not subischial leg length.

A positive correlation exists between Cormic Index and BMI in subjects with sickle cell anaemia and controls, although this correlation is relatively weak (<0.4). The low $r$-values indicate that the Cormic Index is a minor determinant of BMI. This corroborates a study of Nigerians aged between 15 and 56 years in whom weak positive correlation between Cormic Index and BMI was observed [22].

BMI is known to vary with age and body shape. The cut-off used for BMI classification is the same in both children with and children without sickle cell anaemia. There is a marked difference between body shape of children with sickle cell anaemia and that without sickle cell anaemia. In order to account for changes in this documented body shape, the Cormic Index was standardized to compare the BMI of different haemoglobin genotype populations to prevent or reduce the overestimation of prevalence of BMI abnormalities. Upon standardization, the current study showed a 90% reduction in the proportion of subjects otherwise classified as thin. The effect of the standardization was far less felt at the upper end of the BMI spectrum. Indeed, there was only a 17% reduction in the number of subjects classified as overweight. It is thus attractive to argue that the standardization will be more relevant when the objective was to determine proportion of thinness among subjects with sickle cell anaemia.

The extent to which the standardization in the current study applies across races or ethnic groups can only be confirmed by further study. Also, it is plausible that severity of illness may influence the interrelationships between Cormic Index and BMI measurements. Thus, it may be argued that regions with milder or more severe disease expressions may require developing their own standardization models.

In conclusion, the mean Cormic Index decreased with age in both subjects and controls. The mean Cormic Index for children with sickle cell anaemia is comparable with that of HbAA controls except in females older than 10 years that the mean Cormic Index was significantly higher among AA controls than their SS counterparts. The correlation analysis between Cormic Index and height is strongly negative. This may be of great importance for the field of anthropology and forensic medicine. Adjusting for body proportions in classifying BMI drastically reduced the number of sickle cell anaemia subjects who would have been categorized as thin.

## Conflict of Interests

The authors declare that there is no conflict of interests regarding the publication of this paper.

## Authors' Contribution

The study was conceived by all the authors. Data was collected by all authors except Omolara Adeolu Kehinde. Samuel Olufemi Akodu and Olisamedua Fidelis Njokanma analyzed the data, while Samuel Olufemi Akodu wrote the initial draft of the paper. All authors reviewed and approved the final paper for submission.

## References

[1] G. R. Serjeant and B. E. Serjeant, *Sickle Cell Disease*, Oxford University Press, New York, NY, USA, 3rd edition, 2001.

[2] E. M. Barden, D. A. Kawchak, K. Ohene-Frempong, V. A. Stallings, and B. S. Zemel, "Body composition in children with sickle cell disease," *The American Journal of Clinical Nutrition*, vol. 76, no. 1, pp. 218–225, 2002.

[3] A.-W. Al-Saqladi, R. Cipolotti, K. Fijnvandraat, and B. J. Brabin, "Growth and nutritional status of children with homozygous sickle cell disease," *Annals of Tropical Paediatrics*, vol. 28, no. 3, pp. 165–189, 2008.

[4] L. Beker and T. L. Cheng, "Principles of growth assessment," *Pediatrics in Review*, vol. 27, no. 5, pp. 196–198, 2006.

[5] M. C. Ukwuma, "A study of the cormic index in a Southeastern Nigerian population," *The Internet Journal of Biological Anthropology*, vol. 4, no. 1, 2009.

[6] M. Siahkouhian and M. Hedayatneja, "Correlations of anthropometric and body composition variables with the performance of young elite weightlifters," *Journal of Human Kinetics*, vol. 25, no. 1, pp. 125–131, 2010.

[7] N. G. Norgan, "Relative sitting height and the interpretation of the body mass index," *Annals of Human Biology*, vol. 21, no. 1, pp. 79–82, 1994.

[8] B. S. Zemel, D. A. Kawchak, K. Ohene-Frempong, J. I. Schall, and V. A. Stallings, "Effects of delayed pubertal development, nutritional status, and disease severity on longitudinal patterns of growth failure in children with sickle cell disease," *Pediatric Research*, vol. 61, no. 5, pp. 607–613, 2007.

[9] M. T. Ashcroft, G. R. Serjeant, and P. Desai, "Heights, weights, and skeletal age of Jamaican adolescents with sickle cell anaemia," *Archives of Disease in Childhood*, vol. 47, no. 254, pp. 519–524, 1972.

[10] B. A. Woodruff and A. Duffield, "Anthropometric assessment of nutritional status in adolescent populations in humanitarian emergencies," *European Journal of Clinical Nutrition*, vol. 56, no. 11, pp. 1108–1118, 2002.

[11] N. G. Norgan, "Interpretation of low body mass indices: Australian aborigines," *American Journal of Physical Anthropology*, vol. 94, no. 2, pp. 229–237, 1994.

[12] S. Pheasant, "Body space: anthropometry, ergonomics and design," *American Journal of Physical Anthropology*, vol. 4, pp. 331–334, 1986.

[13] O. Awotua-Efebo, E. A. O. Alikor, and K. E. O. Nkanginieme, "Malaria parasite density and splenic status by ultrasonography in stable sickle-cell anaemia (HbSS) children," *Nigerian Journal of Medicine*, vol. 13, no. 1, pp. 40–44, 2004.

[14] M. A. Carpenter, M. S. Tockman, R. G. Hutchinson, C. E. Davis, and G. Heiss, "Demographic and anthropometric correlates of maximum inspiratory pressure: the Atherosclerosis Risk in Communities Study," *American Journal of Respiratory and Critical Care Medicine*, vol. 159, no. 2, pp. 415–422, 1999.

[15] G. A. Oyedeji, "Socio-economic and cultural background of hospitalized children in Ilesha," *Nigerian Journal of Paediatrics*, vol. 12, no. 4, pp. 111–117, 1985.

[16] N. G. Norgan, "Body mass index and nutritional status: the effect of adjusting body mass index for the relative sitting height on estimates of the prevalence of chronic energy deficiency, overweight and obesity," *Asia Pacific Journal of Clinical Nutrition*, vol. 4, no. 1, pp. 137–139, 1995.

[17] M. Sadat-Ali, A. Ammar, J. R. Corea, and A. W. Ibrahim, "The spine in sickle cell disease," *International Orthopaedics*, vol. 18, no. 3, pp. 154–156, 1994.

[18] J. O. Ozoh, M. A. C. Onuigbo, N. Nwankwo, S. O. Ukabam, B. C. Umerah, and C. C. Emeruwa, "'Vanishing' of vertebra in a patient with sickle cell haemoglobinopathy," *British Medical Journal*, vol. 301, no. 6765, pp. 1368–1369, 1990.

[19] M. T. Ashcroft, G. R. Serjeant, and P. Desai, "Heights, weights, and skeletal age of Jamaican adolescents with sickle cell anaemia," *Archives of Disease in Childhood*, vol. 47, no. 254, pp. 519–524, 1972.

[20] P. Dasgupta and S. R. Das, "A cross-sectional growth study of trunk and limb segments of the Bengali boys of Calcutta," *Annals of Human Biology*, vol. 24, no. 4, pp. 363–369, 1997.

[21] J. M. Tanner, R. H. Whitehouse, E. Marubini, and L. F. Resele, "The adolescent growth spurt of boys and girls of the Harpenden growth study," *Annals of Human Biology*, vol. 3, no. 2, pp. 109–126, 1976.

[22] D. O. Adeyemi, O. A. Komolafe, and A. I. Abioye, "Variations in body mass indices among post-pubertal Nigerian subjects with correlation to cormic indices, mid-arm circumferences and waist circumferences," *The Internet Journal of Biological Anthropology*, vol. 2, no. 2, 2009.

# 14

# Sickle Cell Disease Activates Peripheral Blood Mononuclear Cells to Induce Cathepsins K and V Activity in Endothelial Cells

**Philip M. Keegan, Sindhuja Surapaneni, and Manu O. Platt**

*Wallace H. Coulter Department of Biomedical Engineering, Georgia Institute of Technology and Emory University, Atlanta, GA 30332, USA*

Correspondence should be addressed to Manu O. Platt, manu.platt@bme.gatech.edu

Academic Editor: Betty S. Pace

Sickle cell disease is a genetic disease that increases systemic inflammation as well as the risk of pediatric strokes, but links between sickle-induced inflammation and arterial remodeling are not clear. Cathepsins are powerful elastases and collagenases secreted by endothelial cells and monocyte-derived macrophages in atherosclerosis, but their involvement in sickle cell disease has not been studied. Here, we investigated how tumor necrosis alpha (TNF$\alpha$) and circulating mononuclear cell adhesion to human aortic endothelial cells (ECs) increase active cathepsins K and V as a model of inflammation occurring in the arterial wall. ECs were stimulated with TNF$\alpha$ and cultured with peripheral blood mononuclear cells (PBMCs) from persons homozygous for sickle (SS) or normal (AA) hemoglobin. TNF$\alpha$ was necessary to induce cathepsin K activity, but either PBMC binding or TNF$\alpha$ increased cathepsin V activity. SS PBMCs were unique; they induced cathepsin K in ECs without exogenous TNF$\alpha$ ($n = 4$, $P < 0.05$). Inhibition of c-Jun N-terminal kinase (JNK) significantly reduced cathepsins K and V activation by 60% and 51%, respectively. Together, the inflammation and activated circulating mononuclear cells upregulate cathepsin activity through JNK signaling, identifying new pharmaceutical targets to block the accelerated pathology observed in arteries of children with sickle cell disease.

## 1. Introduction

Sickle cell disease is a genetic disorder that causes *in vivo* polymerization of hemoglobin molecules into rigid fibers within red blood cells, deforming them in the canonically described "sickle" shape. Rigid, sickled red blood cells and the byproducts of their hemolysis cause chronic vascular damage and increase systemic levels of inflammatory cytokines, mobilized mononuclear cells [1], and pathological levels of increased monocyte adhesion to the endothelium [2, 3]. Overall, these pathological inflammatory conditions and mononuclear cell-endothelial cell interactions may contribute to intimal thickening, and lumen narrowing seen in pulmonary hypertension and stroke lesions of children; pulmonary hypertension is responsible for 20–30% of sickle-cell-related deaths in adult patients [4, 5] and 11% of children with sickle cell disease will suffer from a major stroke by the age of 16.

Both of these clinical syndromes are characterized by vascular remodeling [6–8]. Vascular remodeling analogous to stroke lesions in sickle cell disease has been observed in atherosclerosis, the major cardiovascular disease, where mononuclear cell infiltration of the subendothelial space, degradation of the elastic lamina, and subsequent smooth muscle cell proliferation mediate lesion progression and luminal narrowing [2]. These similarities suggest that common mechanisms for arterial remodeling may exist between the well-studied, well-characterized atherosclerosis, and the less understood mechanisms of sickle cell disease.

Arterial remodeling can be defined as changes in the composition of proteins, cell types, and even cell phenotypes that induce chronic effects on the structure, mechanical properties, and total health of the artery [6–8]. This includes degradation of old matrix by newly activated proteases as well as synthesis and deposition of new extracellular matrix proteins. Cysteine cathepsins, one such family of proteases upregulated in arterial remodeling [6, 9], belong to the papain superfamily of proteases and contain the most potent human collagenases and elastases [10]. Increased cathepsin activity has been linked to tissue destruction in the cardiovascular system with atherosclerotic elastic lamina degradation [11–13], stent restenosis [14, 15], abdominal aortic aneurysm formation [16], and heart valve remodeling under hypertensive conditions [9].

Two cathepsins in particular have gained significant interest in their role in arterial remodeling in cardiovascular disease. Cathepsin K is the most potent human collagenase yet identified [17], as well as an extremely powerful elastase [18, 19]. Additionally, cathepsin K has been shown to be highly expressed in atherosclerotic lesions where it degrades arterial collagen and subendothelial elastic lamina [12, 13]. Cathepsin V is the most powerful mammalian elastase yet identified and is expressed in human monocyte-derived macrophages [10]. Studies have shown that the human cathepsin V homolog, murine cathepsin L [20, 21], significantly contributes to cardiovascular disease in mouse models [9, 22]. Neither of these two enzymes has been linked to sickle-cell-disease induced vascular wall remodeling and pathology.

In this study, we evaluated the potential involvement of cathepsin-mediated arterial remodeling in sickle cell disease by studying the effects of TNF$\alpha$ stimulation and adhesion of mononuclear cells isolated from whole blood of individuals homozygous for the sickle mutation on endothelial cell expression and activation of cathepsins K and V. We employed a novel, multiplex cathepsin zymography technique to simultaneously quantify the active forms of cathepsins K, L, S, and V in response to the different stimulation and coculture conditions [23]. Furthermore, we investigated the phosphorylation of key kinases to identify intracellular signaling cascades linking TNF$\alpha$ stimulation and mononuclear cell binding to increased levels of active cathepsins K and V as a proposed model for the unique and accelerated tissue remodeling observed in arteries of children and adults living with sickle cell disease.

## 2. Materials and Methods

*2.1. Ethics Statement.* All protocols were reviewed and approved by the Georgia Institute of Technology Institutional Review Board, and informed consent was received from all participants. In the case of minors, assent was provided by parents/guardians.

*2.2. Cell Culture.* Human aortic endothelial cells (HAECs) (Lonza) were cultured in MCDB medium 131 (Mediatech) containing 10% fetal bovine serum (FBS), 1% L-glutamine, 1% penicillin/streptomycin, and 1% endothelial cell growth serum (ECGS). Cells were maintained with 5% $CO_2$ at 37°C.

*2.3. TNF$\alpha$ ELISA.* Whole blood samples were allowed to coagulate for 6 hours, followed by centrifugation at 900 g for 30 minutes to remove platelets and cells. The supernatant was collected, and TNF$\alpha$ levels were quantified using an enzyme-linked immunosorbent assay (ELISA) specific for soluble, human TNF$\alpha$ (R&D Biosystems). Absorbance values were recorded using Synergy 4 (Biotek) at 450 nm with correction readings at 540 nm. Quantification of TNF$\alpha$

protein levels was calculated by generating a four-parameter logistic standard curve using Gen5 software (Biotek).

*2.4. Peripheral Blood Mononuclear Cell Isolation.* Whole blood samples were obtained from males and females homozygous for sickle (SS) or normal (AA) hemoglobin; patients on hydroxyurea, chronic transfusion, or who had experienced a recent crisis were excluded from this study. Whole blood samples were centrifuged against a Ficoll-Paque density gradient (density: 1.077 g/mL; GE Healthcare) for 30 minutes at 2450 rpm to separate the buffy coat layer. After centrifugation, peripheral blood mononuclear cells (PBMCs) were aspirated, washed in PBS, and pelleted by centrifugation for 10 minutes. The isolated cells were then washed with a red blood cell lysis buffer (0.83% ammonium chloride, 0.1% potassium bicarbonate, and 0.0037% EDTA) for seven minutes to remove any contaminating RBCs. Cell number and viability were determined using a Vi-Cell (Beckman Coulter).

*2.5. PBMC Adhesion Assay.* HAECs were preconditioned in normal growth media in the presence or absence of 10 ng/mL recombinant human TNF$\alpha$ (Invitrogen) and cultured for 4 hours prior to the addition of 500,000 PBMCs/mL. Isolated PBMCs were allowed to adhere for 45 minutes prior to washing three times with PBS, and then cocultures were maintained for an additional 20 hours. For JNK inhibition studies, endothelial cells were preconditioned with 10 $\mu$g/mL of SP600125 (EMD Biosciences) for one hour prior to addition of media containing vehicle, 10 ng/mL TNF$\alpha$, and/or 10 $\mu$g/mL of SP600125.

*2.6. Phosphorylated Kinase Screening.* Cell lysates were prepared per BioPlex Suspension Array System instructions (BioRad). Lysates were incubated overnight with fluorescently labeled beads specific for the phosphorylated forms of Akt (Ser473), extracellular signal-regulated kinases 1 and 2 (Thr202/Tyr204, Thr185/Tyr187), c-Jun NH$_2$-terminal kinase (JNK) (Thr 183 /Tyr 185), and c-Jun (Ser63) (BioRad). The samples were then washed and incubated with kinase-specific, biotinylated antibodies for 2 hours, followed by treatment with avidin/streptavidin tagged with phycoerythrin. Phosphorylated kinase levels were measured using a BioPlex 200 System (BioRad).

*2.7. Multiplex Cathepsin Zymography.* Cathepsin zymography was performed as described previously [24]. Determination of cathepsin V band required incubation in acetate buffer, pH 4 [25]. Gels were imaged using an ImageQuant 4010 system (GE Healthcare). Images were inverted in Adobe Photoshop and densitometry was performed using Scion Image.

*2.8. Statistical Analysis.* Each experimental condition was repeated with a minimum of three biological replicates, and each data point is presented as the mean value and standard error of the mean. Representative images are shown.

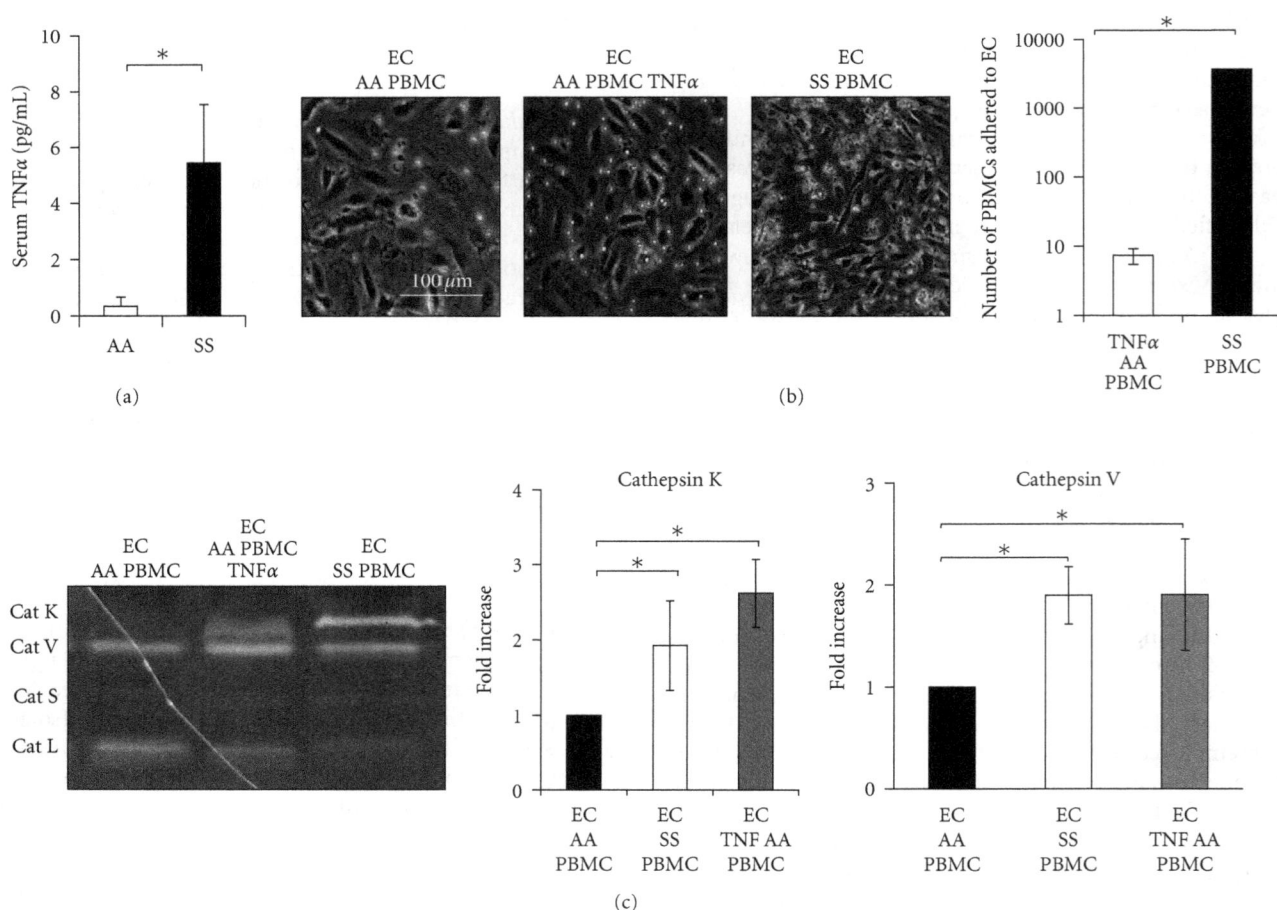

FIGURE 1: Sickle cell disease preconditions circulating peripheral blood mononuclear cells to induce cathepsin K activity. Whole blood samples were obtained from donors homozygous for the normal $\beta$-globin allele (AA) and homozygous for the sickle allele (SS). (a) Baseline serum levels of TNF$\alpha$ were quantified using an ELISA specific for human TNF$\alpha$ ($n = 3$, *$P < 0.05$, SEM bars shown). (b) PBMCs were isolated via differential centrifugation through a density gradient. For cocultures, confluent EC cultures were preconditioned with 10 ng/mL TNF$\alpha$ for 4 hours, prior to the addition of either AA or SS PBMCs. Nonadherent cells were washed away, and cocultures were maintained for an additional 20 hours. Representative images of cocultures were used for mononuclear cell adhesion counts. (c) Cells were lysed and cathepsin K activity was assessed using multiplex cathepsin zymography and quantified via densitometry ($n = 10$, *$P < 0.05$).

Unpaired student $t$-tests were used to determine statistical significance (*$P < 0.05$) between most experimental groups.

## 3. Results

### 3.1. Sickle Cell Disease Preconditions Circulating PBMCs to Induce Cathepsin K Activity.
Whole blood samples were obtained from donors homozygous for normal (AA) or sickle (SS) hemoglobin. First, an ELISA was run to quantify blood serum levels of TNF$\alpha$. SS donors had $5.43 \pm 2.3$ pg/mL of TNF$\alpha$ compared to $0.3 \pm 0.3$ pg/mL of TNF$\alpha$ in AA controls ($n = 3$, $P < 0.05$), an almost 20-fold increase (Figure 1(a)). TNF$\alpha$ stimulation of endothelial cells increased the adhesion of AA PBMCs, compared to unstimulated EC cultures (Figure 1(b)); however, the number of adhered SS PBMCs was 100 times higher than TNF$\alpha$ stimulated AA PBMC cocultures (Figure 1(b); $n = 3$, $P < 0.001$). Cells were cultured together for an additional 20 hours for cathepsin induction, prior to lysing, collection, and multiplex

cathepsin zymography. SS PBMCs significantly increased levels of active cathepsins K and V when cocultured with endothelial cells, and without exogenous TNF$\alpha$ stimulation (Figure 1(c)), suggesting that the SS PBMCs were preconditioned to induce this activity. AA PBMC cocultures in the absence of TNF$\alpha$ lacked detectable bands of active cathepsin K (Figure 1(c), left lane).

### 3.2. TNFa Stimulation and PBMC Interactions with Endothelial Cells Activate JNK Signaling.
To investigate the intracellular signal cascades increasing the levels of active cathepsins K and V downstream of TNF$\alpha$ and PBMC adhesion cues, we measured phosphorylation of JNK, c-jun, Akt, and ERK1/2 using Bioplex/Luminex technology, a quantitative bead-based immunofluorescent assay that allowed measurement of all four signals in one cell extract after 24 hours of coculture. JNK and its downstream signaling protein substrate, c-Jun, showed the greatest activation in response to TNF$\alpha$ stimulation with or without AA or SS PBMCs (Figures 2(a)

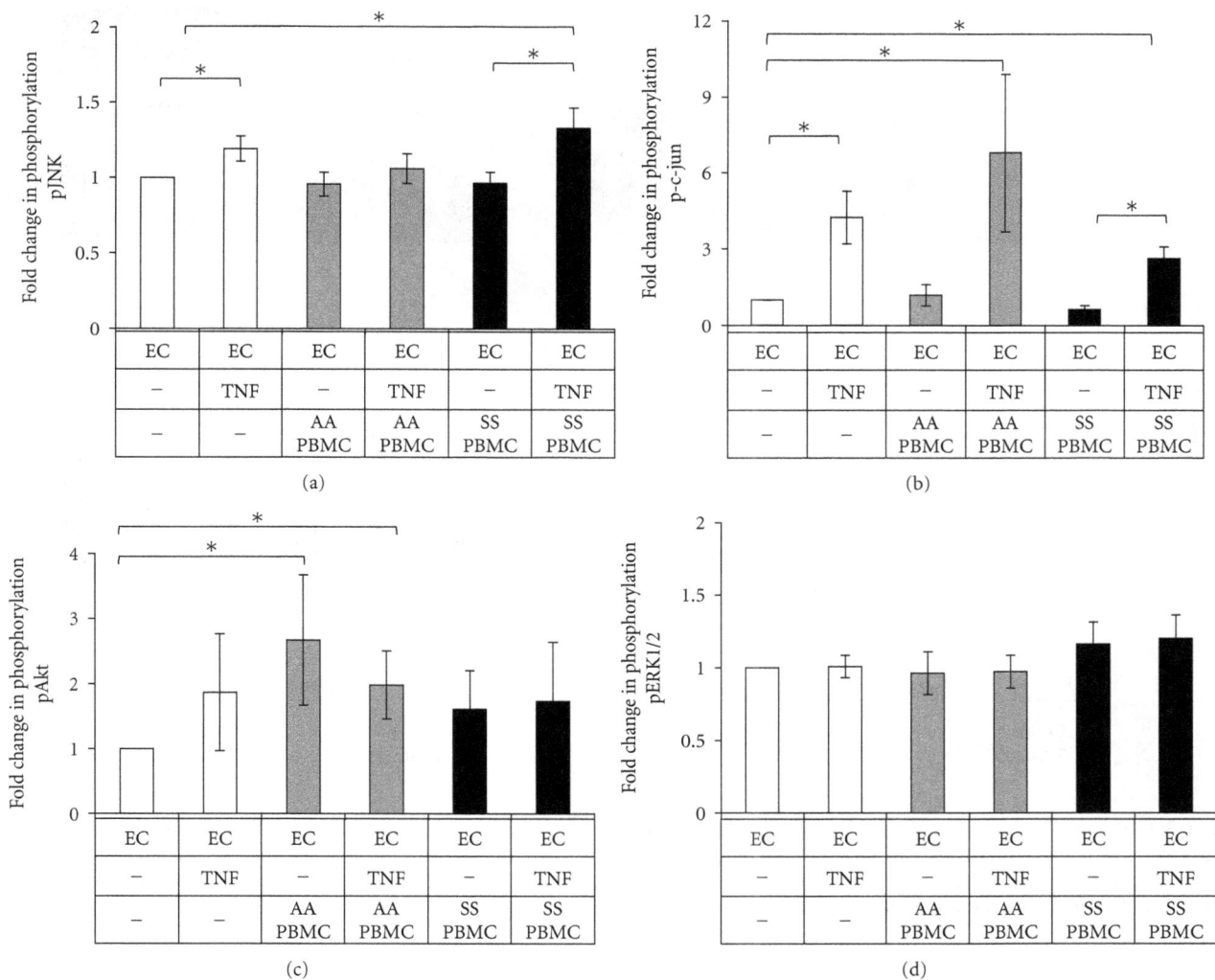

FIGURE 2: TNFα and PBMC interactions increase JNK and Akt phosphorylation. Confluent HAECs were cocultured with peripheral blood mononuclear cells isolated from AA or SS donors, and lysates were collected for kinase analysis. Levels of phosphorylated (a) JNK, (b) c-Jun, (c) Akt, and (d) ERK1/2 were measured, and phosphorylated kinase signals were normalized to unstimulated HAEC control ($n = 3$, *$P < 0.05$, SEM bars shown).

and 2(b), $n = 3$, $P < 0.01$) with c-Jun activation as high as 6-fold that of the EC controls. Akt phosphorylation was significantly increased by AA PBMC binding alone even without TNFα stimulation (Figure 2(c), $n = 3$, $P < 0.01$). There were no changes in ERK 1/2 phosphorylation in any condition for all time points measured (Figure 2(d)).

3.3. Cathepsins K and V Activities Induced by Sickle Cell Disease PBMCs Were Significantly Reduced by JNK Inhibition. Since JNK and c-jun phosphorylation were significantly upregulated, we tested if inhibiting this signal cascade would block the increase in levels of active cathepsins K and V by endothelial cells after adhesion and coculture with SS PBMCs. HAECs were cultured with or without SP600125, a JNK inhibitor, for 1 hour prior to addition of 10 ng/mL TNFα or vehicle. AA or SS PBMCs were subsequently added, and nonadhered cells were washed away. Cell lysates were

collected after 24 hours, and cathepsin activity was assessed through multiplex cathepsin zymography. SP600125 significantly reduced the upregulated cathepsin K and cathepsin V activities of unstimulated SS PBMCs when cocultured with endothelial cells by 48% and 29%, respectively (Figure 3; $n = 5$, $P < 0.05$).

## 4. Discussion

Endothelial cell expression of cathepsins and increased cathepsin-mediated elastase activity are upregulated during atherosclerotic development and induced by inflammation and altered hemodynamics [9, 12, 13, 26, 27], which are both present in sickle cell disease [26], leading to our hypothesis that elevated TNFα and increased circulating mononuclear cells would stimulate increased endothelial cell cathepsin activity. This elevated activity may contribute to arterial

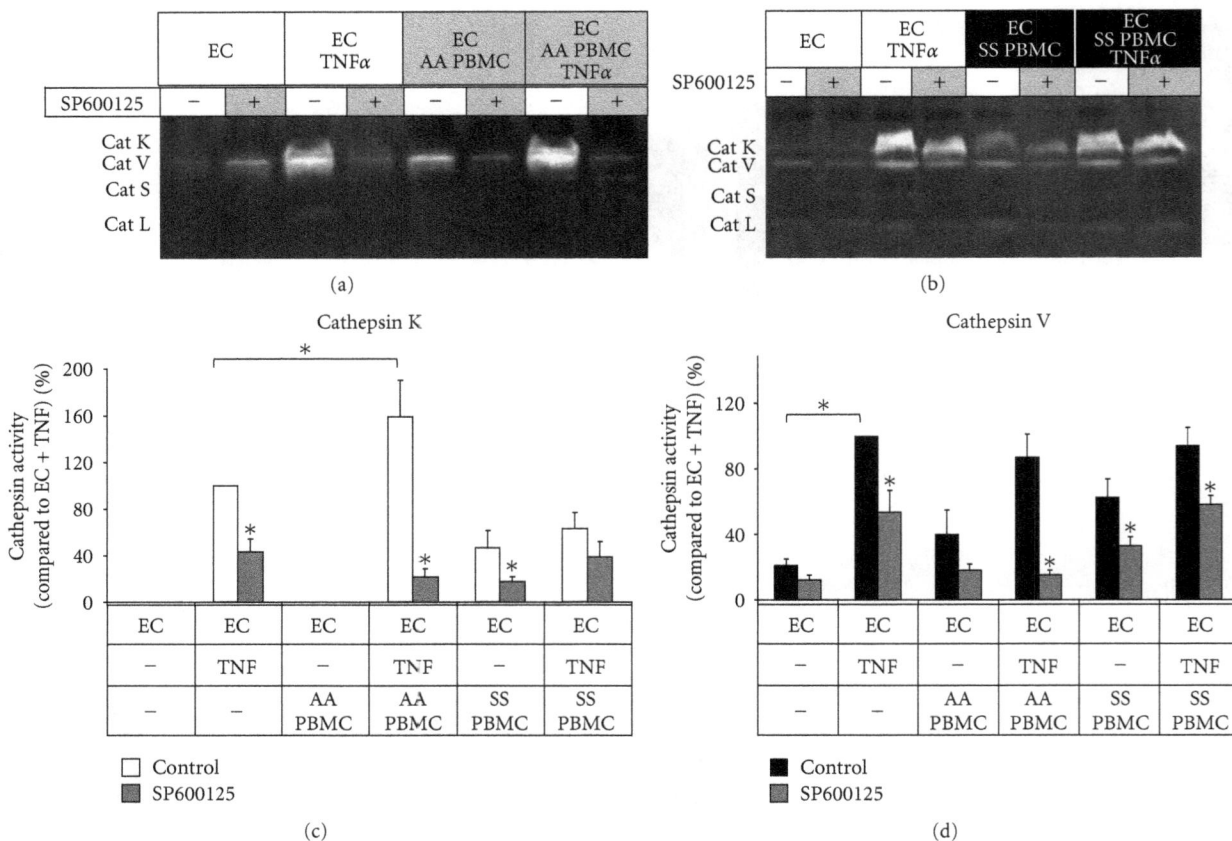

FIGURE 3: Cathepsins K and V activities induced by sickle cell disease PBMCs are significantly reduced by JNK inhibition with SP600125. HAECs were incubated with or without $10\,\mu M$ of the JNK inhibitor, SP600125, 1 hour prior to TNF$\alpha$ stimulation, as described previously. Cocultures with AA or SS PBMCs were maintained for an additional 20 hours. Cell lysates were collected and analyzed via multiplex cathepsin zymography. Densitometric analysis quantified active cathepsins K and cathepsin V ($n = 3$, $^*P < 0.05$, SEM bars shown).

remodeling in sickle cell disease. The findings of this study specifically implicate TNF$\alpha$ and mononuclear cell binding to endothelium as key mediators, and that circulating mononuclear cells in sickle cell disease are predisposed to induce cathepsin proteolytic activity.

Here, we have specifically shown that TNF$\alpha$ stimulation increased the expression and activity of the most potent mammalian collagenase and elastase, cathepsins K and V, respectively (Figure 1). Additionally, SS PBMCs significantly increased cathepsin K activity in endothelial cells in the absence of TNF$\alpha$, suggesting that they were preconditioned in the blood for adhesion to endothelium and cathepsin K induction (Figure 1); AA PBMCs required TNF$\alpha$ stimulation to reach these higher levels of cathepsin K and V (Figure 1). These findings are consistent with reports that circulating sickle erythrocytes increase mononuclear cell activation and adhesion to endothelial cells [28] and support our hypothesis that the blood milieu of people living with sickle cell disease predisposes circulating mononuclear cells to adhere to endothelium and promote arterial remodeling. Previous studies have already established that the circulatory environment in sickle cell disease preconditions peripheral blood mononuclear cells into a pathologically activated state, where these cells produce 139% more TNF$\alpha$ per cell than

control mononuclear cells [28, 29]; these mechanisms may be at play here leading to increased active cathepsins K and V.

Inhibition of JNK signaling with SP600125 reduced the inflammation-induced activation of cathepsins K and V in AA and SS PBMC cocultures with endothelium (Figure 3). These findings highlight the role of JNK signaling as an integration control point and as a therapeutic target to inhibit the initiation of gene and protein expression in response to inflammatory stimuli resulting in endothelial cell upregulation of cathepsins K and V protein and activity. More importantly, the predisposition of SS PBMCs to induce these effects suggests that these novel mechanisms may be occurring constantly in the vasculature of individuals with sickle cell disease. It will be important to continue these studies quantifying cathepsin activation of SS donors with and without stroke or with high transcranial Doppler velocities known to be a risk factor for stroke to parse differential activation mechanisms potentially responsible for the increased risk. Such investigations may reveal novel biomarkers relevant to stroke risk prediction in pediatric patients and open new avenues for pharmaceutical therapies to prevent the arterial remodeling and luminal narrowing that cause cardiovascular complications and death.

## 5. Conclusion

Elevated inflammatory factors and circulating mononuclear cells inherent to sickle cell disease induce pathologically high levels of cathepsins K and V activity when binding to and stimulating endothelial cells, increasing proteolytic activity that may be involved in arterial wall remodeling to increase risk of stroke and pulmonary hypertension. There is a pressing need for novel pharmaceutical targets to inhibit these activities, and from this work, we propose that JNK, cathepsin K, and cathepsin V are three new targets for inhibition to reduce pathological arterial remodeling in sickle cell disease.

## Conflict of Interests

The authors have declared that no competing interests exist.

## Acknowledgments

The authors of this paper would like to thank Eric Kopfle and Alex Miller for assistance with data collection. Additionally, the authors would like to thank the Sickle Cell Foundation of Georgia for collecting and recruiting blood donors for these studies. This paper was funded by Georgia Tech startup funds and NIH New Innovator Grant no. 1DP2OD007433-01 (M. O. Platt) from the Office of the Director, National Institutes of Health. The content is solely the responsibility of the authors and does not necessarily represent the official views of the Office of the Director, National Institutes of Health, or the National Institutes of Health. P. M. Keegan was supported by an NSF graduate research fellowship. The funders had no role in study design, data collection and analysis, decision to publish, or preparation of the paper.

## References

[1] N. Conran, S. T. O. Saad, F. F. Costa, and T. Ikuta, "Leukocyte numbers correlate with plasma levels of granulocyte-macrophage colony-stimulating factor in sickle cell disease," *Annals of Hematology*, vol. 86, no. 4, pp. 255–261, 2007.

[2] J. A. Switzer, D. C. Hess, F. T. Nichols, and R. J. Adams, "Pathophysiology and treatment of stroke in sickle-cell disease: present and future," *Lancet Neurology*, vol. 5, no. 6, pp. 501–512, 2006.

[3] G. A. Barabino, L. V. McIntire, S. G. Eskin, and D. Sears, "Endothelial cell interactions with sickle cell, sickle trait, mechanically injured, and normal erythrocytes under controlled flow," *Blood*, vol. 70, no. 1, pp. 152–157, 1987.

[4] B. Maître, A. Mekontso-Dessap, A. Habibi et al., "Pulmonary complications in adult sickle cell disease," *Revue des Maladies Respiratoires*, vol. 28, no. 2, pp. 129–137, 2011.

[5] L. A. Verduzco and D. G. Nathan, "Sickle cell disease and stroke," *Blood*, vol. 114, no. 25, pp. 5117–5125, 2009.

[6] J. D. Belcher, H. Mahaseth, T. E. Welch et al., "Critical role of endothelial cell activation in hypoxia-induced vasoocclusion in transgenic sickle mice," *American Journal of Physiology*, vol. 288, no. 6, pp. H2715–H2725, 2005.

[7] J. Liu, G. K. Sukhova, J. T. Yang et al., "Cathepsin L expression and regulation in human abdominal aortic aneurysm, atherosclerosis, and vascular cells," *Atherosclerosis*, vol. 184, no. 2, pp. 302–311, 2006.

[8] A. M. Malek, S. L. Alper, and S. Izumo, "Hemodynamic shear stress and its role in atherosclerosis," *Journal of the American Medical Association*, vol. 282, no. 21, pp. 2035–2042, 1999.

[9] M. O. Platt, R. F. Ankeny, and H. Jo, "Laminar shear stress inhibits cathepsin L activity in endothelial cells," *Arteriosclerosis, Thrombosis, and Vascular Biology*, vol. 26, no. 8, pp. 1784–1790, 2006.

[10] Y. Yasuda, Z. Li, D. Greenbaum, M. Bogyo, E. Weber, and D. Brömme, "Cathepsin V, a novel and potent elastolytic activity expressed in activated macrophages," *Journal of Biological Chemistry*, vol. 279, no. 35, pp. 36761–36770, 2004.

[11] G. S. Gacko, "Expression of the elastolytic cathepsins S and K in human atheroma and regulation of their production in smooth muscle cells," *Clinical Chemistry*, vol. 36, pp. 449–452, 1998.

[12] M. O. Platt, R. F. Ankeny, G. P. Shi et al., "Expression of cathepsin K is regulated by shear stress in cultured endothelial cells and is increased in endothelium in human atherosclerosis," *American Journal of Physiology*, vol. 292, no. 3, pp. H1479–H1486, 2007.

[13] G. K. Sukhova, D. I. Simon, H. A. Chapman, and P. Libby, "Expression of the elastolytic cathepsins S and K in human atheroma and regulation of their production in smooth muscle cells," *The Journal of Clinical Investigation*, vol. 102, no. 3, pp. 576–583, 1998.

[14] C. L. Burns-Kurtis, A. R. Olzinski, S. Needle et al., "Cathepsin S expression is up-regulated following balloon angioplasty in the hypercholesterolemic rabbit," *Cardiovascular Research*, vol. 62, no. 3, pp. 610–620, 2004.

[15] A. Garcia-Touchard, T. D. Henry, G. Sangiorgi et al., "Extracellular proteases in atherosclerosis and restenosis," *Arteriosclerosis, Thrombosis, and Vascular Biology*, vol. 25, no. 6, pp. 1119–1127, 2005.

[16] H. Abdul-Hussien, R. G. V. Soekhoe, E. Weber et al., "Collagen degradation in the abdominal aneurysm: a conspiracy of matrix metalloproteinase and cysteine collagenases," *American Journal of Pathology*, vol. 170, no. 3, pp. 809–817, 2007.

[17] P. Garnero, O. Borel, I. Byrjalsen et al., "The collagenolytic activity of cathepsin K is unique among mammalian proteinases," *Journal of Biological Chemistry*, vol. 273, no. 48, pp. 32347–32352, 1999.

[18] W. Kafienah, D. Bromme, D. J. Buttle, L. J. Croucher, and A. P. Hollander, "Human cathepsin K cleaves native type I and II collagens at the N-terminal end of the triple helix," *Biochemical Journal*, vol. 331, part 3, pp. 727–732, 1998.

[19] H. A. Chapman, R. J. Riese, and G. P. Shi, "Emerging roles for cysteine proteases in human biology," *Annual Review of Physiology*, vol. 59, pp. 63–88, 1997.

[20] D. Brömme, Z. Li, M. Barnes, and E. Mehler, "Human cathepsin V functional expression, tissue distribution, electrostatic surface potential, enzymatic characterization, and chromosomal localization," *Biochemistry*, vol. 38, no. 8, pp. 2377–2385, 1999.

[21] E. Tolosa, W. Li, Y. Yasuda et al., "Cathepsin V is involved in the degradation of invariant chain in human thymus and is overexpressed in myasthenia gravis," *The Journal of Clinical Investigation*, vol. 112, no. 4, pp. 517–526, 2003.

[22] M. Yang, Y. Zhang, J. Pan et al., "Cathepsin L activity controls adipogenesis and glucose tolerance," *Nature Cell Biology*, vol. 9, no. 8, pp. 970–977, 2007.

[23] B. Chen and M. O. Platt, "Multiplex zymography captures stage-specific activity profiles of cathepsins K, L, and S in human breast, lung, and cervical cancer," *Journal of Translational Medicine*, vol. 9, pp. 109–2011.

[24] W. A. Li, Z. T. Barry, J. D. Cohen et al., "Detection of femtomole quantities of mature cathepsin K with zymography," *Analytical Biochemistry*, vol. 401, no. 1, pp. 91–98, 2010.

[25] C. L. Wilder and M. O. Platt, "Manipulating substrate and pH in zymography protocols selectively identifies cathepsins K, L, S, and V activity in cells and tissues," *Archives of Biochemistry and Biophysics*, vol. 516, no. 1, pp. 52–57, 2011.

[26] G. A. Barabino, M. O. Platt, and D. K. Kaul, "Sickle cell biomechanics," *Annual Review of Biomedical Engineering*, vol. 12, pp. 345–367, 2010.

[27] G. P. Shi, G. K. Sukhova, A. Grubb et al., "Cystatin C deficiency in human atherosclerosis and aortic aneurysms," *The Journal of Clinical Investigation*, vol. 104, no. 9, pp. 1191–1197, 1999.

[28] R. Zennadi, A. Chien, K. Xu, M. Batchvarova, and M. J. Telen, "Sickle red cells induce adhesion of lymphocytes and monocytes to endothelium," *Blood*, vol. 112, no. 8, pp. 3474–3483, 2008.

[29] J. D. Belcher, P. H. Marker, J. P. Weber, and R. P. Hebbel, "Activated monocytes in sickle cell disease: potential role in the activation of vascular endothelium and vaso-occlusion," *Blood*, vol. 96, no. 7, pp. 2451–2459, 2000.

# 15

# Spatiotemporal Dysfunction of the Vascular Permeability Barrier in Transgenic Mice with Sickle Cell Disease

Samit Ghosh,[1] Fang Tan,[1] and Solomon F. Ofori-Acquah[1,2]

[1] Aflac Cancer and Blood Disorders Center, Division of Hematology/Oncology/BMT, Department of Pediatrics,
  Emory University School of Medicine, Atlanta, GA 30322, USA
[2] Department of Pediatrics, Children's Healthcare of Atlanta, Atlanta, GA 30322, USA

Correspondence should be addressed to Solomon F. Ofori-Acquah, soforia@emory.edu

Academic Editor: Kenneth R. Peterson

Sickle cell disease (SCD) is characterized by chronic intravascular hemolysis that generates excess cell-free hemoglobin in the blood circulation. Hemoglobin causes multiple endothelial dysfunctions including increased vascular permeability, impaired reactivity to vasoactive agonists, and increased adhesion of leukocytes to the endothelium. While the adhesive and vasomotor defects of SCD associated with cell-free hemoglobin are well defined, the vascular permeability phenotype remains poorly appreciated. We addressed this issue in two widely used and clinically relevant mouse models of SCD. We discovered that the endothelial barrier is normal in most organs in the young but deteriorates with aging particularly in the lung. Indeed, middle-aged sickle mice developed pulmonary edema revealing for the first time similarities in the chronic permeability phenotypes of the lung in mice and humans with SCD. Intravenous administration of lysed red blood cells into the circulation of sickle mice increased vascular permeability significantly in the lung without impacting permeability in other organs. Thus, increased vascular permeability is an endothelial dysfunction of SCD with the barrier in the lung likely the most vulnerable to acute inflammation.

## 1. Introduction

Sickle cell disease (SCD) is characterized by the production of red blood cells with increased propensity for lysis and adhesion [1]. Its clinical manifestations fall broadly into two subphenotypes defined by hyperhemolysis and vasoocclusion [2]. At least 30% of the hemolysis in SCD is intravascular [3], which means that the endothelial wall in this disease is persistently exposed to cell-free hemoglobin. The endothelium is a semipermeable barrier that regulates the response of the vascular wall to inflammatory agonists. This response involves activation of adhesion molecule expression, increased permeability of the endothelium, and extravasations of fluid from the blood into interstitial tissue compartments [4]. Increased vascular permeability results from opening of gaps at sites of endothelial cell-cell contacts. There are multiple indicators of systemic inflammation in SCD [5]. In addition, markers of vascular inflammation have also been documented [6–8]. There is increased expression of adhesion molecules in the pulmonary endothelium of the Berkeley sickle mice [9], although the histology of these same mice shows less severe inflammatory and ischemic changes and no evidence of pneumonia [10]. Nonetheless, they spontaneously develop pulmonary hypertension [11], which is a major problem in SCD [12]. Pulmonary edema and the acute chest syndrome implicate increased vascular permeability in both chronic and acute complications of SCD [13, 14]. Despite this significance, there is currently no knowledge of the vascular permeability phenotypes of major organs that are impacted by SCD.

## 2. Materials and Methods

*2.1. Transgenic Sickle Mice.* Experiments were performed using protocols approved by the Institutional Animal Care and Use Committee (IACUC) of Emory University. The Berkeley [15] and Townes [16] transgenic SCD mouse models used have previously been described.

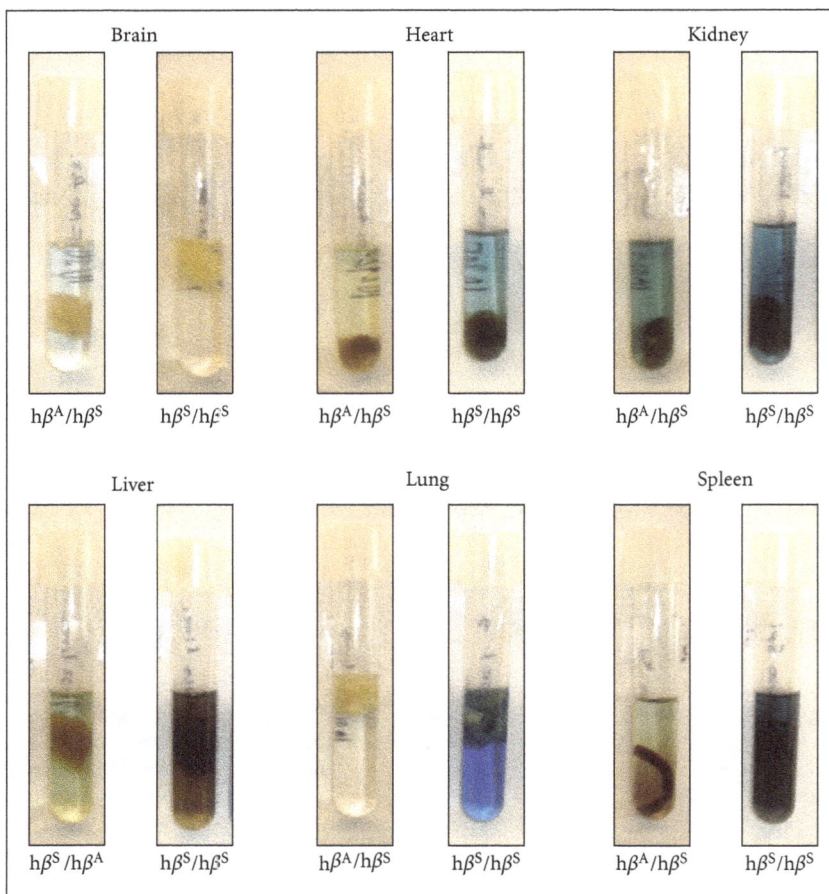

(a)

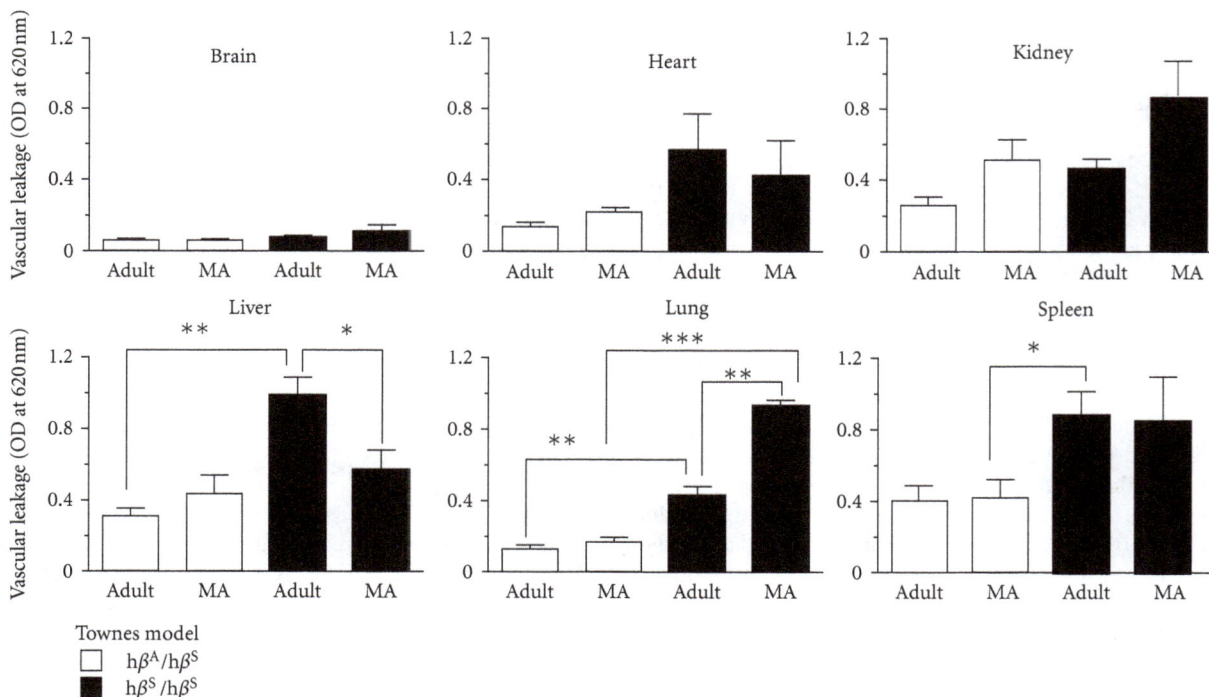

Towbes model

□ hβ$^A$/hβ$^S$
■ hβ$^S$/hβ$^S$

(b)

FIGURE 1: Continued.

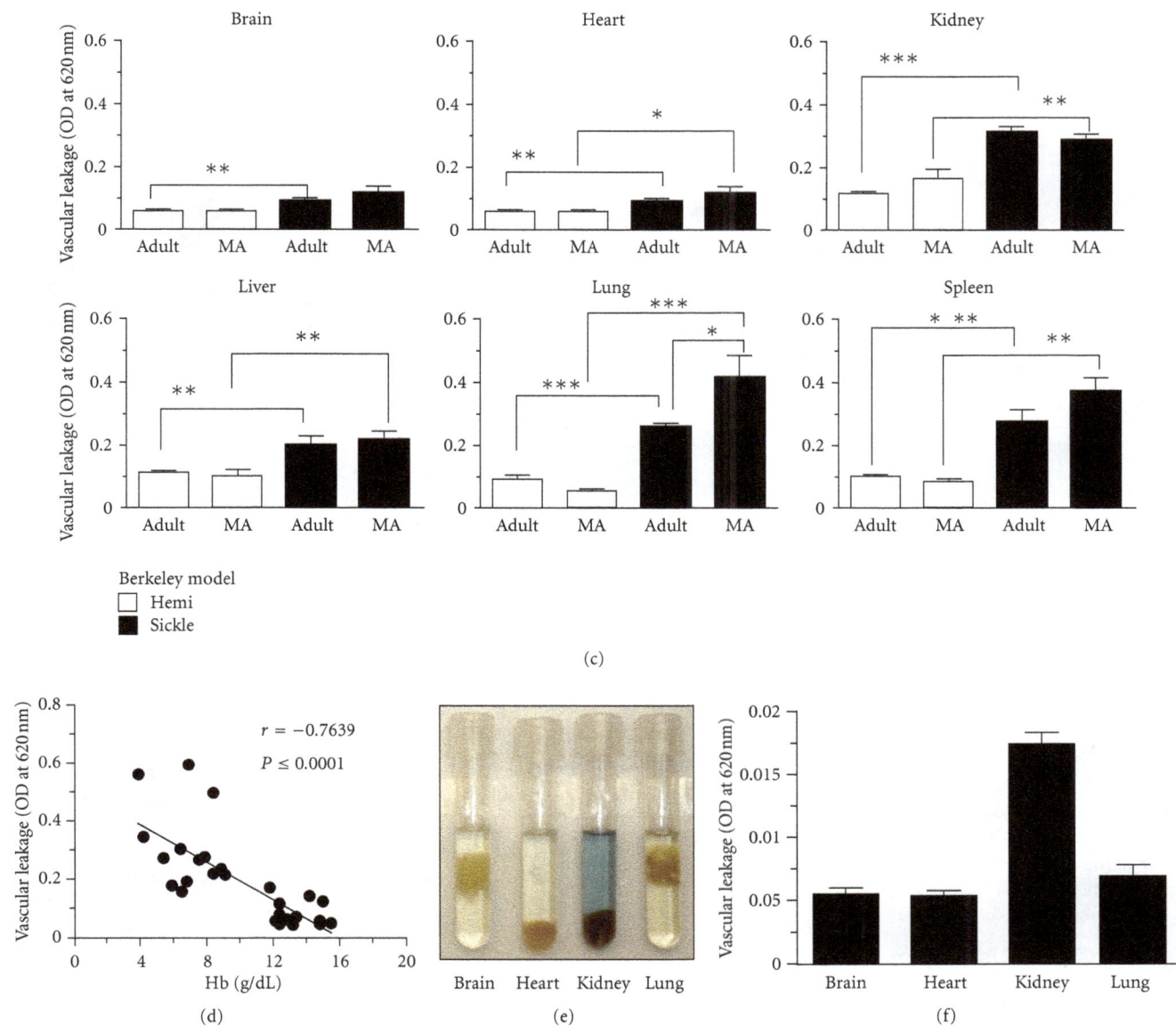

FIGURE 1: Vascular barrier dysfunction in sickle mice. (a) Representative images of organs isolated from sickle mice after injection with Evans blue dye and incubation in formamide for three days. (b, c) Vascular leakage in the indicated organs in adult (3–6 months) and middle-aged (10–13 months) mice of the Townes (heterozygotes-HbAS ($h\beta^A/h\beta^S$) and homozygote sickle-HbSS ($h\beta^S/h\beta^S$)) and Berkeley (hemizygotes and sickle) models. The number of mice studied was as follows: Townes: $n = 3$ for each genotype and age group; Berkeley: Sickle adult, $n = 9$; sickle middle-aged $n = 6$; hemizygote adult, $n = 10$, hemizygote middle-aged $n = 5$. (d) Vascular leakage correlates with hemoglobin. Data shown is the vascular leakage in the lung for a total of 30 mice (15 sickle and 15 hemizygotes) of the Berkeley model. (e) Typical images for the indicated organs isolated from young (4–6 weeks old) Berkeley mice injected with Evans blue dye and incubated in formamide for 3 days. (f) Histogram showing the quantification of Evans blue extravasation of major organs in young sickle mice ($n = 4$). *$P < 0.05$, **$P < 0.01$, and ***$P < 0.001$.

## 2.2. Vascular Leakage and Lung Edema.

Vascular leakage was studied by intravenous injection of cell-impermeable Evan's Blue dye as widely described by several investigators. Mice were injected with 100 μL of 1% cell-impermeable Evans Blue dye (Sigma-Aldrich, St. Louis, MO) in PBS intravenously through tail vein. After 40 min, mice were anesthetized by i.p. injection of avertin (300 mg/kg body weight). To remove the dye from circulation, mice were perfused by injecting 40 mL of PBS containing 2 mM EDTA through left ventricle of the heart allowing the blood to flow out by puncturing renal artery. Organs were harvested and incubated in formamide for 3 days to extract the dye and OD determined at 620 nm. For edema analysis mice were euthanized and the right lobe removed and weighed immediately using an isometric

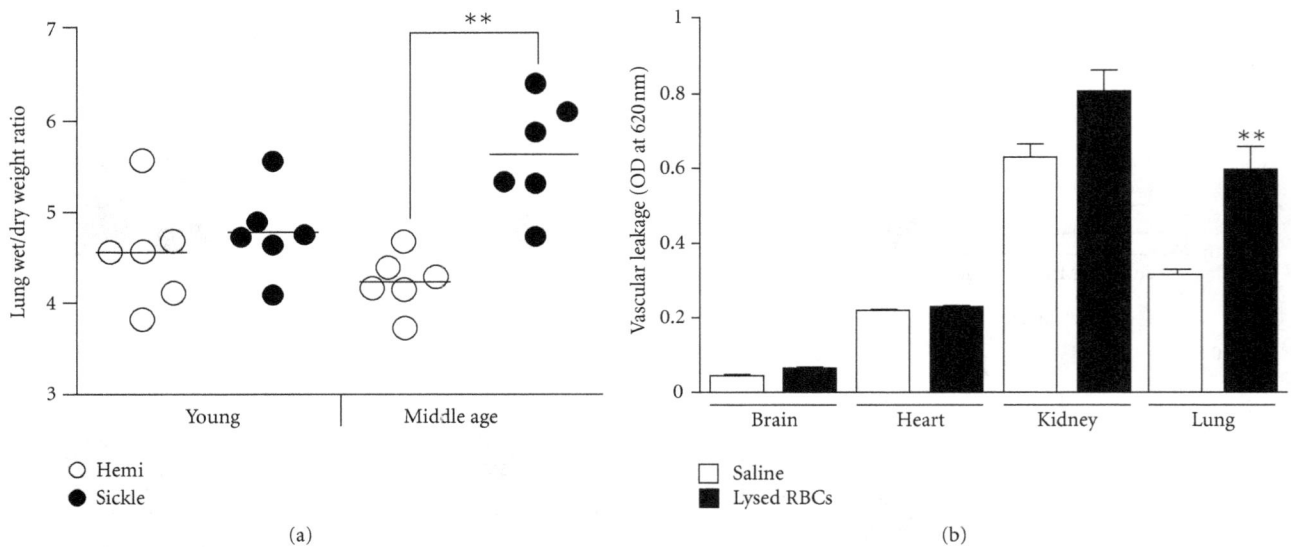

FIGURE 2: Chronic and acute changes in vascular permeability in sickle mouse lungs. (a) Lung edema in middle-aged Berkeley sickle mice as determined by wet/dry weight ratios ($n = 6$). Control groups include young sickle mice ($n = 6$) and young ($n = 6$) and middle-aged ($n = 6$) hemizygotes. (b) Vascular leakage in the indicated organs in Berkeley sickle mice intravenously injected with lysed red blood cells. Note that permeability is significantly increased by lysed red blood cells in the lung but not in other organs. $**P < 0.01$.

transducer (Harvard Apparatus, Holliston, MA). Lungs were dried in an oven at $80°C$ containing desiccant crystals for 24 h, dry weight determined, and ratios calculated.

*2.3. Statistical Analyses.* GraphPad software version 5.0 was used. Differences in vascular leakage and weights were analyzed using $t$-test and correlation studies performed using Pearson's test.

## 3. Results and Discussion

In SCD, the adhesive and vasomotor defects of the vasculature are well defined [17–20], while the vascular permeability remains poorly appreciated. To address this knowledge gap, adult (3–6 months) and middle-aged (10–13 months) mice were injected with 1% Evans blue via the tail vein and the amount of dye that leaked from the circulation into the parenchyma of individual organs examined. Figure 1(a) shows virtually no leakage in the brain contrary to the clear evidence of endothelial barrier breakdown in the other organs. Quantification of vascular leakage revealed that the endothelial barrier is generally more permeable in the sickle mice than in control littermates (Figures 1(b) and 1(c)), despite some differences in the two transgenic models. Indeed, there was a significant correlation between steady-state hemoglobin concentration and lung permeability (Figure 1(d)) ($r = -0.7639$, $P < 0.0001$), indicating that endothelial barrier dysfunction is related to an aspect of SCD. Unlike most organs, vascular permeability in the lung in middle-aged sickle mice was significantly higher than in adult mice, highlighting a role for age in this disease process. This was investigated by extending our study to include

younger mice aged 5-6 weeks. Remarkably, permeability in the heart and lung at this early stage of the disease was identical to that of the brain, which is widely known to have a highly restrictive barrier (Figures 1(e) and 1(f)). Thus, the endothelial barrier in SCD is normal in most organs in the young, becomes abnormal during adulthood, and deteriorates further with aging particularly in the lung.

Pulmonary edema is a common postmortem finding in SCD and yet it has not been appreciated as a chronic lung complication of SCD, probably because of the confounding effect of death [21, 22]. While histology does not reveal evidence of edema in the Berkeley sickle mice [10], we have used a more sensitive approach to clearly demonstrate that vascular permeability in the lungs of both the Berkeley and Townes sickle mice is increased. Our result is in agreement with a recent study that investigated permeability exclusively in the lung of 12–16-weeks-old NY1DD sickle mouse using the same approach [23]. In agreement with these permeability findings, we discovered that the average wet lung weight of middle-aged sickle mice is significantly heavier than that of age-matched hemizygotes (0.64 mg ± 0.04 versus 0.54 mg ± 0.02; $P = 0.03$), and, accordingly, the wet/dry weight ratio, widely used to confirm edema in lungs, was significantly higher ($P = 0.002$) (Figure 2(a)). Taken together, these results show for the first time that middle-aged sickle mice develop pulmonary edema. We cannot exclude the possibility that chronic heart failure contributed to the lung edema reported here; however, the Berkeley mice used in the lung weight measurements were at least three months younger than those reported to have heart failure [11]. Importantly, we show that lung edema correlates with higher vascular permeability in sickle mouse lungs. This concordance advances both conceptual and practical research objectives. It suggests that the permeability phenotypes of the lung in mice and humans with SCD are similar, and it validates, for the first time, the use of the Evans blue extravasation approach to study vascular permeability in transgenic sickle mice.

The permeability phenotypes identified here likely reflect the intrinsic properties of individual organs, as well as of endothelial cell types. For instance, it is well established that heterogeneity of endothelial cell junction contributes to unique permeability attributes [24], and this may account for some of the dramatic differences in permeability phenotypes reported here (e.g., brain and lung). However, endothelial cells in individual organs may also respond differently to barrier disrupting factors found in SCD. Among these factors, cell-free hemoglobin is unique because it is released in abundance during acute intravascular hemolysis, which is a daily event in SCD. We assessed the response of major vascular beds in the sickle mice to acute hemolysis. Leuko-depleted packed red blood cells were lysed by repeated freeze-thaw cycles and intravenously administered to sickle mice via tail vein. Compared to saline, the lysed red blood cells increased vascular permeability by 2-fold in the lungs of adult sickle mice but had a modest or negligible impact on the kidney, brain, and heart (Figure 2(b)). That lysed red blood cells caused morbidity and significantly altered barrier function in the Berkeley sickle mice indicates this and other severe models of SCD can be used to unlock mechanisms of acute hemolysis in SCD. In particular the vulnerability of the lung endothelial barrier to lysed red blood cells highlights acute intravascular hemolysis as a potential trigger of the acute chest syndrome since a decreasing concentration of hemoglobin is invariably associated with this condition [14].

In conclusion, SCD appears to be characterized by weakening of the endothelial barrier, which predisposes some organs, such as the lung to acute loss of barrier function, reminiscent of the acute chest syndrome. Ongoing studies are focused on unraveling the relationship between acute hemolysis and the endothelial barrier in SCD.

## Authors' Contribution

S. Ghosh designed and performed most of the experiments. F. Tan characterized the transgenic mice and performed research. S. F. Ofori-Acquah designed the study and provided overall oversight of the projects.

## Acknowledgments

The authors are grateful to Dr. Townes of the University of Alabama at Birmingham for the knock-in transgenic mice with SCD and to Dr. Archer of Emory University for the Berkeley mice. This work was supported by Grants R01HL077769 awarded to SFOA.

## References

[1] S. Embury, R. P. Hebbel, N. Mohandas, and M. H. Steinberg, *Sickle Cell Disease: Basic Principles and Clinical Practice*, Raven Press, New York, NY, USA, 1995.

[2] G. J. Kato, M. T. Gladwin, and M. H. Steinberg, "Deconstructing sickle cell disease: reappraisal of the role of hemolysis in the development of clinical subphenotypes," *Blood Reviews*, vol. 21, no. 1, pp. 37–47, 2007.

[3] T. A. Bensinger and P. N. Gillette, "Hemolysis in sickle cell disease," *Archives of Internal Medicine*, vol. 133, no. 4, pp. 624–631, 1974.

[4] W. Aird, *Endothelial Biomedicine*, Cambridge University Press, 2007.

[5] M. H. Steinberg, "Sickle cell anemia, the first molecular disease: overview of molecular etiology, pathophysiology, and therapeutic approaches," *TheScientificWorldJournal*, vol. 8, pp. 1295–1324, 2008.

[6] A. J. Duits, R. C. Pieters, A. W. Saleh et al., "Enhanced levels of soluble VCAM-1 in sickle cell patients and their specific increment during vasoocclusive crisis," *Clinical Immunology and Immunopathology*, vol. 81, no. 1, pp. 96–98, 1996.

[7] A. Solovey, Y. Lin, P. Browne, S. Choong, E. Wayner, and R. P. Hebbel, "Circulating activated endothelial cells in sickle cell anemia," *New England Journal of Medicine*, vol. 337, no. 22, pp. 1584–1590, 1997.

[8] A. Solovey, L. Gui, N. S. Key, and R. P. Hebbel, "Tissue factor expression by endothelial cells in sickle cell anemia," *Journal of Clinical Investigation*, vol. 101, no. 9, pp. 1899–1904, 1998.

[9] J. D. Belcher, C. J. Bryant, J. Nguyen et al., "Transgenic sickle mice have vascular inflammation," *Blood*, vol. 101, no. 10, pp. 3953–3959, 2003.

[10] E. A. Manci, C. A. Hillery, C. A. Bodian, Z. G. Zhang, G. A. Lutty, and B. S. Coller, "Pathology of Berkeley sickle cell mice: similarities and differences with human sickle cell disease," *Blood*, vol. 107, no. 4, pp. 1651–1658, 2006.

[11] L. L. Hsu, H. C. Champion, S. A. Campbell-Lee et al., "Hemolysis in sickle cell mice causes pulmonary hypertension due to global impairment in nitric oxide bioavailability," *Blood*, vol. 109, no. 7, pp. 3088–3098, 2007.

[12] M. T. Gladwin, V. Sachdev, M. L. Jison et al., "Pulmonary Hypertension as a Risk Factor for Death in Patients with Sickle Cell Disease," *New England Journal of Medicine*, vol. 350, no. 9, pp. 886–895, 2004.

[13] J. K. Graham, M. Mosunjac, R. L. Hanzlick, and M. Mosunjac, "Sickle cell lung disease and sudden death: a retrospective/prospective study of 21 autopsy cases and literature review," *American Journal of Forensic Medicine and Pathology*, vol. 28, no. 2, pp. 168–172, 2007.

[14] E. P. Vichinsky, L. D. Neumayr, A. N. Earles et al., "Causes and outcomes of the acute chest syndrome in sickle cell disease," *New England Journal of Medicine*, vol. 342, no. 25, pp. 1855–1865, 2000.

[15] C. Pászty, C. M. Brion, E. Manci et al., "Transgenic knockout mice with exclusively human sickle hemoglobin and sickle cell disease," *Science*, vol. 278, no. 5339, pp. 876–878, 1997.

[16] L. C. Wu, C. W. Sun, T. M. Ryan, K. M. Pawlik, J. Ren, and T. M. Townes, "Correction of sickle cell disease by homologous recombination in embryonic stem cells," *Blood*, vol. 108, no. 4, pp. 1183–1188, 2006.

[17] C. D. Reiter, X. Wang, J. E. Tanus-Santos et al., "Cell-free hemoglobin limits nitric oxide bioavailability in sickle-cell disease," *Nature Medicine*, vol. 8, no. 12, pp. 1383–1389, 2002.

[18] M. T. Gladwin, V. Sachdev, M. L. Jison et al., "Pulmonary hypertension as a risk factor for death in patients with sickle cell disease," *New England Journal of Medicine*, vol. 350, no. 9, pp. 886–895, 2004.

[19] R. P. Hebbel, R. Osarogiagbon, and D. Kaul, "The endothelial biology of sickle cell disease: inflammation and a chronic

vasculopathy," *Microcirculation*, vol. 11, no. 2, pp. 129–151, 2004.

[20] B. N. Y. Setty and M. J. Stuart, "Vascular cell adhesion molecule-1 is involved in mediating hypoxia- induced sickle red blood cell adherence to endothelium: potential role in sickle cell disease," *Blood*, vol. 88, no. 6, pp. 2311–2320, 1996.

[21] J. K. Graham, M. Mosunjac, R. L. Hanzlick, and M. Mosunjac, "Sickle cell lung disease and sudden death: a retrospective/ prospective study of 21 autopsy cases and literature review," *American Journal of Forensic Medicine and Pathology*, vol. 28, no. 2, pp. 168–172, 2007.

[22] W. Girard, "Case report: postoperative pulmonary edema and sickle cell crisis," *Clinical Notes on Respiratory Diseases*, vol. 17, no. 4, pp. 13–14, 1979.

[23] K. L. Wallace, M. A. Marshall, S. I. Ramos et al., "NKT cells mediate pulmonary inflammation and dysfunction in murine sickle cell disease through production of IFN-$\gamma$ and CXCR3 chemokines," *Blood*, vol. 114, no. 3, pp. 667–676, 2009.

[24] A. Masedunskas, J. A. King, F. Tan et al., "Activated leukocyte cell adhesion molecule is a component of the endothelial junction involved in transendothelial monocyte migration," *FEBS Letters*, vol. 580, no. 11, pp. 2637–2645, 2006.

# 16

# The Properties of Red Blood Cells from Patients Heterozygous for HbS and HbC (HbSC Genotype)

A. Hannemann,[1] E. Weiss,[1] D. C. Rees,[2] S. Dalibalta,[3] J. C. Ellory,[3] and J. S. Gibson[1]

[1] Department of Veterinary Medicine, University of Cambridge, Madingley Road, Cambridge CB3 0ES, UK
[2] Department of Molecular Haematology, King's College Hospital, London SE5 9RS, UK
[3] Department of Physiology, Anatomy & Genetics, University of Oxford, Parks Road, Oxford OX1 3PT, UK

Correspondence should be addressed to J. S. Gibson, jsg1001@cam.ac.uk

Academic Editor: Maria Stella Figueiredo

Sickle cell disease (SCD) is one of the commonest severe inherited disorders, but specific treatments are lacking and the pathophysiology remains unclear. Affected individuals account for well over 250,000 births yearly, mostly in the Tropics, the USA, and the Caribbean, also in Northern Europe as well. Incidence in the UK amounts to around 12–15,000 individuals and is increasing, with approximately 300 SCD babies born each year as well as with arrival of new immigrants. About two thirds of SCD patients are homozygous HbSS individuals. Patients heterozygous for HbS and HbC (HbSC) constitute about a third of SCD cases, making this the second most common form of SCD, with approximately 80,000 births per year worldwide. Disease in these patients shows differences from that in homozygous HbSS individuals. Their red blood cells (RBCs), containing approximately equal amounts of HbS and HbC, are also likely to show differences in properties which may contribute to disease outcome. Nevertheless, little is known about the behaviour of RBCs from HbSC heterozygotes. This paper reviews what is known about SCD in HbSC individuals and will compare the properties of their RBCs with those from homozygous HbSS patients. Important areas of similarity and potential differences will be emphasised.

## 1. Introduction

Like homozygous HbSS individuals, individuals heterozygous for HbS and HbC (HbSCs) suffer from sickle cell disease (SCD) [1–6]. The condition in HbSC patients (here called HbSC disease cf. HbSS disease in homozygotes) not only has some overlap with that seen in HbSS patients, but also has distinctive laboratory and clinical features identifying it as a separate entity [6–8]. Although HbSC disease is one of the commonest significant genetic diseases worldwide, it is comparatively neglected with very few laboratory or clinical studies addressing the condition directly. Thus, whilst extensive research has been carried out on understanding SCD in HbSS patients, little relates specifically to the pathogenesis in HbSC patients. In clinical trials of potential novel therapies for SCD, HbSC patients are often specifically excluded. Furthermore, most clinical and laboratory features of HbSC disease have been inferred from studies of HbSS, which may not be appropriate. This paper addresses the pathophysiological differences shown by SCD in HbSS and HbSC patients and the diversity in their clinical complications. Particular reference is paid to the transport abnormalities of the RBC membrane.

## 2. Genotypic Variants of SCD

All SCD patients have the abnormal haemoglobin HbS in their red cells instead of the normal adult HbA [9–12]. HbS results from a single base mutation in codon 6 of the $\beta$-globin gene which causes a single amino acid substitution in position $\beta6$ (glutamic acid → valine, with net loss of one negative charge). Homozygous HbSS patients have two copies of the altered gene. The mutation arose in West Africa, where the high prevalence of HbS appears to be due to selection pressure conferred by a relative resistance to malaria. Malaria resistance has also increased the prevalence of a second abnormal Hb, HbC, which like HbS represents one of the most prevalent forms of abnormal human Hb. HbC also has a single mutation/amino acid change at the same position in $\beta$-Hb, but with lysine replacing glutamic acid (hence net loss of two negative charges). These changes in protein charge may alter how the different Hbs interact and modulate transporter function at the RBC membrane [13]. The charge differences are also used for electrophoretic tests for abnormal Hb, although care must be exercised to exclude certain non-SCD haemoglobinopathies which may mimic HbSC. Homozygous HbCC individuals show few disease symptoms apart from a mild haemolytic anaemia [6]. Heterozygotes of HbA with either HbS or HbC are also largely asymptomatic. Coinheritance of HbS and HbC to produce HbSC heterozygotes, however, results in a clinically significant disease similar, but not identical, to that in HbSS individuals [6–8]. Although globally HbSC heterozygotes represent about a third of SCD cases, their distribution is by no means uniform. HbC appears to have originated in Burkina Faso [6] where HbSC cases may outnumber those of HbSS. In other areas, such as the Middle East and India, HbSC cases are rare. In this context, it is worth pointing out that estimates of the frequency of different haemoglobinopathies are likely to be inexact, relying on outdated or incorrect information [14].

## 3. HbSC Disease as a Unique Clinical Entity

All cases of SCD, including those of HbSC disease, are characterised by shortened red cell life span and chronic anaemia, together with recurrent episodes of more acute vaso-occlusion, tissue ischaemia, and increased mortality [12]. Affected individuals have a poor quality of life with numerous complications, for example, pain, cerebrovascular disease (strokes), renal and pulmonary damage, leg ulcers, and priapism [2]. An important feature of SCD is that the clinical scenario is notably heterogeneous—patients may present with mild forms of the disease which rarely require medical intervention or alternatively with more severe complications warranting frequent hospitalisation and aggressive management. Presumably modifier genes and/or environmental factors are significant, but although this area is now receiving considerable attention, it remains poorly understood at present [15–17].

In most cases, HbSC disease is clinically milder than HbSS disease and the various complications of SCD usually occur less often or later in life [8]. For example, leg ulcers and other chronic vascular manifestations occur infrequently. Loss of splenic function is relatively delayed, preserving red cell scavenging and thereby possibly affecting disease complications. Nevertheless, HbSC disease still has a significant impact on patients who show haemolytic anaemia, organ failures (stroke, renal failure, chronic lung disease.), and increased mortality (with a median survival of 60 years for males in USA) [15, 18]. Pregnant women sometimes develop complications having been hitherto asymptomatic [19]. Complications also occur in children with the risk of stroke in childhood being about 100 times greater than

that in the general population [18]. Furthermore, in HbSC heterozygotes, some of the serious complications of SCD (such as osteonecrosis) are as common as for HbSS patients and some (e.g., proliferative sickle retinopathy and possibly acute chest syndrome) occur more frequently [8]. This is also apparent for some central auditory and vestibular problems [19].

Additionally, HbSC is haematologically distinct from HbSS, with higher Hb levels (but lower levels of HbF), lower rates of haemolysis and lower white cell counts [8]. Some of these features are well illustrated in clinical and haematological observations on patients from our clinics (see [20, Table 1]). These distinctive features imply that individuals with HbSC disease should be treated as a discrete subset of SCD patients.

Currently there is very little specific information on the pathophysiology and management of HbSC disease, with much being inferred from studies of HbSS patients. Differences in pathogenesis between HbSC and HbSS disease are expected, however. Understanding them will be important in the management of HbSC patients and may also contribute to a better appreciation of the condition in homozygous individuals.

## 4. Pathogenesis of SCD

Although the underlying molecular defect of SCD is long established, how HbS results in the clinical complications remains poorly understood. The chronic anaemia and acute ischaemic episodes both are associated with altered rheology and increased adhesiveness of both RBCs and vascular endothelium [21]. RBCs are more fragile and more readily scavenged from the circulation, contributing to the chronic anaemia, whilst microvascular occlusion is also encouraged causing the acute ischaemic events characteristic of SCD. Intravascular haemolysis is observed and the consequent release of Hb to circulate freely in plasma contributes to the vasculopathy, probably by scavenging nitric oxide (NO) and causing a functional deficiency of that molecule [22, 23]. Some authors divide the disease complications of SCD into two broad categories, with sequelae caused either predominantly by altered RBC rheology and elevated blood viscosity (e.g., pain, osteonecrosis, and acute chest syndrome) or by intravascular haemolysis and NO scavenging (e.g., pulmonary hypertension, stroke, priapism, and leg ulceration) [24–26]. In any event, polymerisation of HbS on deoxygenation is central to anaemia, vaso-occlusion, and haemolysis—although complete deoxygenation may not be needed, especially in the case of hyperdense RBCs with high cell [Hb], such as some of those found in HbSC individuals. Formation of long rods of HbS distorts RBC shape, reduces deformability, and increases viscosity, thus compromising vascular red cell rheology [27]. Other key events in the pathogenesis have been identified. First, red cell volume is critically important [28]. The increased cation permeability of HbS-containing red cells results in solute loss with water following osmotically. Consequently, [HbS] increases. As the rate of HbS polymerisation upon

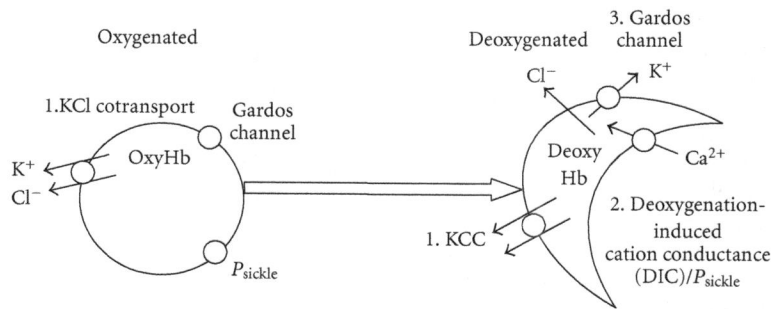

FIGURE 1: Schematic diagram of the main transport pathways activated in red blood cells (RBCs) from sickle cell patients. In RBCs from homozygous HbSS individuals, high cation permeability is accounted for by three main pathways [28, 37]. Under oxygenated conditions, the KCl cotransporter (KCC) is highly active. It is overexpressed in HbSS cells compared to HbAA ones and does not become quiescent as RBCs mature. It is stimulated further by low pH (reduction in extracelluar pH from 7.4 to 7). Under deoxygenated conditions, KCC remains active—again unlike the situation in HbAA RBCs [40]. In addition, two other pathways are observed. The deoxygenation-induced cation conductance (or $P_{sickle}$) is activated as HbS polymerises. It mediates entry of $Ca^{2+}$. Elevation in intracellular $Ca^{2+}$ then leads to activation of the third pathway, the $Ca^{2+}$-activated $K^+$ channel, or Gardos channel. These three pathways result in solute loss, cell shrinkage and dehydration, and consequent increase in [HbS]. They thereby contribute to pathogenesis of sickle cell disease. They are also likely to be involved in solute loss from RBCs of patients heterozygous for HbS and HbC (HbSC genotype), though details are lacking and differences in their behaviour compared to that in HbSS cells are expected.

deoxygenation is proportional to a very high power of [HbS], a small reduction in cell volume and hence increase in [HbS] markedly encourages HbS polymerisation [27]. Second, red cell stickiness is also increased [21, 29–31]. This results, at least in part, from exposure of phosphatidylserine (PS) on the outer bilayer of the membrane [32]. Exposed PS is prothrombotic and increases adherence of red cells to macrophages and endothelium, contributing to chronic anaemia, haemolysis, and vaso-occlusion [33]. Again, the cause of PS exposure is not clear, but sickling-induced $Ca^{2+}$ entry may play an important role [34]. Third, SCD represents an inflammatory state with raised levels of cytokines, chronic elevation of leukocyte counts, shortened leukocyte half-life, and abnormal activation of granulocytes, monocytes, and endothelium [35, 36]. The resulting cytokine stimulation of endothelial cells increases their adhesiveness to sickle RBCs [35, 36]. How these various changes interact to produce the symptoms of SCD represents a major research challenge. In addition, the extent to which these various mechanisms are involved in disease pathogenesis would be expected to differ between HbSS homozygotes and HbSC heterozygotes. For example, reduced intravascular haemolysis in the latter may ameliorate NO scavenging.

## 5. Altered Membrane Transport in Homozygous HbSS Cells

Increased membrane permeability of HbS-containing red cells contributes to SCD pathogenesis by promoting $Ca^{2+}$ entry, KCl loss with water following osmotically, and hence RBC dehydration [28, 34, 37]. In HbSS cells, the involvement of three pathways has been proposed: the KCl cotransporter (KCC), the deoxygenation-induced cation conductance (or $P_{sickle}$), and the $Ca^{2+}$-activated $K^+$ channel

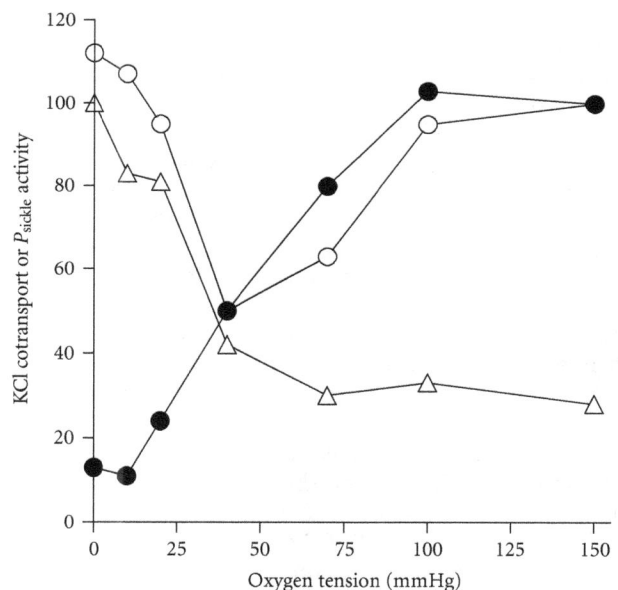

FIGURE 2: Effect of oxygen tension on the activity of KCl cotransport (KCC) or $P_{sickle}$ in red blood cells (RBCs) from normal individuals or patients with sickle cell disease. The activity of each transport pathway is normalised—to the value in oxygenated cells (150 mmHg $O_2$) for KCC activity and for that in deoxygenated RBCs (0 mmHg) in the case of $P_{sickle}$—and given as a percentage. Solid circles give KCC activity in RBCs from normal HbAA individuals; open symbols give KCC activity (open circles) or $P_{sickle}$ activity (open triangles) in RBCs from sickle cell patients (HbSS homozygotes). In these experiments, total magnitude of KCC activity was about 10-fold greater in RBCs from HbSS individuals compared with HbAA ones. Note how the deoxygenation-induced KCC activity and activation of $P_{sickle}$ follow a similar dependence on $O_2$ tension. Data taken from [67].

(or Gardos channel, KCNN4) [28]. These three systems are illustrated schematically in Figure 1.

The first of these, KCC (likely KCC1 and KCC3 isoforms), is more active and abnormally regulated in HbSS cells [38–40]. Mean activity is enhanced >10-fold in unstimulated cells with several stimuli increasing activity further. In normal RBCs, cell swelling is an important trigger of KCC activity [41]. For HbSS cells, however, intracellular pH is probably the most important stimulus *in vivo*, with KCC activity reaching a peak at about pH 7 [38, 42]. The transporter also responds to $O_2$ tension [43]. In normal red cells, high levels of $O_2$ are required for KCC activity, with the transporter becoming inactivated at low $O_2$. By contrast, in HbSS cells, the transporter remains active during full deoxygenation, thereby allowing it to respond to low pH in hypoxic areas (like active muscle beds) [40] (Figures 1 and 2). KCC is regulated by phosphorylation, through cascades of conjugate protein kinases and phosphatases [44], with differences apparent in HbSS cells compared with HbAA ones, but at present these are poorly defined. The relative deficiency of intracellular $Mg^{2+}$ in HbSS cells [45, 46] probably acts to increase KCC activity by altering the activity of these regulatory enzymes.

The second pathway, $P_{sickle}$, is apparently unique to HbS-containing red cells [28, 34]. It is activated to a variable extent by deoxygenation, HbS polymerisation, and shape change [47, 48] (Figures 1 and 2). $P_{sickle}$ has the characteristics of a nonspecific cation channel [34]. An anion permeability is controversial, whilst, more recently, it has been proposed as permeable under certain conditions to nonelectrolytes [49]. The main effect of $P_{sickle}$ is probably the increased $Ca^{2+}$ entry [49, 50] and possibly the $Mg^{2+}$ loss [45]. Raised intracellular $Ca^{2+}$ has several roles which include phospholipid scrambling [51]. It will also activate the third pathway responsible for HbS cell dehydration, the Gardos channel [52] (Figures 1 and 3). The Gardos channel is then capable of mediating very rapid efflux of $K^+$ with $Cl^-$ following for electroneutrality and water osmotically.

These mechanisms cause solute loss and HbSS cell shrinkage. Episodes may be short lived and produce only modest degrees of solute loss. But they may occur repeatedly during the lifetime of the RBCs, often during deoxygenation-induced sickling events. Accordingly, HbSS cells show an increase in MCHC of a few percent compared to normal red cells (c.34 g·dL$^{-1}$ cf. 33 in HbAA cells, density approx 1.085 g·mL$^{-1}$), but importantly there is a large range about this mean with many dense cells (>1.095 g·ml$^{-1}$, MCHC c.38 g·dl$^{-1}$), some of which are exceedingly dense (1.125 g·ml$^{-1}$, c.50 g·dl$^{-1}$) [53]. A significant feature of HbSS RBCs is their marked heterogeneity, with certain subpopulations possibly more important in pathogenesis [28]. The densest HbSS cells are mainly older ones, presumably following repeated episodes of solute loss [54]. Reticulocytes are mostly low density (c.26 g·dl$^{-1}$), as they are in normal individuals [55]. However, there is a small fraction of young, dense HbSS cells, the so-called fast-track reticulocytes, which become rapidly dehydrated on deoxygenation while still young [28, 56].

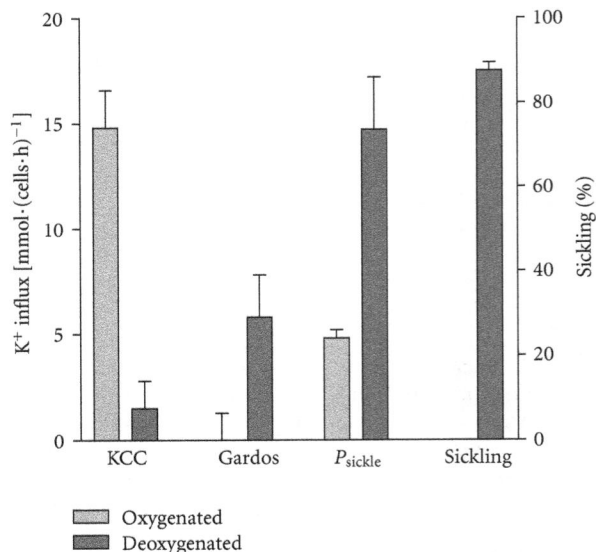

FIGURE 3: Components of $K^+$ transport pathways and sickling in red blood cells (RBCs) from sickle cell disease patients heterozygous for HbS and HbC (HbSC genotype). $K^+$ influxes are given as flux units [mmol·(l cells·h)$^{-1}$] measured at 5 mM $[K^+]_o$ and numbers of sickled cells as a percentage of total RBCs in fully oxygenated (150 mmHg $O_2$) or deoxygenated (0 mmHg) conditions. Although this technique measures a $K^+$ influx, because of the high $K^+$ content of RBCs, net solute movement through the transport systems will be outwards. KCl cotransport activity was calculated as the $Cl^-$-dependent $K^+$ influx, Gardos channel activity as the clotrimazole (5 $\mu$M)-sensitive $K^+$ influx, and $P_{sickle}$ as the $Cl^-$-independent $K^+$ influx ($Cl^-$ substituted with $NO_3^-$). Sickling, $P_{sickle}$, and Gardos channel activation occurs in deoxygenated conditions—as for HbSS RBCs—but KCC activity is low when $O_2$ is removed (as in RBCs from HbAA cells). Data taken from [64].

## 6. Altered Properties of HbSC Cells

RBCs from HbSC patients also show $K^+$ loss, raised MCHC and haemolytic anaemia with reticulocytosis [5, 57–59]. The properties of HbSC RBCs, however, differ in important respects from those of HbSS cells. In HbSC cells, $K^+$ loss and dehydration are markedly more pronounced [58, 59]. MCHC is particularly high, at about 37 g·dl$^{-1}$ (cf. 33 g·dl$^{-1}$ in HbAA individuals; 33-34 g·dl$^{-1}$ for the reversibly sickled fraction of HbSS patients) [57, 58]. Whilst most reticulocytes from normal HbAA and HbSS are characteristically low density (26 g·dl$^{-1}$), HbSC reticulocytes are mainly high density (MCHC c.34 g·dl$^{-1}$) [5, 58]. Usually older RBCs are denser; however the monotonic decrease in reticulocyte count with increasing cell density observed for red cells from HbSS patients (as well as HbAA and HbAS individuals) does not occur in HbSC patients [5, 60]. Instead, HbSC reticulocytes are fairly evenly distributed across the different RBC densities [5], or perhaps even more concentrated in the denser fractions [60]. This has been taken as evidence that a significant proportion of young HbSC cells begin their lives with a high density [5], rather than undergoing a more gradual dehydration observed in HbSS cells upon repeat

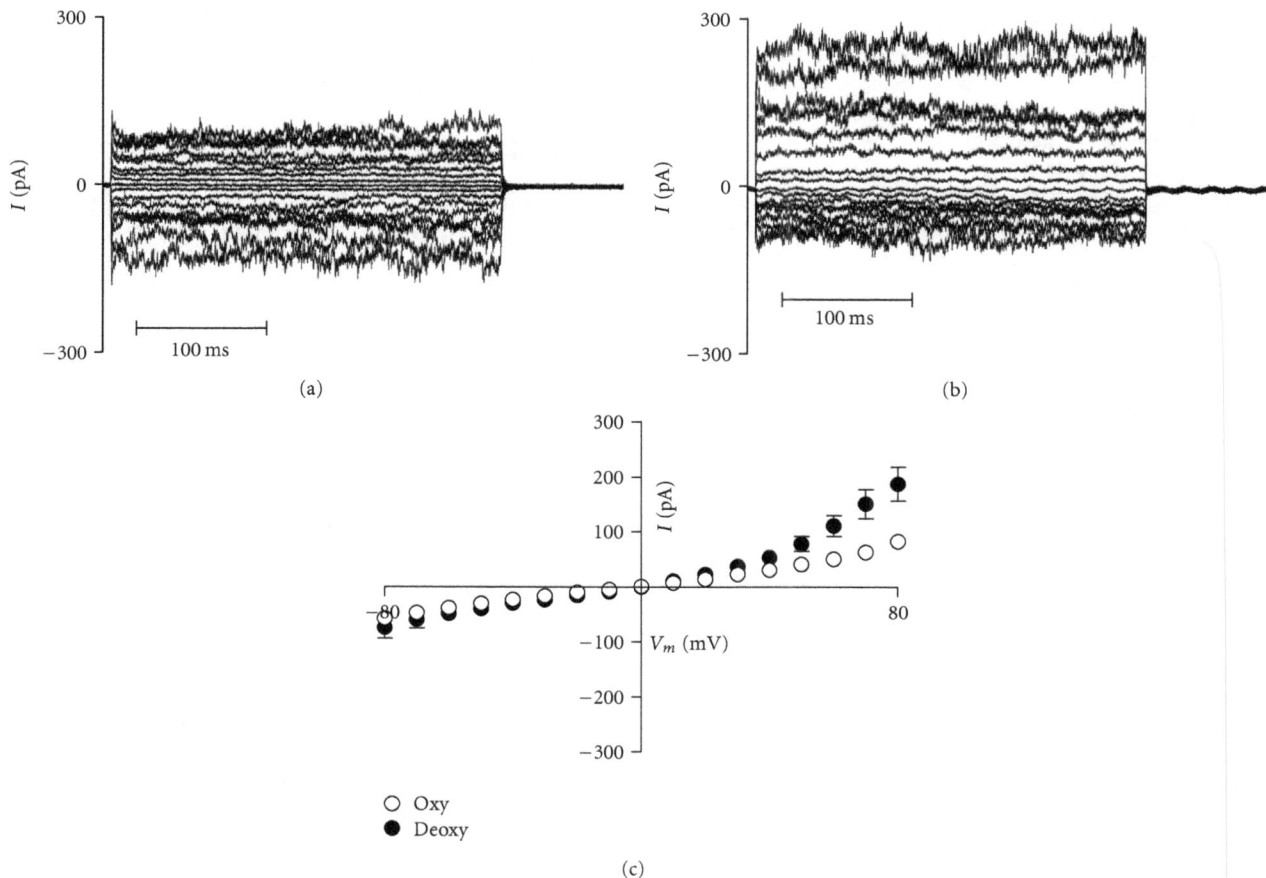

FIGURE 4: Conductance of red blood cells (RBCs) from sickle cell patients heterozygous for HbS and HbC (HbSC genotype). (a), (b) Representative whole-cell recordings from (a) oxygenated and (b) deoxygenated RBCs. (c) Mean whole-cell currents $\pm$ S.E.M., $n = 5$. Test potentials from $-80$ to $+80$ mV were applied for 300 ms in 10 mV increments from a holding potential of $-10$ mV. Measurements were made using $Na^+$-containing bath and pipette solutions. Data taken from [20]. See [66] for experimental details. The conductance of RBCs from HbSC patients is high and increases further on deoxygenation.

episodes of sickling. In this respect, perhaps the majority of HbSC reticulocytes behave like the "fast-track" reticulocytes of HbSS patients [56]—cells which dehydrate rapidly on leaving the bone marrow—but this remains to be established. It also raises the question as to what constitutes RBCs in the less dense HbSC fractions. Can shrunken HbSC cells regain lost solute and increase their volume? If so, what is the mechanism and what are transport systems involved?

As heterozygotes, HbSC cells contain both HbS and HbC, in approximately equal amounts (i.e., 50%). This contrasts with the lower HbS content (c.40%) found in sickle trait HbAS cells [5]. Crystals of HbC are sometimes present in oxygenated RBCs. In contrast to HbS polymers, these deposits are lost on deoxygenation [60]. Because of the high HbS content and polymerisation, HbSC cells also show a deoxygenation-induced sickling shape change. In this case, however, rather than the HbSS sickles and holly leaf forms, deoxygenated HbSC cells show multifolded shapes such as "pita breads" and "tricorns" [60], perhaps because of the high surface area to volume ratio subsequent to their more marked dehydration. How HbS and HbC interact has also

received some attention. Using different Hb mixtures, a direct interaction between the two Hbs appears to only slightly enhance HbS polymerisation. Much more important in HbSC disease is RBC dehydration and consequently the high MCHC [5, 61, 62]. High MCHC and lower levels of HbF may have an effect on the extent and kinetics of HbS polymerisation whilst concurrent Hb mutations (such as $\beta$-thalassaemia) may also play a significant role.

It is therefore critical to understand fully the mechanisms by which these RBCs shrink, but our understanding of the mechanisms involved remains uncertain. Oxygenated HbSC cells have elevated KCC activity that is stimulated by low pH and swelling [13, 60]. Cytoplasmic protein concentration has been suggested as the "volume" sensor of RBCs [63]. It is therefore intriguing to speculate that high KCC activity in oxygenated HbSC cells may result from the presence of HbC crystals which would lower the total concentration of soluble Hb, as occurs in swollen RBCs. In effect, the cells "think" that they are swollen and so activate mechanisms to lose solutes and water, namely, KCC. On the other hand, deoxygenated HbSC cells also show increased $K^+$ efflux, to an extent apparently greater than that observed in deoxygenated HbSS cells [58]. Which pathway mediates the flux in deoxygenated conditions, however, has not been established. If $P_{sickle}$ is involved, given the lower [HbS] of HbSC cells, it is not clear why it should be activated to a greater extent than in HbSS cells. KCC and the Gardos channel represent obvious alternative pathways.

A number of manoeuvres which reduce reticulocyte density may provide evidence for the transport pathways involved in their dehydration. Both $Cl^-$ removal and deoxygenation shift HbSC reticulocytes to lower densities, consistent with solute retention following inhibition of KCC [60]. Hypotonic swelling of HbSC cells also reduces the deoxygenation-induced $K^+$ loss [58], perhaps through reduction in [HbS] removing a $P_{sickle}$-like element of $K^+$ flux.

In preliminary studies, we have observed high KCC activity in oxygenated unfractionated HbSC cells, which was almost completely inhibited on deoxygenation [64]. Thus, KCC in HbSC cells behaved like that in HbSS cells at high $O_2$ tension and like that in HbAA cells when tension was reduced [64] (Figure 3). We also found activation of a deoxygenation-induced $Cl^-$-independent $K^+$ flux [64], a deoxygenation-induced nonelectrolyte permeability [65] and a deoxygenation-induced rise in $K^+$ conductance in patch-clamp experiments [66] (Figure 4), namely, a $P_{sickle}$-like permeability, together with activation of the Gardos channel. In this context, it is interesting that HbC has a higher affinity for the RBC membrane than either HbA or HbS [59] leading to an early suggestion that HbSC interaction is involved in modulating RBC permeability.

It is apparent, however, that our understanding of the permeability of HbSC cells requires further investigation.

## 7. Conclusion: The Importance of Cell Dehydration in HbSC Disease

Understanding dehydration is particularly relevant for HbSC cells. The solubility of deoxygenated HbS is about $17\,g{\cdot}dl^{-1}$ compared to $70\,g{\cdot}dl^{-1}$ for HbA. As HbS represents only about half the total Hbs in HbSC cells, a relatively small decrease in MCHC (from an RBC total of 37 to $33\,g{\cdot}dl^{-1}$) will prevent HbS polymerisation [61] while retaining the functionally important discocyte morphology. As HbS constitutes about half the Hbs in these RBCs, this would mean a fall in [HbS] from 18.5 to 16.5. In comparison, in HbSS cells, a reduction of MCHC to $<25\,g{\cdot}dl^{-1}$ is required, by which time RBCs will be spherocytic, and cell swelling *per se* will adversely affect rheology [58]. Notwithstanding their relevance to dehydration and sickling, the permeability of HbSC cells has not been well studied nor compared in detail with that of HbSS cells. Several areas require more careful investigation. The interaction between different Hbs, membrane target sites regulating permeability, the transport pathways involved, the role of cell density, oxygenation, volume, and pH presents a complex pattern of modalities controlling solute content and hence cell density and MCHC. Control by phosphorylation remains mainly unexplored. The challenge ahead lies to define the most important

stimuli and how they interact to determine cell volume. A major therapeutic goal is the ability to prevent HbSC cell dehydration or to promote rehydration.

## Abbreviations

Here we term red cells from HbSS patients as HbSS cells, those from HbSC individuals as HbSC cells.

## Acknowledgment

The authors thank the Medical Research Council, the British Heart Foundation, and the Wellcome Trust for financial support.

## References

[1] G. R. Serjeant, "Sickle-cell disease," *The Lancet*, vol. 350, no. 9079, pp. 725–730, 1997.

[2] M. H. Steinberg, "Management of sickle cell disease," *The New England Journal of Medicine*, vol. 340, no. 13, pp. 1021–1030, 1999.

[3] M. Hickman, B. Modell, P. Greengross et al., "Mapping the prevalence of sickle cell and beta thalassaemia in England: estimating and validating ethnic-specific rates," *British Journal of Haematology*, vol. 104, no. 4, pp. 860–867, 1999.

[4] NHS sickle cell & thalassaemia screening programme, 2010.

[5] H. F. Bunn, C. T. Noguchi, J. Hofrichter, G. P. Schechter, A. N. Schechter, and W. A. Eaton, "Molecular and cellular pathogenesis of hemoglobin SC disease," *Proceedings of the National Academy of Sciences of the United States of America*, vol. 79, no. 23, pp. 7527–7531, 1982.

[6] R. L. Nagel, M. H. Steinberg, and S. C. Hemoglobin, "disease and HbC disorders," in *Disorders of Hemoglobin*, M. H. Steinberg, B. G. Forget, D. R. Higgs, and R. L. Nagel, Eds., pp. 756–785, Cambridge University Press, Cambridge, UK, 2001.

[7] R. L. Nagel and C. Lawrence, "The distinct pathobiology of sickle cell-hemoglobin C disease: therapeutic implications," *Hematology/Oncology Clinics of North America*, vol. 5, no. 3, pp. 433–451, 1991.

[8] R. L. Nagel, M. E. Fabry, and M. H. Steinberg, "The paradox of hemoglobin SC disease," *Blood Reviews*, vol. 17, no. 3, pp. 167–178, 2003.

[9] L. Pauling, H. A. Itano, S. J. Singer, and I. C. Wells, "Sickle cell anemia, a molecular disease," *Science*, vol. 110, no. 2865, pp. 543–548, 1949.

[10] V. M. Ingram, "Gene mutations in human haemoglobin: the chemical difference between normal and sickle cell haemoglobin," *Nature*, vol. 180, no. 4581, pp. 326–328, 1957.

[11] C. A. Marotta, J. T. Wilson, B. G. Forget, and S. M. Weissman, "Human $\beta$ globin messenger RNA. III. Nucleotide sequences derived from complementary DNA," *The Journal of Biological Chemistry*, vol. 252, no. 14, pp. 5040–5053, 1977.

[12] H. F. Bunn and B. G. Forget, *Hemoglobin: Molecular, Genetic and Clinical Aspects*, WB Saunders, Philadelphia, Pa, USA, 1986.

[13] O. Olivieri, D. Vitoux, F. Galacteros et al., "Hemoglobin variants and activity of the $(K^+Cl^-)$ cotransport system in human erythrocytes," *Blood*, vol. 79, no. 3, pp. 793–797, 1992.

[14] D. J. Weatherall, "The inherited diseases of haemoglobin are an emerging global health burden," *Blood*, vol. 115, pp. 4331–4336, 2010.

[15] M. H. Steinberg, "Genetic etiologies for phenotypic diversity in sickle cell anemia," *TheScientificWorldJournal*, vol. 9, pp. 46–67, 2009.

[16] P. Sebastini, N. Solovieff, S. W. Hartley et al., "Genetic modifiers of the severity of sickle cell anemia idenitified through a genome-wide association study," *American Journal of Hematology*, vol. 85, pp. 29–35, 2010.

[17] S. L. Thein and S. Menzel, "Discovering the genetics underlying foetal haemoglobin production in adults," *British Journal of Haematology*, vol. 145, no. 4, pp. 455–467, 2009.

[18] D. Powars, L. S. Chan, and W. A. Schroeder, "The variable expression of sickle cell disease is genetically determined," *Seminars in Hematology*, vol. 27, no. 4, pp. 360–376, 1990.

[19] K. Ohene-Frempong and M. H. Steinberg, "Clinical aspects of sickle cell anemia in adults and children," in *Disorders of Hemoglobin*, M. H. Steinberg, B. G. Forget, D. R. Higgs, and R. L. Nagel, Eds., pp. 611–670, Cambridge University Press, Cambridge, UK, 2001.

[20] S. Dalibalta, J. C. Ellory, J. A. Browning, R. J. Wilkins, D. C. Rees, and J. S. Gibson, "Novel permeability characteristics of red blood cells from sickle cell patients," *Blood Cells, Molecules, and Diseases*, vol. 45, no. 1, pp. 46–52, 2010.

[21] R. P. Hebbel, "Beyond hemoglobin polymerization: the red blood cell membrane and sickle disease pathophysiology," *Blood*, vol. 77, no. 2, pp. 214–237, 1991.

[22] C. D. Reiter, X. Wang, J. E. Tanus-Santos et al., "Cell-free hemoglobin limits nitric oxide bioavailability in sickle-cell disease," *Nature Medicine*, vol. 8, no. 12, pp. 1383–1389, 2002.

[23] G. J. Kato, V. McGowan, R. F. Machado et al., "Lactate dehydrogenase as a biomarker of hemolysis-associated nitric oxide resistance, priapism, leg ulceration, pulmonary hypertension, and death in patients with sickle cell disease," *Blood*, vol. 107, no. 6, pp. 2279–2285, 2006.

[24] M. J. Stuart and R. L. Nagel, "Sickle-cell disease," *The Lancet*, vol. 364, no. 9442, pp. 1343–1360, 2004.

[25] R. P. Rother, L. Bell, P. Hillmen, and M. T. Gladwin, "The clinical sequelae of intravascular hemolysis and extracellular plasma hemoglobin: a novel mechanism of human disease," *Journal of the American Medical Association*, vol. 293, no. 13, pp. 1653–1662, 2005.

[26] K. C. Wood, L. L. Hsu, and M. T. Gladwin, "Sickle cell disease vasculopathy: a state of nitric oxide resistance," *Free Radical Biology and Medicine*, vol. 44, no. 8, pp. 1506–1528, 2008.

[27] W. A. Eaton and J. Hofrichter, "Hemoglobin S gelation and sickle cell disease," *Blood*, vol. 70, no. 5, pp. 1245–1266, 1987.

[28] V. L. Lew and R. M. Bookchin, "Ion transport pathology in the mechanism of sickle cell dehydration," *Physiological Reviews*, vol. 85, no. 1, pp. 179–200, 2005.

[29] R. Hoover, R. Rubin, G. Wise, and R. Warren, "Adhesion of normal and sickle erythrocytes to endothelial monolayer cultures," *Blood*, vol. 54, no. 4, pp. 872–876, 1979.

[30] R. P. Hebbel, M. A. B. Boogaerts, J. W. Eaton, and M. H. Steinberg, "Erythrocyte adherence to endothelium in sickle-cell anemia. A possible determinant of disease severity," *The New England Journal of Medicine*, vol. 302, no. 18, pp. 992–995, 1980.

[31] D. K. Kaul, X.-D. Liu, X. Zhang et al., "Peptides based on $\alpha$V-binding domains of erythrocyte ICAM-4 inhibit sickle red cell-endothelial interactions and vaso-occlusion in the microcirculation," *American The Journal of Physiology*, vol. 291, no. 5, pp. C922–C930, 2006.

[32] B. N. Yamaja Setty, S. Kulkarni, and M. J. Stuart, "Role of erythrocyte phosphatidylserine in sickle red cell-endothelial adhesion," *Blood*, vol. 99, no. 5, pp. 1564–1571, 2002.

[33] F. A. Kuypers, "Red cell membrane lipids in hemoglobinopathies," *Current Molecular Medicine*, vol. 8, no. 7, pp. 633–638, 2008.

[34] C. H. Joiner, "Cation transport and volume regulation in sickle red blood cells," *American The Journal of Physiology*, vol. 264, no. 2, pp. C251–C270, 1993.

[35] B. N. Yamaja Setty and S. G. Betal, "Microvascular endothelial cells express a phosphatidylserine receptor: a functionally active receptor for phosphatidylserine-positive erythrocytes," *Blood*, vol. 111, no. 2, pp. 905–914, 2008.

[36] B. N. Y. Setty, S. G. Betal, J. Zhang, and M. J. Stuart, "Heme induces endothelial tissue factor expression: potential role in hemostatic activation in patients with hemolytic anemia," *Journal of Thrombosis and Haemostasis*, vol. 6, no. 12, pp. 2202–2209, 2008.

[37] J. S. Gibson and J. C. Ellory, "Membrane transport in sickle cell disease," *Blood Cells, Molecules, and Diseases*, vol. 28, no. 3, pp. 303–314, 2002.

[38] C. Brugnara, H. F. Bunn, and D. C. Tosteson, "Regulation of erythrocyte cation and water content in sickle cell anemia," *Science*, vol. 232, no. 4748, pp. 388–390, 1986.

[39] M. Canessa, A. Spalvins, and R. L. Nagel, "Volume-dependent and NEM-stimulated $K^+, Cl^-$ transport is elevated in oxygenated SS, SC and CC human red cells," *FEBS Letters*, vol. 200, no. 1, pp. 197–202, 1986.

[40] J. S. Gibson, P. F. Speake, and J. C. Ellory, "Differential oxygen sensitivity of the $K^+$-$Cl^-$ cotransporter in normal and sickle human red blood cells," *The Journal of Physiology*, vol. 511, no. 1, pp. 225–234, 1998.

[41] A. C. Hall and J. C. Ellory, "Evidence for the presence of volume-sensitive KCl transport in 'young' human red cells," *Biochimica et Biophysica Acta*, vol. 858, no. 2, pp. 317–320, 1986.

[42] J. C. Ellory, A. C. Hall, and S. A. Ody, "Is acid a more potent activator of KCl co-transport than hypotonicity in human red cells?" *The Journal of Physiology*, vol. 420, p. 149, 1990.

[43] J. S. Gibson, A. R. Cossins, and J. C. Ellory, "Oxygen-sensitive membrane transporters in vertebrate red cells," *Journal of Experimental Biology*, vol. 203, no. 9, pp. 1395–1407, 2000.

[44] J. S. Gibson and J. C. Ellory, "$K^+$-$Cl^-$ cotransport in vertebrate red cells," in *Red Cell Membrane Transport in Health and Disease*, I. Bernhardt and J. C. Ellory, Eds., pp. 197–220, Springer, New York, NY, USA, 2004.

[45] O. E. Ortiz, V. L. Lew, and R. M. Bookchin, "Deoxygenation permeabilizes sickle cell anaemia red cells to magnesium and reverses its gradient in the dense cells," *The Journal of Physiology*, vol. 427, pp. 211–226, 1990.

[46] J. P. Willcocks, P. J. Mulquiney, J. C. Ellory, R. L. Veech, G. K. Radda, and K. Clarke, "Simultaneous determination of low free Mg2+ and pH in human sickle cells using 31P NMR spectroscopy," *The Journal of Biological Chemistry*, vol. 277, no. 51, pp. 49911–49920, 2002.

[47] N. Mohandas, M. E. Rossi, and M. R. Clark, "Association between morphologic distortion of sickle cells and deoxygenation-induced cation permeability increase," *Blood*, vol. 68, no. 2, pp. 450–454, 1986.

[48] V. L. Lew, O. E. Ortiz, and R. M. Bookchin, "Stochastic nature and red cell population distribution of the sickling- induced $Ca^{2+}$ permeability," *The Journal of Clinical Investigation*, vol. 99, no. 11, pp. 2727–2735, 1997.

[49] J. A. Browning, H. C. Robinson, J. C. Ellory, and J. S. Gibson, "Deoxygenation-induced non-electrolyte pathway in red cells from sickle cell patients," *Cellular Physiology and Biochemistry*, vol. 19, no. 1–4, pp. 165–174, 2007.

[50] M. D. Rhoda, M. Apovo, Y. Beuzard, and F. Giraud, "Ca$^{2+}$ permeability in deoxygenated sickle cells," *Blood*, vol. 75, no. 12, pp. 2453–2458, 1990.

[51] L. A. Woon, J. W. Holland, E. P. W. Kable, and B. D. Roufogalis, "Ca$^{2+}$ sensitivity of phospholipid scrambling in human red cell ghosts," *Cell Calcium*, vol. 25, no. 4, pp. 313–320, 1999.

[52] G. Gárdos, "The function of calcium in the potassium permeability of human erythrocytes," *Biochimica et Biophysica Acta*, vol. 30, no. 3, pp. 653–654, 1958.

[53] R. L. Nagel and O. S. Platt, "General pathophysiology of sickle cell anemia," in *Disorders of Hemoglobin*, M. H. Steinberg, B. G. Forget, D. R. Higgs, and R. L. Nagel, Eds., pp. 494–526, Cambridge University Press, Cambridge, UK, 2001.

[54] R. S. Franco, M. Palascak, H. Thompson, and C. H. Joiner, "KCl cotransport activity in light versus dense transferrin receptor- positive sickle reticulocytes," *The Journal of Clinical Investigation*, vol. 95, no. 6, pp. 2573–2580, 1995.

[55] R. S. Franco, M. Palascak, H. Thompson, D. L. Rucknagel, and C. H. Joiner, "Dehydration of transferrin receptor-positive sickle reticulocytes during continuous or cyclic deoxygenation: role of KCl cotransport and extracellular calcium," *Blood*, vol. 88, no. 11, pp. 4359–4365, 1996.

[56] R. M. Bookchin, O. E. Ortiz, and V. L. Lew, "Evidence for a direct reticulocyte origin of dense red cells in sickle cell anemia," *The Journal of Clinical Investigation*, vol. 87, no. 1, pp. 113–124, 1991.

[57] G. R. Serjeant and B. E. Serjeant, "A comparison of erythrocyte characteristics in sickle cell syndromes in Jamaica," *British Journal of Haematology*, vol. 23, no. 2, pp. 205–213, 1972.

[58] M. E. Fabry, D. K. Kaul, and C. Raventos-Suarez, "SC erythrocytes have an abnormally high intracellular hemoglobin concentration. Pathophysiological consequences," *The Journal of Clinical Investigation*, vol. 70, no. 6, pp. 1315–1319, 1982.

[59] S. K. Ballas, J. Larner, E. D. Smith, S. Surrey, E. Schwartz, and E. F. Rappaport, "The xerocytosis of HbSC disease," *Blood*, vol. 69, pp. 124–130, 1987.

[60] C. Lawrence, M. E. Fabry, and R. L. Nagel, "The unique red cell heterogeneity of SC disease: crystal formation, dense reticulocytes, and unusual morphology," *Blood*, vol. 78, no. 8, pp. 2104–2112, 1991.

[61] ME Fabry, J. Harrington, H. Chang, and R. L. Nagel, "Critical contribution of cell density to the pathophysiology of SC cells," *Clinical Research*, vol. 30, article 559a, 1982.

[62] R. M. Bookchin and T. Balazs, "Ionic strength dependence of the polymer solubilities of deoxyhemoglobin S + C and S + A mixtures," *Blood*, vol. 67, no. 4, pp. 887–892, 1986.

[63] A. P. Minton, "Influence of macromolecular crowding on intracellular association reactions: possible role in volume regulation," in *Cellular and Molecular Physiology of Cell Volume Regulation*, K. Strange, Ed., pp. 181–190, CRC Press, Boca Raton, Fla, USA, 1994.

[64] J. S. Gibson, M. C. Muzyamba, S. E. Ball, and J. C. Ellory, "K$^{+}$ transport in HbSC-containing human red blood cells," *The Journal of Physiology*, vol. 535, article S008, p. 27, 2001.

[65] J. C. Ellory, R. Sequeira, A. Constantine, R. J. Wilkins, and J. S. Gibson, "Non-electrolyte permeability of deoxygenated sickle cells compared," *Blood Cells, Molecules, and Diseases*, vol. 41, no. 1, pp. 44–49, 2008.

[66] J. A. Browning, H. M. Staines, H. C. Robinson, T. Powell, J. C. Ellory, and J. S. Gibson, "The effect of deoxygenation on whole-cell conductance of red blood cells from healthy individuals and patients with sickle cell disease," *Blood*, vol. 109, no. 6, pp. 2622–2629, 2007.

[67] J. S. Gibson, A. Khan, P. F. Speake, and J. C. Ellory, "O$_2$ dependence of K$^{+}$ transport in sickle cells: effect of different cell populations and the substituted benzaldehyde 12C79," *The FASEB Journal*, vol. 15, no. 3, pp. 823–832, 2001.

# 17

# Association of Oxidative Stress Markers with Atherogenic Index of Plasma in Adult Sickle Cell Nephropathy

**M. A. Emokpae[1,2] and P. O. Uadia[3]**

[1] Department of Chemical Pathology, Aminu Kano Teaching Hospital, Kano 700001, Nigeria
[2] Department of Medical Laboratory Science, School of Basic Medical Sciences, College of Medical Sciences, University of Benin, Benin City 300001, Nigeria
[3] Department of Biochemistry, University of Benin, Benin City 300001, Nigeria

Correspondence should be addressed to M. A. Emokpae, biodunemokpae@yahoo.com

Academic Editor: Kenneth R. Peterson

This paper evaluates the association of oxidative stress and atherogenic index of plasma in order to assess the cardiovascular risk in Sickle cell nephropathy especially as lipoprotein levels are lower in SCD than non-SCD patients. Antioxidant enzymes, malondialdehyde(MDA), urea, creatinine, and glomerular filtration rate were evaluated in 110 confirmed sickle cell disease patients: 65 males in steady state, aged $21.1 \pm 6.0$ years, 30 males with macroalbuminuria, aged $24.5 \pm 7.0$, years and 15 with chronic kidney disease (CKD), aged $31.8 \pm 2.0$ years. The mean activity levels of glutathione peroxidase (GPx), superoxide dismutase (Cu/ZnSOD), and catalase (CAT) were significantly lower ($P < 0.001$) in SCD with macroalbuminuria and CKD while MDA was higher ($P < 0.001$) in SCD with macroalbuminuria and CKD compared with controls. There was negative correlation between GPx ($P < 0.001$), Cu/ZnSOD ($P < 0.02$), and Atherogenic index of plasma in SCD with CKD, while MDA shows a positive correlation ($P < 0.001$) with AIP in SCD with CKD. There was however no correlation between CAT and AIP. Decreased activity levels of antioxidant enzymes and low HDL-cholesterol concentration were confirmed in adult SCD with CKD in Nigerians. The increase oxidative stress and high atherogenic index in CKD may accelerate the process of cardiovascular complications in adult SCD patients. Atherogenic index of plasma was negatively correlated with antioxidant enzymes and positively with MDA.

## 1. Introduction

Sickle cell disease (SCD) is a haemoglobinopathy which is characterized by red blood cell rigidity, compromised perfusions, and tissue infarction [1]. The kidney of patients with SCD is affected both by haemodynamic changes of chronic and by consequences of vaso-occlusion within the renal medulla [2, 3]. Renal abnormalities in structure and function occur with increasing age of subject with SCD. The pathogenesis of SCD is due to polymerization of sickle red blood cell causing chronic haemolytic anaemia, vaso-occlusive crisis, and intravascular haemolysis. Sickle cell disease patients are susceptible to increased oxidative stress due to constant haemolysis of mutant red blood cells since haemoglobin acts as powerful catalyst for initiation of peroxidative reaction [4, 5]. Proteinuria is common in

adult patients with SCD and we earlier reported a 28% prevalence of proteinuria in this group of patients in Nigeria [6]. Proteinuria is a progression factor in chronic kidney disease heralding a further deterioration in renal function [6]. Metabolic abnormalities, inflammation, and ischaemia may increase oxidative stress in sickle cell nephropathy (SCN). Increased oxidative stress in SCN due to increased pro-oxidative activity may lead to diminished antioxidant system [4, 7]. Increased oxidative stress is considered as an important pathogenic mechanism in the development of cardiovascular, cerebrovascular, and peripheral vascular complications [8, 9]. Autoperoxidation of polyunsaturated fatty acids (PUFAs) is initiated by free radicals, and the products which are oxidized in vivo to form malondialdehyde are capable of damaging membrane of biomolecules [9, 10]. Lipid abnormalities and increased oxidative stress in

TABLE 1: Biochemical and lipid profile of sickle cell disease controls, macroalbuminuria, and chronic kidney disease.

| Variables | SCD controls | SCD macroalbuminuria | SCD CKD | Reference range |
| --- | --- | --- | --- | --- |
| Number of subjects | 65 | 30 | 15 | |
| Age (years) | 21.1 ± 6.0 | 24.5 ± 7.0 | 31.8 ± 2.0* | |
| Urea (mmol/L) | 2.6 ± 0.9 | 8.3 ± 2.0* | 14.2 ± 2.6* | 1.7–8.3 |
| Creatinine ($\mu$mol/L) | 57.3 ± 9.8 | 260 ± 25* | 498 ± 75* | 53–116 |
| eGFR (mL/min) | 101 ± 2.3 | 72 ± 5.0* | 15.1 ± 2.0* | 90–128 |
| Triglyceride (mmol/L) | 1.16 ± 0.4 | 1.20 ± 0.2 | 1.7 ± 0.25* | <1.7 |
| Total cholesterol (mmol/L) | 3.06 ± 0.5 | 3.45 ± 0.6* | 3.9 ± 0.34* | 3.1–6.2 |
| HDL-cholesterol (mmol/L) | 0.72 ± 0.2 | 0.70 ± 0.3 | 0.06 ± 0.08* | 0.8–1.9 |
| LDL-cholesterol (mmol/L) | 1.90 ± 0.5 | 1.8 ± 0.32* | 1.82 ± 0.06* | <3.99 |
| VLDL-cholesterol (mmol/L) | 0.47 ± 0.06 | 0.52 ± 0.06* | 0.74 ± 0.06* | <0.8 |
| AIP | 0.22 | 0.23 | 0.45 | <1.44 |
| TC: HDL | 4.25 | 4.92 | 6.50 | <4.9 |
| LDL: HDL | 2.67 | 2.57 | 3.03 | <2.4 |

eGFR: estimated glomerular filtration rate; AIP: atherogenic index of plasma; *$P < 0.001$.

SCN may accelerate the process of atherosclerosis in patients with SCN. This study evaluates the association of oxidative stress and atherogenic index of plasma in order to assess the cardiovascular risk in SCN especially when lipoprotein levels are lower in SCD than non-SCD patients.

## 2. Materials and Methods

The study population was 110 confirmed SCD patients attending sickle cell disease clinic of Amiru Kano Teaching Hospital. They consisted of 65 males in steady state, aged 21.1±6.0 years, 30 males with macroalbuminuria aged 24.5 ± 7.0 years, and 15 with chronic kidney disease (CKD), aged 31.8 ± 2.0 years. Demographic and clinical examination findings were obtained using structured questionnaires. The study protocol used was approved by the institute's ethical committee and the patients gave informed consent before enrolment in the study. Random urine was obtained for analysis using combi-9 commercial dipstick, which was used to test for biochemical urinalysis. Five milliliter of blood was collected aseptically and dispensed into a plain tube after 12-hour fast. The blood was allowed to clot and serum obtained after centrifugation at 3000 rpm for 10minutes. The sera were stored at −20°C and analysis was done within two weeks of collection. Urea was determined using urease colorimetric technique, creatinine was assayed using sodium hydroxide-picric acid technique, and superoxide dismutase (Cu/ZnSOD), and glutathione peroxidase (GPx) were assayed using ELISA kits supplied by Northwest life science specialities, Vancouver, Canada. Catalase was estimated using kit by SIGMA (St. Louis, Missouri, USA) and malondialdehyde was determined using thiobarbituric acid reacting substance kit supplied by Northwest life science specialties. Total cholesterol and triglyceride (TG) were determined using enzyme-catalyzed colorimetric methods by Randox laboratories, UK. HDL cholesterol was assayed using the supernatant after precipitation with magnesium

chloride-phosphotungstic acid solution, while LDL cholesterol was calculated using Friedewald formula [11]. Cardiovascular risk ratio was calculated using atherogenic index of plasma (AIP) [12], which was defined as log(TG/HDL-c) with TG and HDL-c expressed in molar concentration. Glomerular filtration rate was estimated using Cockroft-Gault formular [13]. Chronic kidney disease was defined as estimated glomerular filtration rate (eGFR) of <60 mL/min and presence of macroalbuminuria. Macroalbuminuria was defined as presence in urine of albumin concentration of ≥300 mg/L. A two-sample $t$-test was used to determine the statistical significance of the means between the different groups. A $P$ value of 0.05 or less was considered statistically significant. Pearson correlation coefficient was used to show the levels of association of antioxidant enzyme levels with AIP in SCD patient with CKD.

## 3. Results

The results are as indicated in Tables 1, 2, and 3. Table 1 shows biochemical and lipoprotein levels of SCD subjects in steady state used as controls, SCD with macroalbuminuria, and CKD. The mean serum urea and creatinine in SCD with macroalbuminuria and CKD were significantly higher ($P < 0.001$) than those of the SCD control subjects while the mean eGFR was significantly lower ($P < 0.001$) in SCD with macroalbuminuria and CKD compared with control subjects. The mean levels of triglyceride, total cholesterol, LDL cholesterol, and VLDL cholesterol were significantly higher ($P < 0.001$) in CKD compared with SCD controls while HDL cholesterol was lower ($P < 0.001$) in CKD compared with control subjects. The atherogenic index significantly increased in SCD patients with CKD compared with SCD with macroalbuminuria and control group.

Table 2 indicates changes in oxidative stress markers in the study group. The mean activity levels of GPx, Cu/ZnSOD, and CAT were significantly lower ($P < 0.001$) in SCD with macroalbuminuria and CKD while MDA was higher

TABLE 2: Oxidative stress markers of sickle cell disease control, macroalbuminuria, and chronic kidney disease.

| Oxidative markers | SCD controls | SCD with macroalbuminuria | SCD with chronic kidney disease | Reference range |
|---|---|---|---|---|
| Number of subjects | 65 | 30 | 15 | |
| Glutathione peroxidase (mU/mL) | $9.2 \pm 0.9$ | $5.54 \pm 3.5^*$ | $3.01 \pm 0.24^*$ | 9.2–19.6 |
| Superoxide dismutase (ng/mL) | $30.6 \pm 5.1$ | $21.3 \pm 5.2^*$ | $18.5 \pm 2.6^*$ | 22.5–103 |
| Catalase ($\mu$mol/min/L) | $154 \pm 7.9$ | $150 \pm 2.58$ | $147 \pm 1.06^*$ | 156–182 |
| Malondialdehyde ($\mu$mol/L) | $2.5 \pm 0.4$ | $3.8 \pm 1.7^*$ | $5.30 \pm 0.3^*$ | 0.025–0.98 |

$^*P < 0.001$.

TABLE 3: Correlation between antioxidant enzymes and atherogenic index of plasma in SCD with chronic kidney disease.

| Correlation between parameters | $R$ value | $P$ value |
|---|---|---|
| GPx and AIP | $-0.760$ | 0.001 |
| Cu/ZnSOD and AIP | $-0.621$ | 0.02 |
| CAT and AIP | $-0.416$ | NS |
| MDA and AIP | 0.943 | 0.001 |

GPx: Glutathione peroxidase; Cu/ZnSOD: Superoxide Dismutase; CAT: Catalase and MDA: Malondialdehyde.

($P < 0.001$) in SCD with macroalbuminuria and CKD compared with controls.

Table 3 shows the levels of association of antioxidant markers with AIP in SCD with CKD. There were negative correlations between GPx ($P < 0.001$), Cu/ZnSOD ($P < 0.02$), and AIP in SCD with CKD, while MDA shows a positive correlation ($P < 0.001$) with AIP in SCD with CKD. The correlation between CAT and AIP was however not significant.

## 4. Discussion

The data showed that there were increases in oxidative stress and lipoprotein levels in SCD patients with macroalbuminuria and CKD. Atherogenic index of plasma was negatively correlated with antioxidant enzymes and positively with MDA in CKD. Studies have shown decreases in the activity levels of antioxidant enzymes in SCD patients in steady state [4] and in non-SCD patients with acute renal failure [14]. The present study associated the decreases in the antioxidant enzyme activity levels with AIP, used as cardiovascular risk, especially as lipoprotein levels in SCD patients are lower than non-SCD individuals in both normal and renal disease. In this study, we observed increased oxidative stress in SCD patients with CKD. Oxidative damage is due to redox imbalance between production of reactive oxygen species (ROS) and the countering effects of the various antioxidants in the body. The increased production of ROS in SCD can be grossly amplified in response to a variety of pathophysiological conditions including renal disorders, inflammation, immunologic disorders, hypoxia, metabolism of drugs or alcohol, and deficiency in antioxidant enzymes [1, 4, 15]. Reactive oxygen species can cause significant damage to biomolecules since membrane lipids readily react with ROS resulting in lipid peroxidation [16–18]. Increased oxidative

stress has been reported to mediate most of the risk factors involved in kidney disease [19]. Free radical mediated injury is the primary event leading to renal injury and progressive renal insufficiency and may lead to increased levels of lipid peroxidation. This occurs because cell membrane contains large quantity of PUFAs. These PUFAs react with ROS to form peroxide derivatives [20, 21]. Oxidative damage may alter both structure and function of the glomerulus due to its effects on mesangial and endothelial cells. Overexpression of ROS by both enzymatic and nonenzymatic pathways (Fenton chemistry) promotes intravascular oxidant stress that can disrupt nitric oxide homeostasis and produce the highly oxidative peroxynitrite [22]. Previous reports have showed that renal disease in SCD has the capacity to diminish arginine bioavailability through the loss of de novo arginine synthesis from citrulline which occurs primarily in the kidneys. Renal insufficiency may impair the major route for endogenous arginine biosynthesis [23] since it plays some roles in the regulation of nitric oxide production [24]. Adults with SCD are arginine deficient even at steady state [25, 26].

The observed increases ($P < 0.001$) in the levels of serum triglyceride, LDL, VLDL, and decrease ($P < 0.001$) of HDL-cholesterol levels in SCD patients with CKD are consistent with other studies elsewhere and in Nigeria [27–30]. The lipid profile of SCD patients is quite lower than that in subjects with normal haemoglobin and SCD patients in Nigeria have even lower levels than SCD patients in America and the Middle East [27–29]. Several reasons have been proposed as to why there are inconsistencies between lipid studies; these include differences in age, diet, weight, smoking, gender, small sample sizes, different ranges of disease severity, and treatment regimen [31–33]. Shores et al. [28] proposed the reasons why lipoprotein levels are lower in SCD than nonSCD even in the same environmental condition to be partly due to a decrease in red blood cell volume leading to a dilution effect on plasma constituents. It may also result from strong downregulation of the synthetic pathways or downregulation of the enzymes in lipid biosynthesis. Others suggested that it is the haemolytic stress in SCD patients that is associated with a significant reduction in plasma lipids in SCD patients [29, 34].

## 5. Conclusion

Decreased activity levels of antioxidant enzymes and low HDL-cholesterol concentration were confirmed in adult SCD with CKD in Nigerians. The increase oxidative stress and high atherogenic index in CKD may accelerate the process of cardiovascular complications in adult SCD patients. Atherogenic index of plasma was negatively correlated with antioxidant enzymes and positively with MDA.

## References

[1] M. A. Emokpae, P. O. Uadia, and A. A. Gadzama, "Correlation of oxidative stress and inflammatory markers with the severity of sickle cell nephropathy," *Annals of African Medicine*, vol. 9, no. 3, pp. 141–146, 2010.

[2] I. Batinic-Haberle, J. S. Reboucas, and I. Spasojevic, "Superoxide Dismutase mimics: chemistry, pharmacology and Therapeutic potential," *Antioxid Redox Signal*, vol. 13, no. 6, pp. 877–918, 2010.

[3] G. R. Serjeant, "Renal manifestation in sickle cell disease," in *Oxford Textbook of Clinical Nephrology*, pp. 261–281, Oxford University Press, London, UK, 2nd edition, 1992.

[4] A. M. Emokpae, P. O. Uadia, and A. Kuliya-Gwarzo, "Antioxidant enzymes and acute phase proteins correlate with marker of lipid peroxide in adult Nigerian sickle cell disease patients," *Iranian Journal of Basic Medical Sciences*, vol. 13, no. 4, pp. 177–182, 2010.

[5] E. S. Klings and H. W. Farber, "Role of free radicals in the pathogenesis of acute chest syndrome in sickle cell disease," *Respiratory Research*, vol. 2, no. 5, pp. 280–285, 2001.

[6] A. Abdu, M. Emokpae, P. Uadia, and A. Kuliya-Gwarzo, "Proteinuria among adult sickle cell anemia patients in Nigeria," *Annals of African Medicine*, vol. 10, no. 1, pp. 34–37, 2011.

[7] M. H. Steinberg, "Pathophysiologically based drug treatment of sickle cell disease," *Trends in Pharmacological Sciences*, vol. 27, no. 4, pp. 204–210, 2006.

[8] R. P. Hebbel, J. W. Eaton, M. Balasingam, and M. H. Steinberg, "Spontaneous oxygen radical generation by sickle erythrocytes," *Journal of Clinical Investigation*, vol. 70, no. 6, pp. 1253–1259, 1982.

[9] J. Yam, L. Frank, and R. J. Roberts, "Oxygen toxicity: comparison of lung biochemical responses in neonatal and adult rats," *Pediatric Research*, vol. 12, no. 2, pp. 115–119, 1978.

[10] I. Fridovich and B. Freeman, "Antioxidant defenses in the lung," *Annual Review of Physiology*, vol. 48, pp. 693–702, 1986.

[11] W. T. Friedewald, R. I. Levy, and D. S. Fredrickson, "Estimation of the concentration of low-density lipoprotein cholesterol in plasma, without use of the preparative ultracentrifuge," *Clinical Chemistry*, vol. 18, no. 6, pp. 499–502, 1972.

[12] D. W. Cockcroft and M. H. Gault, "Prediction of creatinine clearance from serum creatinine," *Nephron*, vol. 16, no. 1, pp. 31–41, 1976.

[13] V. Manfredini, L. L. Lazzaretti, I. H. Griebeler, A. P. Santin, V. D. Brandao, and S. Wagner, "Blood antioxidant parameters in sickle cell anaemia patients in steady state," *National Medical Association*, vol. 100, pp. 897–902, 2008.

[14] G. Ramani, G. Kavitha, P. K. Dhass, and R. M. Aruna, "Oxidative stress and its association with cardiovascular risk in acute renal failure," *International Journal of Pharma and Bio Sciences*, vol. 2, no. 3, pp. B329–B334, 2011.

[15] G. Remuzzi and T. Bertani, "Pathophysiology of progressive nephropathies," *New England Journal of Medicine*, vol. 339, no. 20, pp. 1448–1456, 1998.

[16] K. Pawlak, D. Pawlek, and M. Mysliwice, "Cu/Zn superoxide dismutase plasma level as a new useful chemical biomarker of oxidative stress in patients with end stage renal disease," *Clinical Biochemistry*, vol. 38, pp. 700–705, 2005.

[17] O. G. Arinola, J. A. Olaniyi, and M. O. Akiibinu, "Evaluation of antioxidant levels and trace element status in Nigerian sickle cell disease patients with Plasmodium parasitaemia," *Pakistan Journal of Nutrition*, vol. 7, no. 6, pp. 766–769, 2008.

[18] T. A. Sutton, H. E. Mang, S. B. Campos, R. M. Sandol, M. C. Yoder, and B. A. Molitoris, "Injury of the renal microvascular endothelium alters banner function after ischemia," *American Journal of Physiology*, vol. 285, pp. F191–F198, 2003.

[19] R. E. Ratych and G. B. Bulkley, "Free-radical-mediated postischemic reperfusion injury in the kidney," *Journal of Free Radicals in Biology and Medicine*, vol. 2, no. 5-6, pp. 311–319, 1986.

[20] S. P. Mark, R. H. John, and F. F. Thomas, "Oxygen free radicals in Ischaemic acute renal failure in the rat," *Journal of Clinical Investigation*, vol. 74, pp. 1156–1164, 1984.

[21] E. L. Greene and M. S. Paller, "Oxygen free radicals in acute renal failure," *Mineral and Electrolyte Metabolism*, vol. 17, no. 2, pp. 124–132, 1991.

[22] M. A. Emokpae, O. H. Uwumarongie, and H. B. Osadolor, "Sex dimorphism in serum lecithin: cholesterol acyltransferase and lipoprotein lipase activities in adult sickle cell anaemia patients with proteinuria," *Indian Journal of Clinical Biochemistry*, vol. 26, no. 1, pp. 57–61, 2011.

[23] K. C. Wood, L. L. Hsu, and M. T. Gladwin, "Sickle cell disease vasculopathy: a state of nitric oxide resistance," *Free Radical Biology and Medicine*, vol. 44, no. 8, pp. 1506–1528, 2008.

[24] C. R. Morris, "Mechanisms of vasculopathy in sickle cell disease and Thalassemia. Current and Future Therapies of sickle cell anemia," *Hematology*, vol. 1, pp. 177–185, 2008.

[25] C. R. Morris, C. Teehanke, and G. Kato, "Decreased arginine bioavailability contributes to the pathogenesis of pulmonary artery hypertension," in *Proceedings of the Annual Meeting of American College of Cardiology*, Orlando, Fla, USA, 2005.

[26] C. O. Enwonwu, "Increased metabolic demand for arginine in sickle cell anaemia," *Medical Science Research*, vol. 17, no. 23, pp. 997–998, 1989.

[27] M. A. Emokpae, A. Abdu, P. O. Uadia, and M. M. Borodo, "Lipid profile in sickle cell disease patients with chronic kidney disease," *Sahel Medical Journal*, vol. 13, no. 1, pp. 20–23, 2010.

[28] J. Shores, J. Peterson, D. VanderJagt, and R. H. Glew, "Reduced cholesterol levels in African-American adults with sickle cell disease," *Journal of the National Medical Association*, vol. 95, no. 9, pp. 813–817, 2003.

[29] Z. Rahimi, A. Merat, M. Haghshenass, H. Madani, M. Rezaei, and R. L. Nagel, "Plasma lipids in Iranians with sickle cell disease: hypocholesterolemia in sickle cell anemia and increase of HDL-cholesterol in sickle cell trait," *Clinica Chimica Acta*, vol. 365, no. 1-2, pp. 217–220, 2006.

[30] C. R. Morris, F. A. Kuypers, S. Larkin, E. P. Vichinsky, and L. A. Styles, "Patterns of arginine and nitric oxide in patients with sickle cell disease with vaso-occlusive crisis and acute chest syndrome," *Journal of Pediatric Hematology/Oncology*, vol. 22, no. 6, pp. 515–520, 2000.

[31] M. Z. Zailaie, Z. M. Marzouki, and S. M. Khoja, "Plasma and red blood cells membrane lipid concentration of sickle cell disease patients," *Saudi Medical Journal*, vol. 24, no. 4, pp. 376–379, 2003.

[32] E. Choy and N. Sattar, "Interpreting lipid levels in the context of high-grade inflammatory states with a focus on rheumatoid arthritis: a challenge to conventional cardiovascular risk actions," *Annals of the Rheumatic Diseases*, vol. 68, no. 4, pp. 460–469, 2009.

[33] A. P. H. Gotto, *Manual of Lipid Disorders: Reducing the Risk for Coronary Heart Disease*, Lippincott, Williams and Wilkins, Philadelphia, Pa, USA, 2003.

[34] S. Zorca, L. Freeman, M. Hildesheim et al., "Lipid levels in sickle-cell disease associated with haemolytic severity, vascular dysfunction and pulmonary hypertension," *British Journal of Haematology*, vol. 149, no. 3, pp. 436–445, 2010.

# 18

# Sickle-Cell Disease Healthcare Cost in Africa: Experience of the Congo

**L. O. Ngolet,**[1] **M. Moyen Engoba,**[2] **Innocent Kocko,**[1] **Alexis Elira Dokekias,**[1] **Jean-Vivien Mombouli,**[3] **and Georges Marius Moyen**[1]

[1]*Clinical Hematology Unit, Brazzaville Teaching Hospital, Auxence Ickonga Avenue, P.O. Box 32, Brazzaville, Congo*
[2]*Pediatric Intensive Care Unit, Brazzaville Teaching Hospital, Brazzaville, Congo*
[3]*National Laboratory of Public Health, Brazzaville Teaching Hospital, Brazzaville, Congo*

Correspondence should be addressed to L. O. Ngolet; lngolet@yahoo.fr

Academic Editor: Duran Canatan

*Background.* Lack of medical coverage in Africa leads to inappropriate care that has an impact on the mortality rate. In this study, we aimed to evaluate the cost of severe acute sickle-cell related complications in Brazzaville. *Methods.* A retrospective study was conducted in 2014 in the Paediatric Intensive Care Unit. It concerned 94 homozygote sickle-cell children that developed severe acute sickle-cell disease related complications (average age 69 months). For each patient, we calculated the cost of care complication. *Results.* The household income was estimated as low (<XAF 90,000/<USD 158.40) in 27.7%. The overall median cost for hospitalization for sickle-cell related acute complications was XAF 65,460/USD 115.21. Costs were fluctuating depending on the generating factors of the severe acute complications ($p = 0.041$). They were higher in case of complications generated by bacterial infections (ranging from XAF 66,765/USD 117.50 to XAF 135,271.50/USD 238.07) and lower in case of complications associated with malaria (ranging from XAF 28,305/49.82 to XAF 64,891.63/USD 114.21). The mortality rate was 17% and was associated with the cost of the case management ($p = 0.006$). *Conclusion.* The case management cost of severe acute complications of sickle-cell disease in children is high in Congo.

## 1. Introduction

Sickle-cell disease is the most frequent haemoglobin disorder in the world, mostly in sub-Saharan Africa where 75% of the 300, 000 babies are born each year with haemoglobin disorders live [1, 2]. Homozygous form of SCD is associated with very high child mortality, but reliable data are lacking. WHO estimates that 70% of deaths are avoidable by putting in place "preventive" measures [3]. These measures encompass early diagnosis, information, education, and prophylaxis of infections [4–6]. In sub-Saharan Africa, medical coverage program like Medicaid that supports patients in the expenses generated by medical management of their disease does not exist or is very insufficient. In Congo where 1% of the population is affected by the homozygous form of the disease,

such program does not exist [7]. The nonaccessibility to care and medicines is linked in 54.61% to financial challenges [8]. This inaccessibility is higher at the tertiary level of medical facilities such as the teaching hospital where the costs of care are far higher. The consequence of this is the arrival of patients at an advanced stage of the disease. Overall, in Africa and in Congo, contrary to the Western countries, morbidity and mortality are associated with the costs of sickle-cell disease (SCD) care. Although hospitalization appears to drive the majority of SCD treatment cost [9–11], only one study published in Africa has examined the hospitalization cost of SCD [12]. That small study was conducted on adult in the Hematology Unit in Congo in 2012. None studies report the cost of care for SCD children inpatient hospitalization. The purpose of this study is to report the cost of severe acute complications of SCD related care for pediatric inpatients hospitalization in the Emergency Department of the Brazzaville Teaching Hospital in Congo.

## 2. Material and Methods

Brazzaville Teaching Hospital has a total of 4 pediatric departments: Intensive Care, Neonatology, Infant Care, and Toddler/Teenager care where a total of 5,657 children were admitted during the period of our study. This study was conducted from January 1 to December 31, 2014, in the Pediatric Intensive Care Unit (PICU) of Brazzaville Teaching Hospital. PICU manages all medical emergencies that involve immediate vital prognostic of children aged 1 month to 16 years old.

*2.1. Data Collection and Assessment Procedures.* We enrolled in the study all pediatric patients that were developing severe acute SCD related complications. SCD children with no severe SCD related complications were not included in the study. We defined as severe acute complications all life threatening sickle-cell disease related acute complications. These are

(1) acute exacerbation of anemia due to acute splenic sequestration or acute hyperhemolysis;

(2) major acute pain syndromes;

(3) acute chest syndrome;

(4) stroke;

(5) mixed severe acute crisis that combines acute exacerbation of anemia and major pain syndromes;

(6) severe infection: in the context of functional asplenia, a temperature over 38, 5°C with or without a source is an emergency and considered as severe infection.

*Generated Factors.* Generated factors are factors that trigger acute exacerbation anemia, pain syndromes, acute chest syndrome, stroke, and mixed crisis. These factors are infectious or physical such as environmental heat, stress, wearing heat retaining clothing, and dehydration.

Thus, 94 sickle-cell disease children presenting one severe acute complication have been included in the study.

*2.2. Cost Assessment of the Case Management of Severe Acute Complications.* Costs generated correspond to the fees encountered for the diagnosis and treatment of acute complications and generating factors. The global cost was calculated by adding costs of medicines, hospitalization and diagnosis tests.

Hospitalization fees depend on the length of admission of the patient. Patients are charged XAF 25,000/USD 42.64 for the total of 5 days (first five days at the hospital) and then XAF 5,000/USD 11.72 for each day from the 6th day of hospitalization. Costs of medicines and diagnostic tests have been calculated from the fares displayed by the teaching hospital. The consumables, dressing, syringes, and infusion sets as well as the hospitalization or physician visits fees before the patient's admission to the PICU, were not included.

Income of the family was interpreted based on the official lowest salary fixed by the government (XAF 90,000/USD 153.53). The income was low when it was lower than XAF 90,000/USD 153.53, middle when it was between XAF 90,000/USD 153.53 and XAF 500,000/USD 852.96, and high when it was above USD XAF 500,000/USD 852.96.

The data were computed on Microsoft Excel 2013 and processed and analyzed with the software STATA (version 12, Texas, USA). For the description of each quantitative variable, the mean/average value, median, and standard deviation were calculated. For the comparison of qualitative data, the ANOVA and Student tests were used. The tests were significantly significant when $p$ value $<0.05$. The different costs have been calculated in XAF and then converted into USD using the exchange rate of USD $1 = $ XAF 568.19.

## 3. Results

*3.1. Characteristics of the Population.* 1278 children were admitted in PICU during our study. Among them, 136 (10.64%) had sickle-cell disease and 94 (69.11%) had developed severe acute complications. These were 48 boys (51.1%) and 46 girls (48.9%) making a sex ratio of 1.04. the patients were aged from 6 to 192 months with an average age of $69 \pm 50$ months. Fifty-eight patients (61.7%) were coming to the hospital from their homes whereas 24 children (25.5%) were referred by primary and secondary health facilities. Twelve children (12.8%) were from other teaching hospital departments. It had been possible to determine the income of 50 families (53.2%). Among them, 26 (52%) had low status income while 18 (36%) had middle and 6 (12%) had high one (Table 1).

*3.2. Costs of Hospital Expenses.* The average length of hospitalization has been 5.5 days (extremes of 1 and 16 days) generating a median cost of XAF 30,000/USD 52.79 (range XAF 25,000/USD 42.64 and XAF 80,000/USD 136.47). Sixteen children (17%) died during their hospitalization. The mortality rate was significantly higher in the age group older than 120 months with no influence of referral origin of the patient ($p = 0.004$).

The median global cost care of SCD related acute complications was XAF 65.460/USD 111.67 (range XAF 28,305/USD 49.81 and XAF 365,740/USD 643.69). Diagnostic tests, hospitalizations, and medicines represented, respectively, 16%, 38%, and 49% of the global cost (Table 2).

Bacterial infections were the most frequent acute complication associated with SCD related crisis with 50 cases (53.2%). Care of bacterial infections whatever the type of sickle-cell crisis they were triggering was the most expensive since the quotation for their care was the highest (range: XAF 62,800/USD 107.13 and XAF 135271.5/USD 230.76), followed by malaria (range: XAF 28.305/USD 48.28 and XAF 99,944/USD 170.49). Vascular complications were represented by acute chest syndrome and stroke with respective costs care of XAF 42,800/USD 73.01 and XAF 103,492/USD 176.55 ($p = 0.041$) Table 3.

TABLE 1: Characteristics of the population.

| | n (%) |
|---|---|
| *Gender* | n (%) |
| Female | 46 (48.9) |
| Male | 48 (51.1) |
| Sex ratio | 1.04 |
| *Age (months)* | |
| Mean ± Ecart type | 69.26 ± 50.40 |
| Min–max | 6–192 |
| *Referred by* | n (%) |
| Teaching hospital's departments | 12 (12.8) |
| Primary and secondary public offices | 14 (14.9) |
| Private offices | 10 (10.6) |
| Home | 58 (61.7) |
| *Hospitalization length (days)* | n (%) |
| 1-2 | 44 (46.8) |
| 3–8 | 34 (36.2) |
| 9–16 | 16 (17) |
| *Income* | n (%) |
| Low | 26 (27.7) |
| Middle | 6 (6.4) |
| High | 18 (19.1) |
| Unknown | 44 (46.8) |
| *Death* | n (%) |
| Yes | 78 (83.0) |
| No | 16 (17.0) |
| *Age of death** | n (%) |
| 0–24 | 1 (12.5) |
| 25–60 | 0 (00) |
| 61–120 | 6 (37.5) |
| >120 | 8 (50) |

*$p = 0.004$.

## 4. Discussion

This first study has allowed estimating the cost of care of severe acute complications SCD related in pediatric population admitted in intensive care. The global cost borne by families is high since it is on average XAF 65,460/USD 111.67 per episode, representing 2/3 of the minimum wage salary in Congo officially set at XAF 90,000/USD 153.53. Our study has several limits. First, the analysis of these results does not take into account the fees generated by consumables (syringes, infusion sets, and dressings). They are also to be paid by the patient, as well as fees for preadmission physician visit or hospitalization in different hospitals or units that concerned 38.3% of our sample population. The second limitation is the care costs estimations. Estimated costs were calculated from the teaching hospital costing that has the lowest fees. Nevertheless, fees displayed by the teaching hospital do not allow a real cost recovery, limiting a sustainable procurement in reagents but also in medicines. Referring to a WHO study, availability of medicines is limited. Only 60% of essential

medicines are available in public pharmacies [8]. These parameters, which are difficult to evaluate since many medicines and tests are bought and used out of the teaching hospital, could contribute to underestimating the real care cost of SCD related acute complications. A similar study conducted on adults in the clinical hematology department reported a comparable average global cost care: XAF 88,365/USD 155.520 [12]. Nevertheless, some reservation must be expressed in comparing these costs, since the hospitalization fees in the clinical hematology department are fixed at XAF 10,000/USD 17.05 no matter the length of hospitalization. Consequently, the fees for hospitalization represented only 8.8% of the global expense in that study compared to 38% in ours [12].

Bacterial infections are the first cause of admission of sickle-cell disease children and adults in Africa [13–16]. The cost of care for their management is higher whatever the type of associated severe acute complications (XAF 66,765/USD 113.89 to XAF 135,271/USD 230.78). This is the consequence of the high cost of antibiotics in the continent [8, 17, 18]. Despite an ambitious essential medicines policy (with antibiotics in priority position) in Congo that aims to reduce the cost of medicines, these medicines remain inaccessible for the majority of the population [8]. Additionally, only 57% of antibiotics are prescribed by their international nonpropriety name (INN) [9]. This trend seems similar in sub-Saharan Africa as a study in private pharmacies in Mali showed that only 48.2% of antibiotics were prescribed in INN [18]. Also, procurement challenges at the hospital pharmacy, limited availability of essential medicines, and presence of fake antibiotics on the market are some elements pushing for prescription and purchase of branded medicines. Besides, microbiologic proof of infections barely provided by our laboratories is responsible of an overprescription of antibiotics and then an over cost care. Lastly, the absence of standard therapeutic chart has a perceptible impact on the cost of the prescription by irrational use of antibiotics.

Malaria represented the second cause of admission of sickle-cell disease children with a total of 29.8%. Malaria is widely considered a major cause of illness and death in SCD patients [14, 19, 20]. Even though we find in our study strong association between hyperhemolysis crisis and malaria, the association of this comorbidity is controversial. Some investigators have associated it with the anemic hyperhemolysis crisis while others suggest that patients living with SCD are protected from malaria [21, 22]. Despite the fact that the National Programme on Malaria has chosen the combination of artesunate and amodiaquine as first-line treatment, quinine is still used in first intention in almost 85% of health facilities [9].

The additional costs of the prescription in our study come from the purchase of pain killers and labile blood products. Blood transfusion is a major therapeutic element in the treatment of sickle-cell disease crisis since it is performed on 47% of sickle-cell disease children [14]. The supply cost for a bag of erythrocyte concentrate is XAF 7,500/USD 12.79, whereas the effective expenses for its preparation are estimated at XAF 65,000/USD 110.88. This causes supply challenges as mentioned earlier.

TABLE 2: Acute severe sickle-cell complications global treatment cost in XAF (USD).

|  | Hospitalization cost | Diagnosis test cost | Medicines cost | Global cost care |
|---|---|---|---|---|
| Mean | 33,085.1 (58.23) | 12,068.18 (21.23) | 53,647.67 (94.41) | 93,889.21 (165.24) |
| Ecart type | 16,535.4 (29.1) | 10,493.76 (18.46) | 59,461.21 (104.65) | 78,622.47 (138.37) |
| Median | 30,000 (52.79) | 10,500 (18.47) | 32,267.5 (56.79) | 65,460 (111.67) |
| Min–max | 25,000–80,000 (42.64–136.47) | 0–48,000 (0–84.47) | 3,305–272,740 (5.81–480.02) | 28,305–365,740 (49.81–643.69) |

$t = 2028$, $p = 0.026$.

TABLE 3: Severe acute sickle-cell complications and its generated factors treatment cost.

| Diagnostic | $n$ | % | Global management care XAF (USD) | $p$ value |
|---|---|---|---|---|
| Major acute pain + bacterial infections | 12 | 12.8 | 66,765 (117.50) |  |
| Hyperhemolysis + bacterial infections | 18 | 19.2 | 103,492 (182.14) | $p = 0.041$ |
| Mixed severe acute crisis + bacterial infections | 28 | 29.8 | 135,271 (238.07) |  |
| Major acute pain + malaria | 4 | 4.2 | 28,305 (49.82) |  |
| Hyperhemolysis + malaria | 16 | 17,1 | 64,891.63 (114.21) |  |
| Mixed severe acute crisis + malaria | 8 | 8.5 | 99,944 (175.90) |  |
| Major acute pain + acute chest syndrome | 2 | 2.1 | 42,800 (75.33) |  |
| Hyperhemolysis + acute chest syndrome | 2 | 2.1 | 62,800 (110.52) |  |
| Mixed severe acute crisis + stroke | 4 | 4.2 | 130,333 (229.38) |  |
| Total | 94 | 100 |  |  |

## 5. Conclusion

This study has examined the cost of severe acute SCD related complications in intensive care. Severe acute SCD related complications remain worrisome not only due to their graveness, but mainly due to the expenses that families must bear for their care. This study is the first to examine the cost of all components of care for pediatrics population with SCD admitted in intensive care. It is an important input to SCD treatment strategies, health care planning, and research prioritization. This study has also shown that infections and malaria remain persistently high. Additional research is needed to better understand infectious pattern of children with SCD.

## Conflict of Interests

The authors declare that there is no conflict of interests regarding the publication of this paper.

## Acknowledgment

The authors are grateful to Dr. Lapnet Mustapha to his assistance in the translation.

## References

[1] World Health Organisation, *Management of Birth Defects and Hemoglobin Disorders: Report of a Joint Who-March of Dimes Meeting*, World Health Organization, Geneva, Switzerland, 2006.

[2] B. Modell and M. Darlison, "Global epidemiology of haemoglobin disorders and derived service indicators," *Bulletin of the World Health Organization*, vol. 86, no. 6, pp. 480–487, 2008.

[3] D. C. Rees, T. N. Williams, and M. T. Gladwin, "Sickle-cell disease," *The Lancet*, vol. 376, no. 9757, pp. 2018–2031, 2010.

[4] T. N. William and S. K. Obaro, "Sickle cell disease and malaria morbidity: a tale with two tails," *Trends in Parasitology*, vol. 27, no. 7, pp. 315–320, 2011.

[5] A. B. John, A. Ramlal, H. Jackson, G. H. Maude, A. W. Sharma, and G. R. Serjeant, "Prevention of pneumococcal infection in children with homozygous sickle cell disease," *British Medical Journal*, vol. 288, no. 6430, pp. 1567–1570, 1984.

[6] M. H. Gaston, J. I. Verter, G. Woods et al. et al., "Prophylaxis with oral penicillin in children with sickle cell anemia," *The New England Journal of Medicine*, vol. 314, no. 25, pp. 1593–1599, 1986.

[7] A. B. Mpemba Loufoua, P. Makoumbou, J. R. Mabiala Babela et al., "Dépistage néonatal de la drépanocytose au Congo Brazzaville," *Annales de l'Université Marien Ngouabi*, vol. 11, no. 5, pp. 21–25, 2010.

[8] *Rapport: Evaluation du Secteur Pharmaceutique du Congo*, OMS, Juillet, 2006.

[9] S. Lanzkron, C. Haywood Jr., J. B. Segal, and G. J. Dover, "Hospitalization rates and costs of care of patients with sickle-cell anemia in the state of Maryland in the era of hydroxyurea," *American Journal of Hematology*, vol. 81, no. 12, pp. 927–932, 2006.

[10] H. Davis, R. M. Moore Jr., and P. J. Gergen, "Cost of hospitalizations associated with sickle cell disease in the United States," *Public Health Reports*, vol. 112, no. 1, pp. 40–43, 1997.

[11] R. D. Moor, S. Charache, M. L. Terrin et al., "The costs of children with sickle cell anemia. Preparing for managed care,"

*Journal of Pediatric Hematology/Oncology*, vol. 20, no. 6, pp. 528–533, 1998.

[12] L. O. Ngolet, H. Ntsiba, and A. Elira Dokekias, "Le coût de la prise en charge hospitalière des crises drépanocytaires," *Annales de l'Université Marien Ngouabi*, vol. 14, no. 5, pp. 14–19, 2013.

[13] E. Barett-Connor, "Bacterial infection and sickle cell anemia," *Medicine*, vol. 50, pp. 94–112, 1971.

[14] J. R. Mabiala-Babela, T. Nkanza-Kaluwako, P. S. Ganga-Zandzou, S. Nzingoula, and P. Senga, "Causes d'hospitalisation des enfants drépanocytaires : influence de l'âge (C.H.U. de Brazzaville, Congo)," *Bulletin de la Société de Pathologie Exotique*, vol. 98, no. 5, pp. 392–393, 2005.

[15] G. R. Serjeant, "Mortality from sickle cell disease in Africa," *British Medical Journal*, vol. 330, no. 7489, pp. 432–433, 2005.

[16] S. D. Grosse, I. Odame, H. K. Atrash, D. D. Amendah, F. B. Piel, and T. N. Williams, "Sickle cell disease in Africa. A neglected cause of early childhood mortality," *American Journal of Preventive Medicine*, vol. 41, no. 6, supplement 4, pp. S398–S405, 2011.

[17] Y. Coulibaly, A. Konate, D. Done, and F. Bougoudogo, "Étude de la prescription des antibiotiques en milieu hospitalier malien," *Revue Malienne D'infectiologie et de Microbiologie*, vol. 3, pp. 2–8, 2014.

[18] IFMT, "Antibiotiques dans les pays en développement," MS.IFMT//M05, 2004.

[19] D. Diallo and G. Tchernia, "Sickle cell disease in Africa," *Current Opinion in Hematology*, vol. 9, no. 2, pp. 111–116, 2002.

[20] A. Elira Dokekias, "Etude analytique des facteurs d'aggravation de la maladie drépanocytaire au Congo," *Médecine d'Afrique Noire Électronique*, vol. 43, no. 5, pp. 279–285, 1996.

[21] I. Diagne, G. M. Soares, A. Gueye et al., "Infections in Senegalese children and adolescent with sickle cell anemia presenting with severe anaemia in a malarious area," *Tropical Doctor*, vol. 45, no. 1, pp. 55–58, 2000.

[22] A. I. Juwah, A. Nlemadim, and W. Kaine, "Clinical presentation of severe anemia in pediatric patients with sickle cell anemia seen in Enugu, Nigeria," *American Journal of Hematology*, vol. 72, no. 3, pp. 185–191, 2003.

# 19

# Musculoskeletal Manifestations of Sickle Cell Anaemia

**A. Ganguly, W. Boswell, and H. Aniq**

*Department of Radiology, Royal Liverpool University Hospital, Prescot Street, Liverpool L7 8XP, UK*

Correspondence should be addressed to A. Ganguly, drakash_ganguly@yahoo.co.uk

Academic Editor: Maria Stella Figueiredo

Sickle cell anaemia is an autosomal recessive genetic condition producing abnormal haemoglobin HbS molecules that result in stiff and sticky red blood cells leading to unpredictable episodes of microvascular occlusions. The clinical and radiological manifestations of sickle cell anaemia result from small vessel occlusion, leading to tissue ischemia/infarction and progressive end-organ damage. In this paper we discuss and illustrate the various musculoskeletal manifestations of sickle cell disease focusing primarily on marrow hyperplasia, osteomyelitis and septic arthritis, medullary and epiphyseal bone infarcts, growth defects, and soft tissue changes.

## 1. Introduction

Sickle cell anaemia is an autosomal recessive genetic condition due to a mutation in the beta-globin gene resulting in replacement of glutamic acid in position 6 of the beta-globin chain by valine resulting in an abnormal haemoglobin HbS molecule. The term sickle cell disease applies to those patients who have at least one abnormal HbS chain and another abnormal beta chain. If the second abnormal chain is also an HbS chain then the patient is considered to be homozygous Hb SS-defined as sickle cell anaemia. Alternatively, other abnormal haemoglobin chains like Hb C or thalassemia result in Hb SC and Hb S-thal, respectively. The combination of an abnormal HbS chain and a normal beta-globin chain is called sickle cell trait.

The abnormal HbS protein chain polymerizes reversibly in deoxygenated environment into a gelatinous network of fibrous polymers that stiffen the RBC membrane, increases the viscosity, and causes dehydration resulting in a sickle shape. These abnormal cells lose there pliability and are abnormally sticky provoking unpredictable episodes of microvascular occlusions and premature haemolysis. The clinical and radiological manifestations of sickle cell anaemia are manifold; however, pathophysiologically all of them result from rigid adherent cells cogging small vessels, leading to tissue ischemia/infarction and gradual end-organ damage.

In this paper we discuss and illustrate the various musculoskeletal manifestations of sickle cell disease. For the benefit of the reader we have subdivided the paper into the following sections.

## 2. Marrow Replacement and Hyperplasia

In a normal healthy adult haematopoietic red marrow is found in the axial skeleton (spine, sternum, pelvis, ribs, and proximal long bones) with yellow marrow conversion in the rest of the appendicular skeleton. As the sickle cell patient is chronically anaemic there is persistence of red marrow in both the axial and appendicular skeleton into adulthood together with bone marrow hyperplasia. On T1W MRI, normal fatty marrow shows high signal intensity, while haematopoietic red marrow is low in signal (Figures 1(a) and 1(b)). Marrow hyperplasia results in widening of the medulla and subsequent cortical thinning, resulting in coarsening of the normal trabecular pattern with loss of corticomedullary differentiation in both long and flat bones (Figure 2). This process may also cause the bone to appear osteopaenic and make the bone prone to softening and fracture [1]. The best example of bone softening is seen in the vertebral bodies, where the end plates assume a smooth concavity described as fish mouth vertebra (Figure 1(a)).

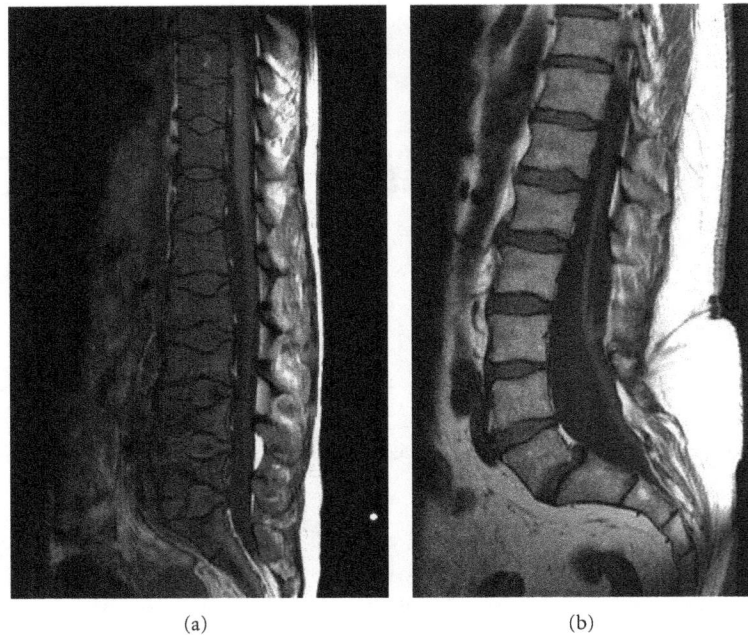

(a)                                                        (b)

FIGURE 1: (a) shows a T1W sagittal MRI spine of a patient with sickle cell anaemia with diffuse low signal from the vertebral bodies consistent with hyperplastic haematopoietic red marrow replacing the normal bright fatty marrow. Note smooth concavity of the vertebral endplates at multiple levels from bone softening (fish mouth vertebra). Normal appearance of marrow is depicted on (b) for comparison.

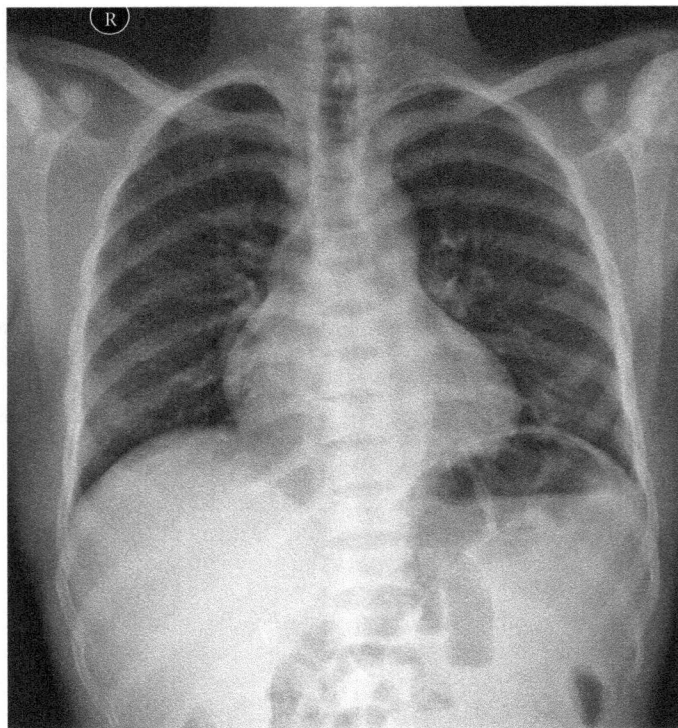

FIGURE 2: Chest radiograph showing coarsening of trabecular pattern with loss of corticomedullary differentiation of the ribs subject to haematopoietic marrow replacement in a patient with sickle cell disease. Note avascular necrosis involving the humeral heads bilaterally and colonic gas replacing splenic shadow in the left upper quadrant (secondary sign of autosplenectomy/small spleen subject to previous infarcts).

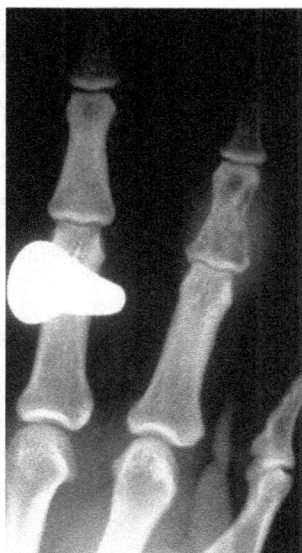

FIGURE 3: Plain radiograph of the hand of a patient with sickle cell anaemia showing patchy lucency and associated soft tissue swelling consistent with osteomyelitis of the middle phalanx of the index finger.

Although less common in sickle cell disease, widening of the diploic space in the skull results in "hair on end" appearances, which is classically described in other forms of haemoglobinopathy-like thalassemia [2].

A further form of marrow hyperplasia is extramedullary haematopoiesis (although this is relatively uncommon in sickle cell anaemia, being more usually associated with sickle cell variants like HbS-thal, hereditary spherocytosis and thalassemia) [3]. Potential sites include the liver and spleen and paraspinal soft tissues. Rarer locations include the middle ear [4]. Radionuclide imaging with sulphur colloid imaging can confirm the haematopoietic nature of these masses [5]. Foci of extramedullary haematopoiesis are seen as well defined focal mass lesions and show intermediate signal weighting on T1 and T2 weighted MR images and are of soft tissue attenuation at CT [1].

Patients with sickle cell anaemia who have received multiple transfusions may develop secondary haemosiderosis, with excess iron collecting in the reticuloendothelial system. Classically it shows diffuse low signal on T2W gradient echo images, involving the liver and spleen, subject to the increased sensitivity of GRE images to magnetic susceptibility artefact of Iron.

## 3. Osteomyelitis

Osteomyelitis occurs in 18% while septic arthritis occurs in 7% of patients with sickle cell disease according to a study [6]. Patients with sickle cell anaemia have an increased incidence of septic arthritis and osteomyelitis as compared to the general population due to the abnormal red blood cells reducing flow in the small vessels, resulting in relative ischemic zones [7]. The body's own immunological response is less effective in areas of impaired vascularity. Hyposplenism due to autosplenectomy also results in a degree of immunocompromise. Osteomyelitis is most common in the diaphyses of long bones [8]. There is an increased incidence of salmonella osteomyelitis in sickle cell patients [9], where it is believed to be the most common pathogen: staph. aureus being the second most common organism [9].

The classical clinical findings of pain, fever, and raised inflammatory markers can also be seen in infarction, which can cause diagnostic difficulty [3].

Plain film findings of osteomyelitis include osteopaenia, periosteal reaction with or without associated cortical destruction, sinus tract formation, and soft tissue extension (Figure 3). Features such as osteopaenia and periosteal reaction are not specific to osteomyelitis and can also be seen in acute bone infarction. As in osteomyelitis in nonsickle cell patients, the plain film findings lag behind the clinical picture and the plain film may be normal for up to 10 days [1]. Isotope bone scan and labelled white cell scans may be helpful, with triple phase bone scan showing increased activity in all 3 phases [1]. Labelled white cell scans can show increased uptake in infection with reduced uptake in areas of infarction, but the diffuse marrow abnormality present can hinder interpretation (Figure 4) [10, 11].

MR scanning is the preferred method of assessment [3]. On T2 weighted images, areas of osteomyelitis will be of increased signal intensity [12]. On T1 weighting, osteomyelitis is of low signal intensity (although areas of red marrow will also be of low signal intensity). Focal fluid collections and associated soft tissue abnormalities can also be demonstrated. Osteomyelitis will also show areas of enhancement postgadolinium. This will tend to be more diffuse than in infarction. Rim enhancement may also be seen but is not specific as it is also seen in bone infarction [13]. Soft tissue enhancement is again not specific for infection and can be seen in both.

(a)

(b)

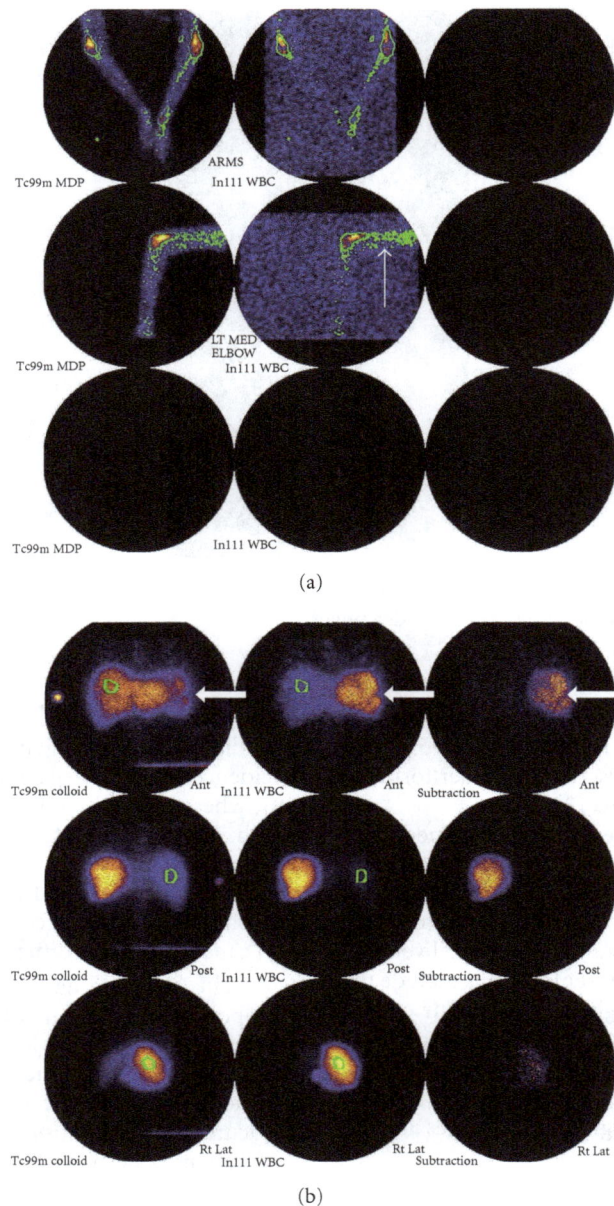

FIGURE 4: (a) In111 WBC and Tc99m colloid scan images in a patient with sickle cell anaemia showing abnormal increased activity in the distal left humerus on the WBC scan (white arrows) consistent with osteomyelitis. (b) Note also that multiple photopenic areas in the splenic tissue, seen on both WBC and colloid images (thick white arrows) suggest multiple splenic infarcts.

In the spine particularly, high signal is seen on T2 weighted images in the affected disc or vertebral body in the case of infective discitis and vertebral osteomyelitis with enhancement of the abnormal areas postgadolinium injection (Figures 5(a), 5(b) and 5(c)).

As well as osteomyelitis, patients with sickle cell disease have an increased incidence of septic arthritis [1]. Joint effusion will be seen (although this can also be seen with bone infarction). Ultrasound may be used to confirm or refute the presence of effusion and also to guide joint aspiration. MR may also demonstrate joint fluid. Synovium enhances vividly postgadolinium and there may be bone marrow oedema surrounding the joint.

## 4. Bone Infarcts: Epiphyseal and Medullary

Abnormal red cell shape blocking capillaries result in bone infarction in both the diaphyses, causing medullary infarcts and in the epiphyses, causing the appearances of avascular necrosis. This can present as the classical painful bone crisis.

Medullary bone infarcts are far more common than osteomyelitis in patients with sickle cell disease [14], but

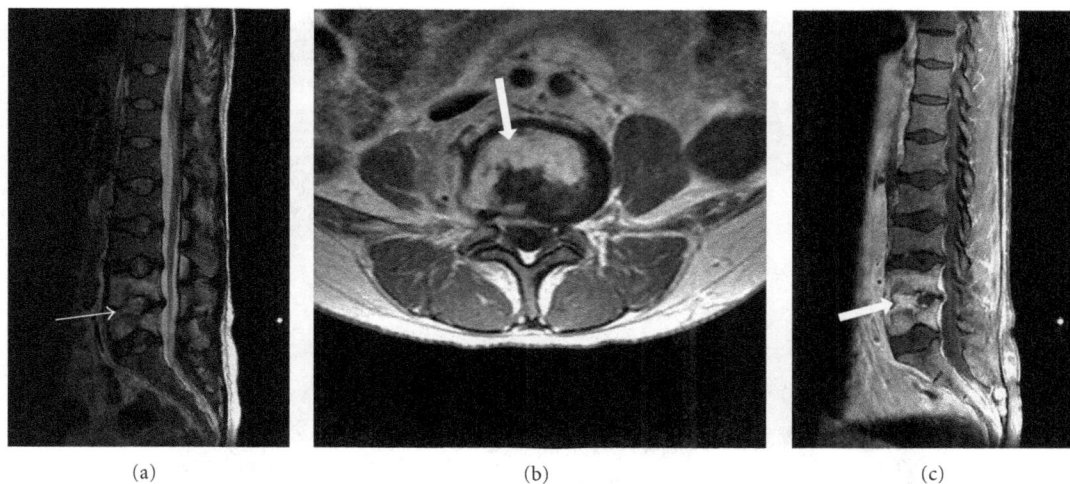

FIGURE 5: (a), (b), and (c) T2W sagittal, T1W axial and sagittal postgadolinium images in a patient with sickle cell anaemia, showing high signal in the anterior aspect of the L4/5 disc on T2W sequence (thin arrow) and enhancement on the post contrast images (thick arrows) consistent with discitis.

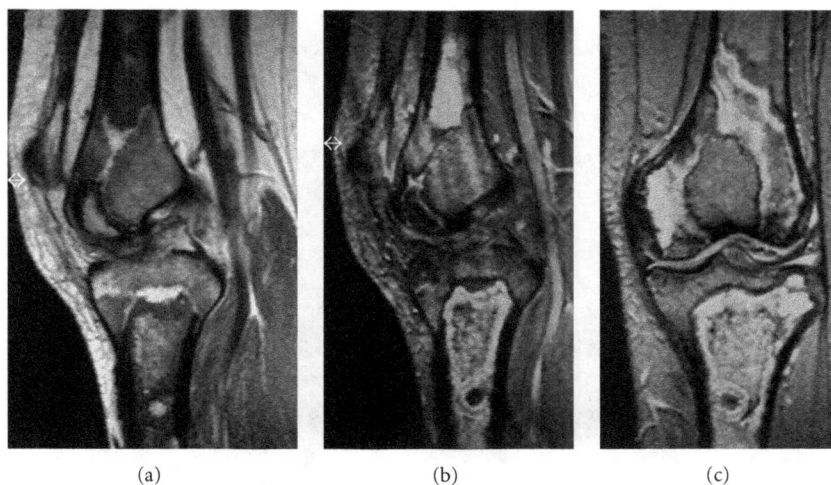

FIGURE 6: (a), (b) and (c) T1W sagittal, T2W sagittal, and coronal MRI knee in a patient with sickle cell anaemia showing, low signal change on T1W images with corresponding areas of solid and serpiginous high signal change on T2W sequence consistent with medullary infarcts involving the femur and tibia.

clinical differentiation can be difficult [7]. Initial radiographs are usually normal with an acute infarction [12]. Later films show patchy lucency, possibly with periosteal reaction [3]. As the condition becomes more chronic sclerosis develops. Bone scintigraphy may show initial photopenia, but as the bone revascularises uptake may return to normal or even be increased. This makes interpretation of the radioisotope imaging difficult as the relevance of the imaging findings is related to the length of time since the infarction [1]. On T2 weighted MR scanning, infarction is seen as an area of high signal intensity (as in osteomyelitis) [13]. Infarcts may also show peripheral enhancement postgadolinium and soft tissue change, further complicating diagnosis [15] (Figures 6(a), 6(b), and 6(c)).

A further pattern of bone infarction is involving the epiphysis. This is more usually referred to as avascular necrosis (Figures 2, 7, 8, and 9). Again, initial radiographs are normal. Later typical appearances of sclerosis, subchondral collapse, and flattening can be appreciated. It is stated that about 40% of patients with sickle cell disease would develop AVN by their mid 50s [16]. T2 weighted MR scanning shows high signal intensity (fat suppressed sequences are particularly sensitive). A serpiginous low signal intensity line is classically seen. As the necrosis progresses, sclerosis develops, and there is collapse of the affected epiphysis (Figures 10(a), 10(b), and 10(c)).

In the spine, AVN of the end plate produces a sharp central step in the vertebral body end plate, causing the

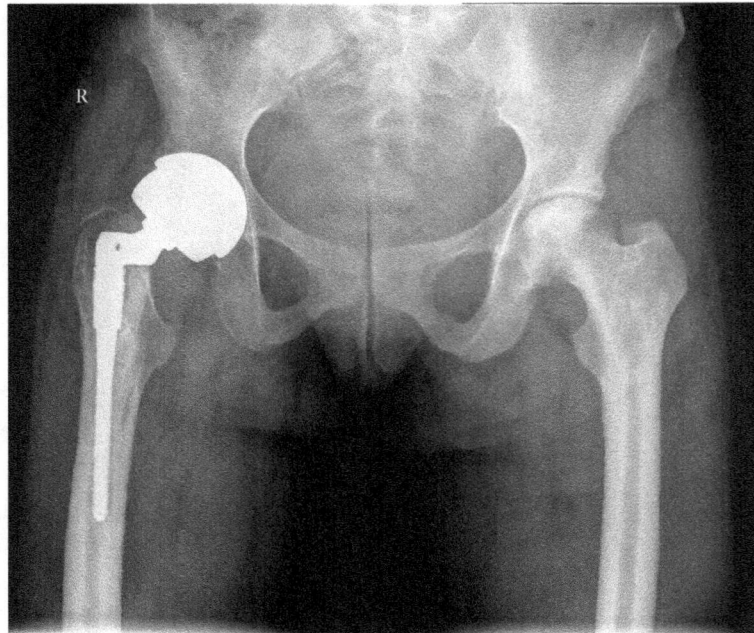

FIGURE 7: Plain radiograph of the pelvis showing sclerosis of the left femoral head consistent with avascular necrosis. Note total hip replacement due to premature secondary osteoarthritis secondary to avascular necrosis on the right.

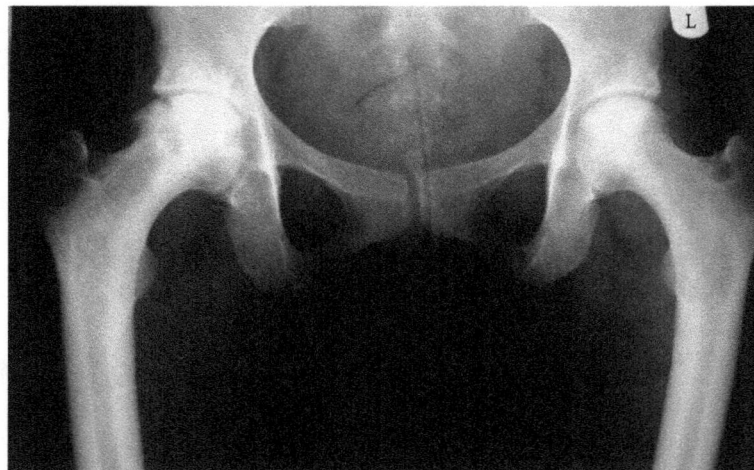

FIGURE 8: Plain radiograph of the pelvis in another patient with sickle cell anaemia more advanced avascular necrosis with sclerosis and subchondral collapse of the right femoral head. Less severe changes are seen on the left.

H-shaped vertebra (Figures 11(a) and 11(b)). This can be easily differentiated from the smooth concavity seen with bone softening.

In children, infarction within the small bones of the hand and feet result in painful dactylitis termed "hand-foot" syndrome; as red marrow does not persist in the hands and feet into later childhood, the syndrome is not seen in children beyond the age of 5 [17]. It presents with painful extremities and radiologically shows soft tissue swelling, periosteal new bone, and patchy areas of sclerosis and lucency [1].

## 5. Soft Tissue Abnormalities

Occlusion of vessels leads to inflammation and myonecrosis resulting in areas of fluid collection, haematoma, infarction, or abscess formation in the muscles. Abnormal areas show high signal on T2 weighted and fluid sensitive sequences on MRI. Areas of infection can occur independently or in conjunction with osteomyelitis where it again shows high signal on T2 weighted images and postgadolinium ring enhancement [1].

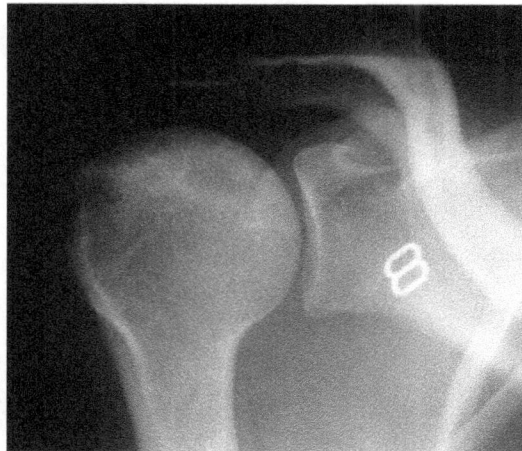

FIGURE 9: Plain radiograph of the shoulder showing early patchy sclerosis of the right humeral head consistent with early avascular necrosis (snow storm appearance).

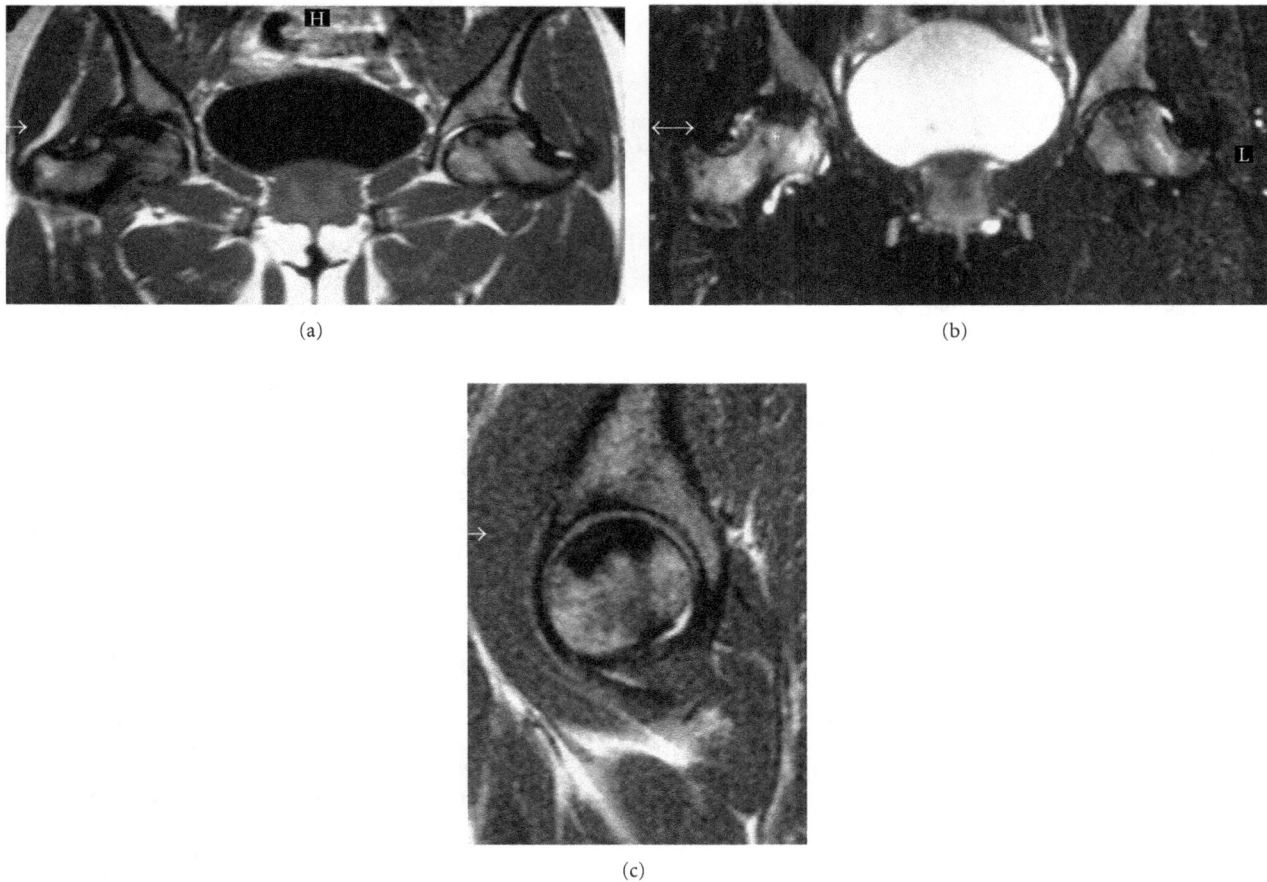

(a)

(b)

(c)

FIGURE 10: (a), (b), and (c) T1W coronal, T2FS (fat saturated) coronal and T1W sagittal MRI of the pelvis and right hip of a patient with sickle cell anaemia. Advanced avascular necrosis with subchondral collapse is seen superiorly in the femoral heads as evidenced by low signal areas on both T1W and T2W images. Additional areas of high signal, particularly in the right femoral neck on the T2FS images depict further areas of ischemia.

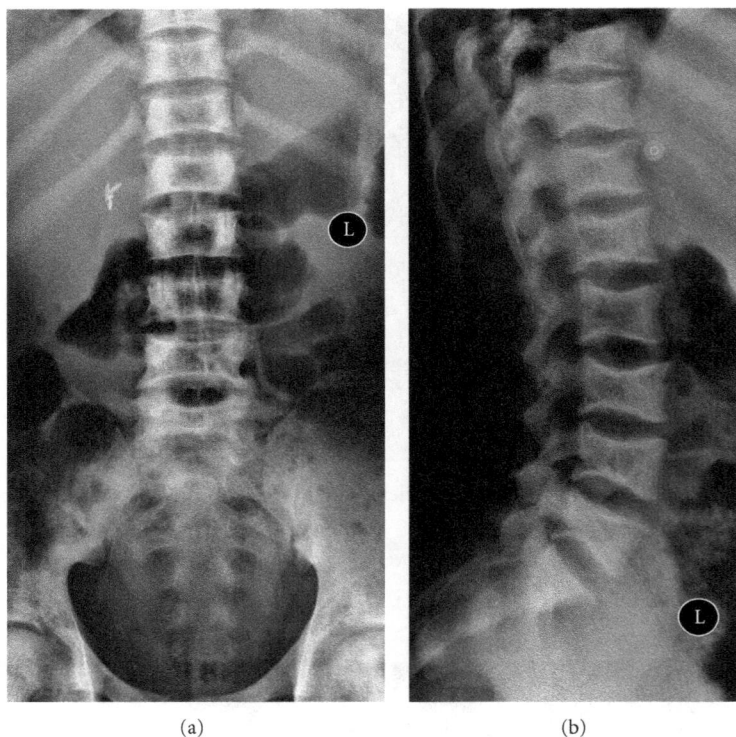

(a)                                                                    (b)

FIGURE 11: (a) and (b) AP and lateral plain radiographs of the lumbar spine showing sharp end plate depressions due to central end-plate infarction resulting in classic H-shaped vertebrae. On the other hand bone softening results in smooth concavity described as fish mouth vertebra. Also note cholecystectomy clips from previous surgery for pigmented stones and patchy sclerosis of the pelvic bones from medullary infarction.

Leg ulcers are also common, particularly over bony prominences subject to tissue ischemia.

## 6. Growth Effects

Patients with sickle cell anaemia have reduced height [18]. This is believed to be due to bone marrow hyperplasia [7]. Bones are generally shorter due to epiphyseal shortening subject to ischemia/infarction and vascular compromise to the growth plate. Premature closure of growth plates also occurs.

## References

[1] V. C. Ejindu, A. L. Hine, M. Mashayekhi, P. J. Shorvon, and R. R. Misra, "Musculoskeletal manifestations of sickle cell disease," Radiographics, vol. 27, no. 4, pp. 1005–1021, 2007.

[2] J. I. Sebes and L. W. Diggs, "Radiographic changes of the skull in sickle cell anemia," American Journal of Roentgenology, vol. 132, no. 3, pp. 373–377, 1979.

[3] G. J. Lonergan, D. B. Cline, and S. L. Abbondanzo, "From the archives of the AFIP: sickle cell anemia," Radiographics, vol. 21, no. 4, pp. 971–994, 2001.

[4] E. L. Applebaum and A. Frankel, "Extramedullary hematopoiesis of the middle ear," American Journal of Otolaryngology, vol. 10, no. 4, pp. 287–290, 1989.

[5] F. L. Datz and A. Taylor, "The clinical use of radionuclide bone marrow imaging," Seminars in Nuclear Medicine, vol. 15, no. 3, pp. 239–259, 1985.

[6] J. Bahebeck, R. Atangana, A. Techa, M. Monny-Lobe, M. Sosso, and P. Hoffmeyer, "Relative rates and features of musculoskeletal complications in adult sicklers," Acta Orthopaedica Belgica, vol. 70, no. 2, pp. 107–111, 2004.

[7] A. Almeida and I. Roberts, "Bone involvement in sickle cell disease," British Journal of Haematology, vol. 129, no. 4, pp. 482–490, 2005.

[8] J. E. Stark, C. M. Glasier, R. D. Blasier, J. Aronson, and J. J. Seibert, "Osteomyelitis in children with sickle cell disease: early diagnosis with contrast-enhanced CT," Radiology, vol. 179, no. 3, pp. 731–733, 1991.

[9] M. W. Burnett, J. W. Bass, and B. A. Cook, "Etiology of osteomyelitis complicating sickle cell disease," Pediatrics, vol. 101, no. 2, pp. 296–297, 1998.

[10] C. J. Palestro, C. Love, G. G. Tronco, M. B. Tomas, and J. N. Rini, "Combined labeled leukocyte and technetium 99m sulfur colloid bone marrow imaging for diagnosing musculoskeletal infection," Radiographics, vol. 26, no. 3, pp. 859–870, 2006.

[11] C. J. Palestro, P. Roumanas, A. J. Swyer, C. K. Kim, and S. J. Goldsmith, "Diagnosis of musculoskeletal infection using combined In-111 labeled leukocyte and Tc-99m SC marrow imaging," Clinical Nuclear Medicine, vol. 17, no. 4, pp. 667–670, 1992.

[12] G. Madani, A. M. Papadopoulou, B. Holloway, A. Robins, J. Davis, and D. Murray, "The radiological manifestations of sickle cell disease," Clinical Radiology, vol. 62, no. 6, pp. 528–538, 2007.

[13] H. Umans, N. Haramati, and G. Flusser, "The diagnostic role of gadolinium enhanced MRI in distinguishing between

acute medullary bone infarct and osteomyelitis," *Magnetic Resonance Imaging*, vol. 18, no. 3, pp. 255–262, 2000.

[14] K. Keeley and G. R. Buchanan, "Acute infarction of long bones in children with sickle cell anemia," *Journal of Pediatrics*, vol. 101, no. 2, pp. 170–175, 1982.

[15] V. Bonnerot, G. Sebag, M. De Montalembert et al., "Gadolinium-DOTA enhanced MRI of painful osseous crises in children with sickle cell anemia," *Pediatric Radiology*, vol. 24, no. 2, pp. 92–95, 1994.

[16] H. E. Ware, A. P. Brooks, R. Toye, and S. I. Berney, "Sickle cell disease and silent avascular necrosis of the hip," *Journal of Bone and Joint Surgery*, vol. 73, no. 6, pp. 947–949, 1991.

[17] S. S. Babhulkar, K. Pande, and S. Babhulkar, "The hand-foot syndrome in sickle-cell haemoglobinopathy," *Journal of Bone and Joint Surgery*, vol. 77, no. 2, pp. 310–312, 1995.

[18] O. S. Platt, W. Rosenstock, and M. A. Espeland, "Influence of sickle hemoglobinopathies on growth and development," *New England Journal of Medicine*, vol. 311, no. 1, pp. 7–12, 1984.

# 20

# Attitudes toward Management of Sickle Cell Disease and Its Complications: A National Survey of Academic Family Physicians

Arch G. Mainous III,[1,2] Rebecca J. Tanner,[1] Christopher A. Harle,[1] Richard Baker,[3] Navkiran K. Shokar,[4] and Mary M. Hulihan[5]

[1]Department of Health Services Research, Management and Policy, University of Florida, P.O. Box 100195, Gainesville, FL 32610, USA
[2]Department of Community Health and Family Medicine, University of Florida, P.O. Box 100237, Gainesville, FL 32610-0237, USA
[3]Department of Health Sciences, University of Leicester, 22-28 Princess Road West, Leicester LE1 6TP, UK
[4]Department of Family and Community Medicine, Texas Tech University Health Science Center at El Paso, 9849 Kenworthy Street, El Paso, TX 79924, USA
[5]Division of Blood Disorders, CDC, National Center on Birth Defects and Developmental Disabilities, Mail-Stop E87, 1600 Clifton Road, Atlanta, GA 30333, USA

Correspondence should be addressed to Arch G. Mainous III; arch.mainous@ufl.edu

Academic Editor: Duran Canatan

*Objective.* Sickle cell disease (SCD) is a disease that requires a significant degree of medical intervention, and family physicians are one potential provider of care for patients who do not have access to specialists. The extent to which family physicians are comfortable with the treatment of and concerned about potential complications of SCD among their patients is unclear. Our purpose was to examine family physician's attitudes toward SCD management. *Methods.* Data was collected as part of the Council of Academic Family Medicine Educational Research Alliance (CERA) survey in the United States and Canada that targeted family physicians who were members of CERA-affiliated organizations. We examined attitudes regarding management of SCD. *Results.* Overall, 20.4% of respondents felt comfortable with treatment of SCD. There were significant differences in comfort level for treatment of SCD patients depending on whether or not physicians had patients who had SCD, as well as physicians who had more than 10% African American patients. Physicians also felt that clinical decision support (CDS) tools would be useful for treatment (69.4%) and avoiding complications (72.6%) in managing SCD patients. *Conclusions.* Family physicians are generally uncomfortable with managing SCD patients and recognize the utility of CDS tools in managing patients.

## 1. Introduction

Sickle cell disease (SCD) affects millions of people throughout the world and is particularly common among those whose ancestors came from sub-Saharan Africa; Spanish-speaking regions in the Western Hemisphere (South America, the Caribbean, and Central America); Saudi Arabia; India; and Mediterranean countries such as Turkey, Greece, and Italy. It is estimated that SCD affects 90,000 to 100,000 Americans, and sickle cell trait occurs among 1 in 12 African Americans [1].

Patients with sickle cell disease require comprehensive care including preventive interventions, pain management, hydroxyurea, and blood transfusions [2]. Further, complications of transfusions like iron overload are common and have significant consequences like cirrhosis, heart failure, and death [3, 4]. Due to the complex and disabling nature of sickle cell disease, appropriate ambulatory management is critical to avoid acute pain and vasoocclusive episodes and hospitalizations. One estimate has suggested that annually, United States' average hospitalization costs for SCD are $6,223 per hospitalization [5]. Interventions designed to prevent SCD complications and avoid hospitalizations are estimated to have substantial economic benefits, as the discounted lifetime cost of care averages $460,151 per patient with SCD [6].

Translation of evidence from clinical trials into health care delivery for patients with sickle cell disease needs to happen. For example, hydroxyurea, the only currently available FDA-approved medication for preventing complications of sickle cell disease, is effective. The Multicenter Study of Hydroxyurea in Patients with Sickle Cell Anemia, a multicenter landmark randomized controlled trial, clearly demonstrated that use of hydroxyurea by adult patients with sickle cell anemia resulted in a significant reduction in the frequency of pain crises, hospitalizations, and red blood cell transfusions [7]. A nine-year follow-up observational study revealed a reduction in mortality for patients taking hydroxyurea compared to study participants not taking the medication [8]. However, hydroxyurea is underused [9]. In one study at three teaching hospitals in the southeastern United States only 42% of adult SCD patients were taking hydroxyurea [10].

The extent to which family physicians are comfortable implementing such advances in treatment for SCD in clinical practice is unclear. Little information exists on current practice and use of therapies for children and adults with SCD in this setting. There are many factors that could influence a physician's attitudes toward SCD. For example, SCD is more prevalent among African Americans, and so physicians whose practices are comprised of larger proportions of African Americans might be more attuned to issues such as SCD that disproportionately affect their patient population. Physicians who have active patients with SCD may be more familiar and more comfortable with SCD patients and the disease. Physician age is another factor that may influence comfort with managing and treating SCD patients. Younger physicians may have a greater recall of details regarding less common diseases that are infrequently seen in practice. In addition, age may influence interest in use of technology in the clinical encounter. Because of the significant impact on morbidity and mortality and health care costs associated with inappropriate management of SCD [11–14], it is important to better understand current practice. A better understanding of sickle cell management and complication knowledge deficits of physicians will help to drive interventions like clinical decision support CDS systems [15, 16] and primary-specialty physician comanagement programs to improve care for the vulnerable population of people with SCD. Less common diseases such as SCD are prime candidates for CDS tools, as they can support physician knowledge and management of diseases that they do not encounter regularly in practice.

## 2. Methods

This study is an analysis of a survey conducted as part of the Council of Academic Family Medicine Educational Research Alliance (CERA). CERA is a joint initiative of all four major US academic family medicine organizations (Society of Teachers of Family Medicine (STFM), North American Primary Care Research Group (NAPCRG), Association of

Departments of Family Medicine (ADFM), and Association of Family Medicine Residency Directors (AFMRD)).

The investigators submitted questions related to SCD practice and treatment for inclusion in the CERA survey. The survey was designed as an omnibus survey incorporating several distinct subprojects focusing on different topic areas. Practicing physician members of the CERA-affiliated organizations in the United States were identified for participation. Although these organizations are all headquartered in the United States, there are some members from outside the United States. This survey was limited to US based members. Since some individuals were members of multiple organizations, unique individuals were selected for the sampling frame. The study was approved by the American Academy of Family Physicians Institutional Review Board.

The survey was conducted between November, 2013, and January, 2014, and sent to 3158 physicians who are members of Council of Academic Family Medicine organizations. The potential respondents were surveyed electronically with an initial email invitation for participation. The survey was conducted through the infrastructure of STFM. The survey was introduced in an email that included a personalized greeting, a letter signed by the presidents of each of the four participating organizations urging participation, and a link to the survey. Nonrespondents were sent two follow-up emails encouraging participation. As the survey was structured as an omnibus survey, with several subprojects contained within the overall survey, it was possible for respondents to skip questions.

The survey questions for this study were developed following a review of the literature to identify key concepts and issues suggesting the need for additional knowledge. The attitudinal outcomes of interest were physicians' responses to questions related to their "comfort managing sickle cell disease patients," "complication concerns," "willingness to manage patients," and "usefulness of CDS tools".

*2.1. Comfort Managing Patients.* Comfort with overall management and pain management of SCD patients was assessed using a Likert scale (somewhat/very uncomfortable, neutral, and somewhat/very comfortable). Comfort with managing SCD patients with specific treatment options (red blood cell transfusions, hematopoietic stem cell transplant (HSCT), and hydroxyurea) was assessed as well. These options represent the main treatments available for SCD patients and represent a wide range of usage in practice, from relatively common pain management to the less frequently used HSCT.

*2.2. Complication Concerns.* Concern for SCD complications was assessed using physician's stated level of concern (somewhat/very unconcerned, neutral, and somewhat/very concerned) for known complications of SCD, including iron overload, stroke, atherosclerosis, and pneumonia.

*2.3. Willingness to Comanage Patients with a Specialist.* Willingness to comanage an SCD patient was assessed for pediatric and adult patients (somewhat/very likely, neutral, and somewhat/very unlikely).

*2.4. Use of Clinical Decision Support Tools on SCD Care.* The willingness of a physician to self-manage care of SCD patients with the assistance of a CDS tool was assessed for pediatric and adult patients (somewhat/very unlikely, neutral, and somewhat/very likely). The perceived utility of CDS tools was assessed for diagnosis of SCD, treatment of SCD, and the avoidance of complications (somewhat/very useful, neutral, and somewhat/very not useful).

*2.5. Demographics.* We collected data on age, race/ethnicity, academic rank, primary physician duty, patient time, time in clinic, proportion of patients who are African American, number of patients with SCD, and proportion of patients with SCD who are under 19 years of age from all survey participants (Table 1).

## 3. Analysis

We computed descriptive statistics to understand the general practice patterns of the survey respondents and their overall attitudes toward SCD and SCD treatment. We collapsed all of the Likert scale questions into two categories, examining the difference between those who answered the questions with a positive answer (somewhat and very comfortable, likely, and concerned) and respondents who felt neutral or responded negatively. Next, we conducted bivariate analyses with chi-square tests to compare attitudes based on respondents' proportion of African American patients (less than 10% versus 10% or greater), as well as by the presence of SCD patients in the physician's practice, and by physician age (younger than 50 versus 50 and older). We judged statistical significance at $P \leq 0.05$.

## 4. Results

The overall number of surveys returned was 1060 for a 34% response rate. We analyzed data from the 1042 physicians who responded to at least one question on the SCD section of the survey. Table 1 shows demographic information about these physician respondents. The majority of physicians had no SCD patients, and only 15.9% had more than five SCD patients. Slightly less than half of the surveyed physicians spent 3 or more half-days in clinic. Overall, few physicians had a substantial proportion of African American patients, with only 25.7% reporting 25% or more African American patients. Table 2 shows the bivariate analysis for comfort managing patients, complications concerns, willingness to comanage patients, and thoughts on CDS tools for the full population. Table 3 shows differences between physicians with <10% African American patients and physicians with 10% or more African American patients. Table 4 shows differences between physicians with no active SCD patients and those with active SCD patients. There were no significant differences between groups in relation to perceived utility of CDS for helping direct treatment or avoiding complications. A majority of all groups felt that CDS would be useful.

There were several significant differences between physicians under age 50 and those aged 50 and older. A smaller

TABLE 1: Respondent demographics.

| | |
|---|---|
| Sample size | 1042 |
| Male, % | 56.6 |
| Age, % | |
| Under 40 | 21.9 |
| 40–49 | 28.8 |
| 50–59 | 30.0 |
| 60+ | 19.3 |
| Race/ethnicity, % | |
| White | 84.2 |
| African American | 3.6 |
| Hispanic | 3.5 |
| Asian/other | 8.8 |
| Rank, % | |
| Assistant professor | 31.9 |
| Associate professor | 32.5 |
| Full professor | 24.6 |
| Not applicable | 11.0 |
| Terminal degree, % | |
| M.D. | 93.5 |
| D.O. | 5.7 |
| Other | 0.8 |
| Primary duty, % | |
| Administration | 26.4 |
| Clinical teaching | 51.5 |
| Research | 5.9 |
| Faculty development | 1.7 |
| Clinical care | 9.6 |
| Nonacademic physician | 0.6 |
| Other | 4.4 |
| Patient time ≥50%, % | 22.8 |
| Time in clinic, % | |
| <3 half days | 50.4 |
| 3–6 half days | 44.6 |
| 7+ half days | 5.1 |
| % of patients who are African American, % | |
| <10% | 46.8 |
| 10–24% | 27.5 |
| 25–49% | 18.4 |
| 50+% | 7.3 |
| Number of patients with SCD | |
| 0 patients | 59.6 |
| 1–4 patients | 34.5 |
| 5–10 patients | 14.5 |
| 11+ patients | 1.4 |
| % of SCD patients who are under 19 years of age, % | |
| <10% | 56.8 |
| 10–24% | 18.1 |
| 25–49% | 14.0 |
| 50+% | 11.1 |

percentage of younger physicians were comfortable with overall management of SCD patients (15.7%) compared to

TABLE 2: Physician perceptions of SCD, full sample.

|  | Full sample |
| --- | --- |
| Comfort managing patients | Comfortable |
| Overall management, % | 20.4 |
| RBC transfusions, % | 30.8 |
| HSCT, % | 0.6 |
| Hydroxyurea treatment, % | 20.5 |
| Pain management, % | 47.8 |
| Complication concerns | Concerned |
| Iron overload, % | 60.9 |
| Stroke, % | 77.6 |
| Atherosclerosis, % | 45.9 |
| Pneumonia, % | 71.4 |
| Willing to comanage patient with specialist | Likely |
| Pediatric patients, % | 79.7 |
| Adult patients, % | 67.8 |
| Impact of CDS on willingness to manage SCD patients | Likely |
| Pediatric patients, % | 25.6 |
| Adult patients, % | 34.1 |
| Perceived utility of CDS for SCD patient care | Useful |
| Diagnosis | 22.9 |
| Treatment | 69.4 |
| Avoiding complications | 72.6 |

older physicians (25.1%, $P = 0.0002$). A larger percentage of physicians who were older expressed concern for iron overload, with 66.1% expressing concern, in contrast to 55.8% of younger physicians ($P = 0.0009$). A greater percentage of younger physicians were more willing to comanage adult SCD patients (70.8%) than older physicians (64.3%, $P = 0.03$). A greater percentage of younger physicians were willing to independently manage adult SCD patients with the assistance of a CDS tool, with 38.1% of younger physicians indicating an increased likelihood, compared to 29.9% of older physicians ($P = 0.007$). A larger percentage of younger physicians saw the utility of CDS tools, with 72.5% indicating that CDS tools would be useful for the treatment of patients, compared with 66.6% of older physicians ($P = 0.04$). In addition, a greater percentage of younger physicians considered CDS tools useful for avoiding complications than older physicians (77.7% versus 67.2%, $P = 0.0002$).

## 5. Discussion

The results of this study indicate that academic family physicians have few SCD patients in their patient panel. More importantly, the results indicate that there are concerns among these primary care physicians regarding their ability to manage SCD and its complications. That said, there seems to be general agreement that a CDS tool may play a beneficial role in managing these patients especially among younger physicians.

As might be expected, more frequent interaction with SCD patients or African American patients, those at higher risk for SCD, was associated with greater comfort in managing SCD patients. Age of the physician was related to comfort managing these patients in several important ways. Older physicians appeared more comfortable with treatment and management of a complication like iron overload, potentially reflecting lifetime exposure to this patient population, while younger physicians were more likely to embrace tools that would assist them in managing patients independently.

A CDS for managing SCD received significant endorsement from this sample of academic family physicians. CDS tools have been successfully utilized in the management of care for a number of conditions [15, 16]. It appears that a CDS would have utility for both managing treatment and complications. Younger physicians were more likely to see a CDS to be particularly useful. As electronic health records become more commonplace in primary care the ability to implement a CDS for less common diseases is increased. Although there is evidence of alert fatigue with CDS for common conditions [17], the use of a CDS for SCD would not likely be perceived as an annoyance but rather as a benefit.

This study is the first study to report on family physician's comfort and attitudes with managing SCD. In addition to this strength, there are several limitations to this study. The first is that although the survey is based on a national sample of family physicians, a group that would likely encounter SCD child and adult patients, the group under study is all in academic settings. Consequently, in terms of clinical practice most academic family physicians do not practice full time. This amount of clinical practice may potentially affect their comfort with SCD. Second, even though the sample size allows us to examine responses to more than 1,000 respondents, the response rate of 34% is not exceptionally high. Thus, there may be some bias in the participants based on their comfort and interest in the questions. The low response rate may have been a result of the time of year the survey was sent out, as it was administered during the holiday season. As was clear from the practice characteristics, SCD patients are not common in the patient panels of the respondents. It is possible that individuals with no SCD patients were less likely to participate in a study on managing SCD patients. Finally, the level of training that physicians received for SCD was not assessed. Physician attitudes regarding SCD management are likely to be influenced not only by SCD patients in their care, but also by the amount of SCD-specific training they received.

In conclusion, although academic family physicians recognize issues in their comfort and ability to manage SCD patients they endorse the potential utility of CDS. Future studies could evaluate whether a CDS system could improve the quality of care and control of complications like iron overload for this vulnerable population.

## Disclaimer

The findings and conclusions in this report are those of the authors and do not necessarily represent the official position of the Centers for Disease Control and Prevention.

TABLE 3: Physician perceptions of SCD by percentage of patients who are African American.

| | Physicians with <10% African American patients | Physicians with ≥10% African American patients | P value |
|---|---|---|---|
| Comfort managing patients | Comfortable | Comfortable | |
| Overall management, % | 12.7 | 27.0 | <0.0001 |
| RBC transfusions, % | 25.4 | 35.6 | 0.0006 |
| HSCT, % | 0.2 | 1.0 | 0.14 |
| Hydroxyurea treatment, % | 16.1 | 24.3 | 0.002 |
| Pain management, % | 42.4 | 52.6 | 0.001 |
| Complication concerns | Concerned | Concerned | |
| Iron overload, % | 58.6 | 62.8 | 0.18 |
| Stroke, % | 75.3 | 79.5 | 0.12 |
| Atherosclerosis, % | 43.5 | 48.0 | 0.15 |
| Pneumonia, % | 68.0 | 74.3 | 0.03 |
| Willing to comanage patient with specialist | Likely | Likely | |
| Pediatric patients, % | 78.2 | 80.9 | 0.31 |
| Adult patients, % | 69.8 | 66.0 | 0.20 |
| Impact of CDS on willingness to manage SCD patients | Likely | Likely | |
| Pediatric patients, % | 24.0 | 27.0 | 0.27 |
| Adult patients, % | 31.3 | 36.6 | 0.08 |
| Perceived utility of CDS for SCD patient care | Useful | Useful | |
| Diagnosis | 27.2 | 19.2 | 0.003 |
| Treatment | 68.1 | 70.4 | 0.45 |
| Avoiding complications | 70.2 | 74.5 | 0.13 |

TABLE 4: Physician perceptions of SCD by number of patients with SCD.

| | Physicians with no SCD patients | Physicians with 1 or more SCD patients | P value |
|---|---|---|---|
| Comfort managing patients | Comfortable | Comfortable | |
| Overall management, % | 9.8 | 36.1 | <0.0001 |
| RBC transfusions, % | 21.8 | 45.1 | <0.0001 |
| HSCT, % | 0.2 | 1.3 | 0.026 |
| Hydroxyurea treatment, % | 14.2 | 30.4 | <0.0001 |
| Pain management, % | 39.0 | 61.7 | <0.0001 |
| Complication concerns | Concerned | Concerned | |
| Iron overload, % | 58.5 | 64.3 | 0.07 |
| Stroke, % | 75.3 | 80.7 | 0.04 |
| Atherosclerosis, % | 45.4 | 46.7 | 0.70 |
| Pneumonia, % | 67.3 | 77.6 | 0.0004 |
| Willing to comanage patient with specialist | Likely | Likely | |
| Pediatric patients, % | 76.5 | 84.1 | 0.003 |
| Adult patients, % | 70.1 | 64.5 | 0.07 |
| Impact of CDS on willingness to manage SCD patients | Likely | Likely | |
| Pediatric patients, % | 23.5 | 28.8 | 0.06 |
| Adult patients, % | 30.8 | 38.7 | 0.01 |
| Perceived utility of CDS for SCD patient care | Useful | Useful | |
| Diagnosis | 26.9 | 17.0 | 0.0003 |
| Treatment | 68.9 | 70.1 | 0.71 |
| Avoiding complications | 72.2 | 73.2 | 0.72 |

## Conflict of Interests

The authors declare that there is no conflict of interests regarding the publication of this paper.

## Acknowledgments

The authors would like to acknowledge Richard Lottenberg, M.D., for his assistance. This study is funded in part by Cooperative Agreement 1U01DD000754-01 from the Centers for Disease Control and Prevention. The findings and conclusions in this report are those of the authors and do not necessarily represent the official position of the Centers for Disease Control and Prevention.

## References

[1] National Heart, Lung, and Blood Institute, *Disease and Conditions Index. Sickle Cell Anemia: Who Is at Risk?* US Department of Health and Human Services, National Institutes of Health, National Heart, Lung, and Blood Institute, Bethesda, Md, USA, 2009.

[2] National Institutes of Health, *The Management of Sickle Cell Disease*, Department of Health and Human Services, National Institutes of Health, National Heart, Lung, and Blood Institute, Bethesda, Md, USA, 2002.

[3] M. A. Blinder, F. Vekeman, M. Sasane, A. Trahey, C. Paley, and M. S. Duh, "Age-related treatment patterns in sickle cell disease patients and the associated sickle cell complications and healthcare costs," *Pediatric Blood and Cancer*, vol. 60, no. 5, pp. 828–835, 2013.

[4] J. Porter and M. Garbowski, "Consequences and management of iron overload in sickle cell disease," *Hematology/the Education Program of the American Society of Hematology*, vol. 2013, no. 1, pp. 447–456, 2013.

[5] C. A. Steiner and J. L. Miller, "Sickle cell disease patients in U.S. hospitals, 2004," HCUP Statistical Brief #21, Agency for Healthcare Research and Quality, Rockville, Md, USA, 2006, http://www.hcup-us.ahrq.gov/reports/statbriefs/sb21.pdf.

[6] T. L. Kauf, T. D. Coates, L. Huazhi, N. Mody-Patel, and A. G. Hartzema, "The cost of health care for children and adults with sickle cell disease," *American Journal of Hematology*, vol. 84, no. 6, pp. 323–327, 2009.

[7] S. Charache, M. L. Terrin, R. D. Moore et al., "Effect of hydroxyurea on the frequency of painful crises in sickle cell anemia. Investigators of the Multicenter Study of Hydroxyurea in Sickle Cell Anemia," *The New England Journal of Medicine*, vol. 332, no. 20, pp. 1317–1322, 1995.

[8] M. H. Steinberg, F. Barton, O. Castro et al., "Effect of hydroxyurea on mortality and morbidity in adult sickle cell anemia: risks and benefits up to 9 years of treatment," *The Journal of the American Medical Association*, vol. 289, no. 13, pp. 1645–1651, 2003.

[9] S. Lanzkron, C. Haywood Jr., J. B. Segal, and G. J. Dover, "Hospitalization rates and costs of care of patients with sickle-cell anemia in the state of Maryland in the era of hydroxyurea," *American Journal of Hematology*, vol. 81, no. 12, pp. 927–932, 2006.

[10] H. Elmariah, M. E. Garrett, L. M. de Castro et al., "Factors associated with survival in a contemporary adult sickle cell disease cohort," *The American Journal of Hematology*, vol. 89, no. 5, pp. 530–535, 2014.

[11] E. Jacob and American Pain Society, "Pain management in sickle cell disease," *Pain Management Nursing*, vol. 2, no. 4, pp. 121–131, 2001.

[12] J. Kanter and R. Kruse-Jarres, "Management of sickle cell disease from childhood through adulthood," *Blood Reviews*, vol. 27, no. 6, pp. 279–287, 2013.

[13] B. Aygun, S. Padmanabhan, C. Paley, and V. Chandrasekaran, "Clinical significance of RBC alloantibodies and autoantibodies in sickle cell patients who received transfusions," *Transfusion*, vol. 42, no. 1, pp. 37–43, 2002.

[14] C. H. Pegelow, R. J. Adams, V. McKie et al., "Risk of recurrent stroke in patients with sickle cell disease treated with erythrocyte transfusions," *The Journal of Pediatrics*, vol. 126, no. 6, pp. 896–899, 1995.

[15] M. S. Player, J. M. Gill, A. G. Mainous III et al., "An electronic medical record-based intervention to improve quality of care for gastro-esophageal reflux disease (GERD) and atypical presentations of GERD," *Quality in Primary Care*, vol. 18, no. 4, pp. 223–229, 2010.

[16] A. G. Mainous III, C. A. Lambourne, and P. J. Nietert, "Impact of a clinical decision support system on antibiotic prescribing for acute respiratory infections in primary care: quasi-experimental trial," *Journal of the American Medical Informatics Association*, vol. 20, no. 2, pp. 317–324, 2013.

[17] A. S. Kesselheim, K. Cresswell, S. Phansalkar, D. W. Bates, and A. Sheikh, "Clinical decision support systems could be modified to reduce "alert fatigue" while still minimizing the risk of litigation," *Health Affairs*, vol. 30, no. 12, pp. 2310–2317, 2011.

# 21

# Role of Extracellular Hemoglobin in Thrombosis and Vascular Occlusion in Patients with Sickle Cell Anemia

**Zhou Zhou, Molly Behymer, and Prasenjit Guchhait**

*Thrombosis Research Division, Cardiovascular Research Section, Department of Medicine, Baylor College of Medicine, One Baylor Plaza, N1319, Houston, TX 77030, USA*

Correspondence should be addressed to Prasenjit Guchhait, guchhait@bcm.tmc.edu

Academic Editor: Fernando F. Costa

Sickle cell anemia (SCA) is a common hemolytic disorder caused by a gene mutation in the $\beta$-globin subunit of hemoglobin (Hb) and affects millions of people. The intravascular hemolysis releases excessive amount of extracellular hemoglobin (ECHb) into plasma that causes many cellular dysfunctions in patients with SCA. ECHb scavenges NO which promotes crisis events such as vasoconstriction, thrombosis and hypercoagulation. ECHb and its degradation product, heme, are known to cause oxidative damage to the vessel wall and stimulate the expression of adhesive protein ligands on vascular endothelium. Our study shows that ECHb binds potently to VWF—largest multimeric glycoprotein in circulation—through the A2-domain, and significantly inhibits its cleavage by the metalloprotease ADAMTS13. Furthermore, a subpopulation of VWF multimers bound to ECHb exists in significant amount, accounting for about 14% of total plasma VWF, in SCD patients. The Hb-bound VWF multimers are resistant to ADAMTS13, and are hyperactive in aggregating platelets. Thus, the data suggest that Hb-bound VWF multimers are ultralarge and hyperactive because they are resistant to the protease. The Hb-bound VWF multimers are elevated parallely with the level of ECHb in patients' plasma, and is associated with the pathogenesis of thrombosis and vascular occlusion in SCA.

## 1. Introduction

Sickle cell anemia (SCA) is a hemolytic disorder first described by Herrick in 1910 [1]. In 1949, Pauling and his team first demonstrated the molecular basis of SCA, showing that the disease is caused by a small difference in the molecular structure of hemoglobin, an oxygen-carrying protein in plasma [2]. In 1957, Ingram discovered that the disease was caused by a single amino acid substitution (Glutamic acid → Valine) in the $\beta$-globin subunit of hemoglobin [3].

Sickle cell anemia affects millions of people worldwide and is associated with significant morbidity and mortality. An estimated 2% of the world's population carries genes responsible for SCA. Each year about 300,000 infants are born with SCA, including more than 200,000 cases in Africa [4]. More than 33% of deaths in SCA patients are caused by vascular occlusions and related crises, such as strokes and transient ischemic attacks [5, 6]. It is estimated that stroke alone results in 20% mortality in such patients between the ages of 5 to 10 years, with 70% of those patients having a motor deficit and significant neurocognitive deficits; 70% have a recurrent stroke within the next 3 years [7, 8].

It is known that under hypoxic conditions, deoxygenation triggers a hydrophobic interaction between the mutated hemoglobin (HbS) molecules, resulting in the polymerization of HbS and sickling of the RBCs. Sickling alters the cell membrane properties, which reduce cellular flexibility and lead to unusual cell adherence to vascular endothelium [5, 6]. Studies further suggest that sickling alters the RBCs' membrane properties including a significant expression/exposure of different adhesive molecules, which mediate the adhesion of sickle RBCs to endothelium and subendothelial matrix [9–16]. Previous studies, including our own, suggest that exposure of a membrane lipid such as sulfated glycosphingolipid or sulfatide on sickle RBCs promotes sickle cell adhesion to endothelial ligands (such as $\alpha_v\beta_3$ and ULVWF) and subendothelial matrix proteins (such as VWF, TSP, LN and FN) [17–19]. Furthermore, the data also demonstrate that sickle RBCs express a significant quantity of phosphatidylserine (PS) on the cell surface and promote the adhesion to the endothelium through binding to $\alpha_v\beta_3$ [20]. Besides the increase of expression/exposure of adhesive molecules on sickle RBCs, which is associated with increased cell adhesion to the vessel wall, sickling also causes the release of excessive extracellular hemoglobin (ECHb) into plasma from the sickle RBCs during intravascular hemolysis.

## 2. Extracellular Hemoglobin Causes Cellular Dysfunctions

Hemoglobin is a heme-containing globular protein in RBCs that can deliver oxygen and remove carbon dioxide to/from cells and tissues. In hemolytic conditions such as SCA, RBCs release an excessive amount of ECHb into plasma, ranging from $20$–$330\,\mu g/mL$ in patients, which can exceed $410\,\mu g/mL$ during vasoocclusive crisis [21–23]. Upon release, ECHb forms a complex with the hemoglobin-scavenger, haptoglobin, in circulation and is cleared by binding to CD163 on macrophage or leukocyte surfaces [24, 25]. Haptoglobin can bind approximately $70$–$150\,\mu g/mL$ of ECHb depending on the haptoglobin allotype [26]. Once the capacity of haptoglobin is exceeded, an elevated level of ECHb accumulates in plasma, causing many cellular dysfunctions. In severe hemolytic diseases such as PNH and SCA, serum haptoglobin is typically undetectable [27].

The accumulation of excessive ECHb in plasma intensifies the consumption of endogenous nitric oxide (NO), resulting in several cellular dysfunctions such as vasoconstriction and systemic and pulmonary hypertension in patients with hemolytic disorders including SCA. It has been shown that the ECHb could scavenge NO, an important endogenous vasodilator, and impair the vasodilatory response to infusions of the direct-acting NO donor to patients [28]. Consistently, patients with plasma ECHb levels higher than $100\,\mu g/ml$ have shown an 80% reduction in NO-dependent blood flow responses [28]. Other *in vivo* studies further show that nitroglycerin-induced vasodilation is impaired in SCA patients [29] and the diminished vasomotor response to NO donors is observed in transgenic SCA mice [30].

Excessive ECHb also causes other cellular dysfunctions in SCA. The elevated ECHb in patients' plasma impairs renal function. Plasma ECHb is normally filtered through the glomerulus and actively reabsorbed in proximal tubule cells where it is catabolized with release of iron in the form of hemosiderin. When the capacity of kidney's reabsorption is exceeded, crises events such as renal dysfunction and failure occur [31]. Second, excessive plasma ECHb may also contribute to platelet activation and thrombosis. An *in vitro* experiment shows that the addition of ECHb to human serum at concentrations of $0.2$–$2\,mg/mL$ dose-dependently inhibits the activity of metalloprotease ADAMTS13, an enzyme critical in limiting platelet thrombus formation [32]. It is also suggested that the major untoward effects of ECHb on platelet function are most likely mediated by NO scavenging. NO has been shown to inhibit platelet aggregation, induce disaggregation of aggregated platelets, and

inhibit platelet adhesion through increasing cyclic guanine monophosphate (cGMP) levels [33]. In addition, NO is also known to interact with components of the coagulation cascade (such as factor XIII and fibrin) to downregulate clot formation [34, 35]. Thus, NO scavenging by ECHb or the reduction of NO generation may result in an increase in intravascular coagulopathy.

## 3. Extracellular Hemoglobin Blocks Cleavage of VWF Multimers

Our investigation shows that excessive ECHb significantly inhibits the cleavage of VWF [23], a multimeric protein in circulation that normally serves in hemostatic functions. However, under pathophysiological conditions such as in SCA patients, the hyperactive VWF multimers play a significant role in cell adhesion and prothrombotic complications. This is particularly significant given that VWF multimers secreted from endothelial cells or platelets may accumulate as ultralarge (UL) multimers in plasma if not properly cleaved by the metalloprotease ADAMTS13. As evident in SCA, inflamed endothelium constitutively secretes ULVWF, maintaining a high VWF antigen level in plasma. Studies, including our own, suggest that elevated VWF levels, particularly ultralarge multimers, exist in SCA patients' plasma, and are associated with increased sickle cell and platelet adhesion to vascular endothelium [23, 36–39]. Several studies have also suggested that ULVWF multimers contain all the determinants necessary for blood cells (including platelets, sickled-RBCs, and neutrophils) to tether and stably adhere to endothelium spontaneously [40–42].

Considering the implicated role of VWF in SCD pathophysiology, we have investigated the function of the plasma metalloprotease ADAMTS13 that determines the length and activity of VWF. Though SCD patients have an elevated level of higher molecular weight or ultralarge VWF multimers in plasma than normal, they have a very mild [23] or no [36] deficiency in ADAMTS13 activity. This is important given that ULVWF multimers freshly secreted from endothelial cells are accumulated in plasma due to impaired cleavage by ADAMTS13, as seen in patients with thrombotic thrombocytopenic purpura (TTP). Severe TTP patients have very low ADAMTS13 activity (<5% of normal) caused by a genetic mean or autoantibody inhibition, resulting in the accumulation of ULVWF multimers and the development of thrombotic microangiopathy [43–45]. We therefore suggested that such a mild deficiency in ADAMTS13 in SCD patients (70% of normal) is probably insufficient to cause any similar effects on the VWF axis. Consistent with that notion, we have shown that ECHb does interact with VWF to inhibit its cleavage by ADAMTS13, and the mechanism is independent of the metalloprotease activity [23]. We have further demonstrated that ECHb binds to the ADAMTS13 cleavage site on the A2 domain of VWF multimers to block its cleavage by the metalloprotease. The study shows that the presence of $100\,\mu g/mL$ of ECHb in buffer completely inhibited the VWF cleavage by ADAMTS13 under physiological flow shear conditions [23]. Since the SCA patients

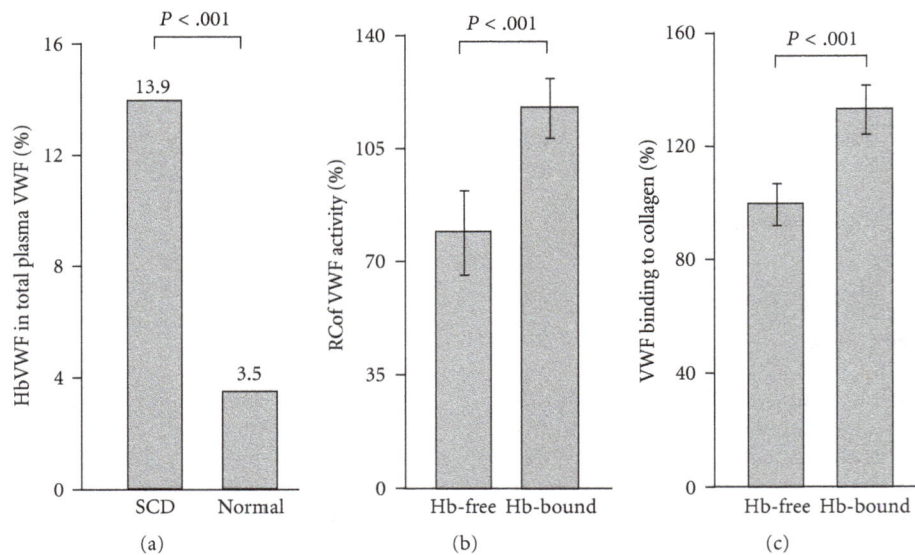

FIGURE 1: Hb-bound VWF multimers are prevalent in SCD patients and are hyperactive. (a): the VWF was purified from plasma (1 mL) of SCD patients or normal individuals by a Superose gel filtration column. The 1st protein peak (at 280 nm UV) was collected for VWF. Further, the Hb-bound VWF was isolated from above VWF fraction using an Ni-NTA affinity column. The VWF antigen level was measured using a commercial kit. The Hb VWF multimers existed as about 14% of total VWF in patients compared to only about 3.5% in normals ($n = 5$). (b): the ristocetin cofactor VWF activity assay shows that the Hb-bound VWF multimers are 35% more activity than the Hb-free counterparts. (c), The collagen binding assay also shows that the Hb-bound VWF multimers are 33% more adhesive to collagen than the Hb-free multimers.

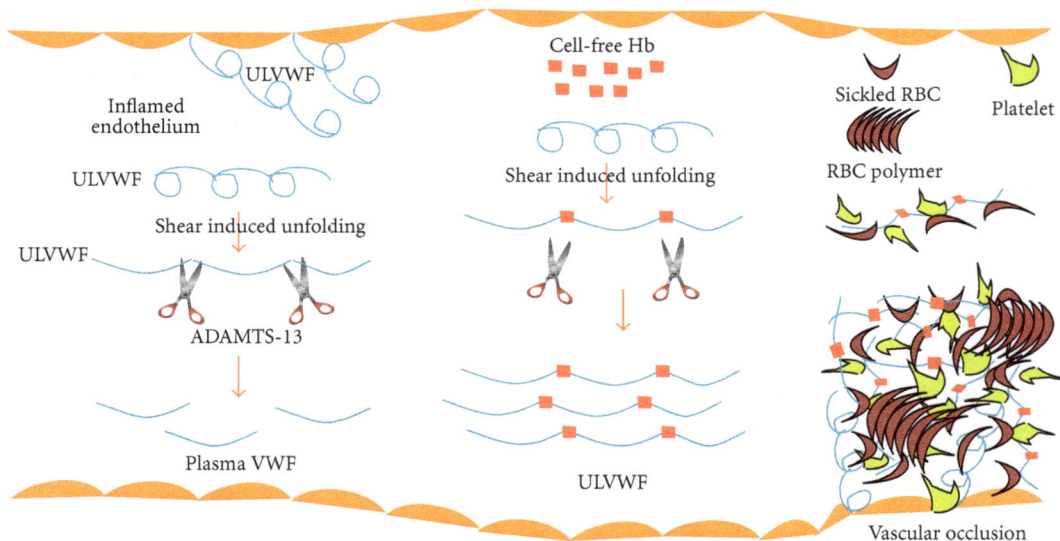

FIGURE 2: The schematic diagram shows that upon activation of the vascular endothelium, ultralarge VWF is released and is cleaved by ADAMTS13 to smaller fragments that circulate in plasma as an inactive form. Under pathophysiological conditions such as SCA, excessive extracellular Hb blocks the cleavage of a subpopulation of VWF multimers. The uncleaved Hb-bound VWF multimers accumulate in plasma, which are hyperactive in binding to platelets or sickled/fragmented-RBCs to promote cell adhesion and events such as thrombosis and vascular occlusion.

have elevated ECHb in plasma, as estimated up to 410 $\mu$g/mL during their vasoocclusive crisis [21–23], we speculated that excessive ECHb could impair VWF cleavage by ADAMTS13 in vivo and promote accumulation of hyperactive VWF multimers in patients' plasma. Accordingly, we have isolated

a subpopulation of VWF multimers from plasma that are bound to ECHb [46]. The Hb-bound VWF multimers exist in SCA patients' plasma, accounting for 14% of total plasma VWF, which is about 4-folds more than normal individuals (Figure 1). Though the interaction between

ECHb and VWF and their relationship *in vivo* is still not clearly un-derstood, our data have shown that increased Hb-bound VWF multimers parallely coexisted with the high ECHb level in patients' plasma (mean $\pm$ SE $\sim$ 263.8 $\pm$ 41.7 (SCA) versus 46.2 $\pm$ 9.6 (Normal, $n$ = 5)) [46]. Furthermore, we have observed that ECHb preferentially binds to the endothelial cell-purified ULVWF over the plasma-purified VWF multimers. It is possible that ECHb binds to ULVWF multimers that are freshly released into plasma and have their A2-domains exposed. As evident, the A2-domain of ULVWF multimers has unique features such as a lack of protection by disulfide bonds within VWF and low resistance to unfolding that help the domain to be exposed easily [47]. When exposed to intravascular hydrodynamic shear forces, the tensile force on the ULVWF multimers increases by the square of the multimer length, providing an efficient mechanism for unfolding of the A2 domain on ULVWF [48]. The similar mechanism in which shear force induced exposure of the A2 domain in freshly released (UL)VWF multimers could probably facilitate the binding of ECHb to VWF, which prevents the cleavage of ULVWF multimers by ADAMTS13. As expected, we found that Hb-bound VWF multimers are 30–35% more adhesive to platelets and subendothelial matrix collagen and less cleavable by ADAMTS13 compared to their Hb-free counterparts [46].

We have speculated that elevated plasma Hb-bound VWF, parallely with increased ECHb, might play an important role in the culmination of blood cell (including platelets, sickle RBCs, and neutrophils) adhesion to vascular endothelium and development of related crises events such as thrombosis, thromboembolism, ischemic strokes, and myocardial infarctions in patients with SCA. This mechanism is not only limited to SCA, but also occurs in other hemolytic disorders including thalassemia, and hemolytic uremic syndrome. This mechanism is shown through a schematic diagram in Figure 2.

# References

[1] J. B. Herrick, "Peculiar elongated and sickle-shaped red blood corpuscles in a case of severe anemia," *Archives of Internal Medicine*, vol. 6, no. 5, pp. 517–521, 1910.

[2] L. Pauling, H. A. Itano, S. J. Singer, and I. C. Wells, "Sickle cell anemia, a molecular disease," *Science*, vol. 110, no. 2865, pp. 543–548, 1949.

[3] V. M. Ingram, "Gene mutations in human hæmoglobin: the chemical difference between normal and sickle cell hæmoglobin," *Nature*, vol. 180, no. 4581, pp. 326–328, 1957.

[4] "WHO report on sickle cell anemia and thalassemia," 2006.

[5] M. J. Stuart and R. L. Nagel, "Sickle-cell disease," *Lancet*, vol. 364, no. 9442, pp. 1343–1360, 2004.

[6] W. A. Eaton and J. Hofrichter, "Hemoglobin S gelation and sickle cell disease," *Blood*, vol. 70, no. 5, pp. 1245–1266, 1987.

[7] B. Balkaran, G. Ghar, J. S. Morris, P. W. Thomas, B. E. Serjeant, and G. R. Serjeant, "Stroke in a cohort of patients with homozygous sickle cell disease," *Journal of Pediatrics*, vol. 120, no. 3, pp. 360–366, 1992.

[8] W. C. Wang, J. W. Langston, R. G. Steen et al., "Abnormalities of the central nervous system in very young children with sickle cell anemia," *Journal of Pediatrics*, vol. 132, no. 6, pp. 994–998, 1998.

[9] J. M. Harlan, "Introduction: anti-adhesion therapy in sickle cell disease," *Blood*, vol. 95, no. 2, pp. 365–367, 2000.

[10] R. P. Hebbel, M. A. B. Boogaerts, J. W. Eaton, and M. H. Steinberg, "Erythrocyte adherence to endothelium in sickle-cell anemia. A possible determinant of disease severity," *New England Journal of Medicine*, vol. 302, no. 18, pp. 992–995, 1980.

[11] N. Mohandas, E. Evans, B. Kukan, and A. Leung, "Sickle erythrocyte adherence to vascular endothelium. Morphology correlates and the requirement for divalent cations and collagen-binding plasma proteins," *Journal of Clinical Investigation*, vol. 76, no. 4, pp. 1605–1612, 1985.

[12] D. K. Kaul and M. E. Fabry, "In vivo studies of sickle red blood cells," *Microcirculation*, vol. 11, no. 2, pp. 153–165, 2004.

[13] M. Udani, Q. Zen, M. Cottman et al., "Basal cell adhesion molecule/lutheran protein: the receptor critical for sickle cell adhesion to laminin," *Journal of Clinical Investigation*, vol. 101, no. 11, pp. 2550–2558, 1998.

[14] R. A. Swerlick, J. R. Eckman, A. Kumar, M. Jeitler, and T. M. Wick, "$\alpha\beta$-integrin expression on sickle reticulocytes: vascular cell adhesion molecule-1-dependent binding to endothelium," *Blood*, vol. 82, no. 6, pp. 1891–1899, 1993.

[15] K. Sugihara, T. Sugihara, N. Mohandas, and R. P. Hebbel, "Thrombospondin mediates adherence of CD36 sickle reticulocytes to endothelial cells," *Blood*, vol. 80, no. 10, pp. 2634–2642, 1992.

[16] C. A. Hillery, M. C. Du, R. R. Montgomery, and J. P. Scott, "Increased adhesion of erythrocytes to components of the extracellular matrix: isolation and characterization of a red blood cell lipid that binds thrombospondin and laminin," *Blood*, vol. 87, no. 11, pp. 4879–4886, 1996.

[17] D. D. Roberts, S. B. Williams, H. R. Gralnick, and V. Ginsburg, "von Willebrand factor binds specifically to sulfated glycolipids," *Journal of Biological Chemistry*, vol. 261, no. 7, pp. 3306–3309, 1986.

[18] D. D. Roberts, C. N. Rao, and J. L. Magnani, "Laminin binds specifically to sulfated glycolipids," *Proceedings of the National Academy of Sciences of the United States of America*, vol. 82, no. 5, pp. 1306–1310, 1985.

[19] P. Guchhait, J. A. López, and P. Thiagarajan, "Characterization of autoantibodies against sulfatide from a V-gene phage-display library derived from patients with systemic lupus erythematosus," *Journal of Immunological Methods*, vol. 295, no. 1-2, pp. 129–137, 2004.

[20] P. Guchhait, S. K. Dasgupta, A. Le, S. Yellapragada, J. A. López, and P. Thiagarajan, "Lactadherin mediates sickle cell adhesion to vascular endothelial cells in flowing blood," *Haematologica*, vol. 92, no. 9, pp. 1266–1267, 2007.

[21] H. N. Naumann, L. W. Diggs, L. Barreras, and B. J. Williams, "Plasma hemoglobin and hemoglobin fractions in sickle cell crisis," *American Journal of Clinical Pathology*, vol. 56, no. 2, pp. 137–147, 1971.

[22] C. D. Reiter, X. Wang, J. E. Tanus-Santos et al., "Cell-free hemoglobin limits nitric oxide bioavailability in sickle-cell disease," *Nature Medicine*, vol. 8, no. 12, pp. 1383–1389, 2002.

[23] Z. Zhou, H. Han, M. A. Cruz, J. A. López, J. F. Dong, and P. Guchhait, "Haemoglobin blocks von Willebrand factor proteolysis by ADAMTS-13: a mechanism associated with sickle cell disease," *Thrombosis and Haemostasis*, vol. 101, no. 6, pp. 1070–1077, 2009.

[24] P. Philippidis, J. C. Mason, B. J. Evans et al., "Hemoglobin scavenger receptor CD163 mediates interleukin-10 release and

heme oxygenase-1 synthesis: antiinflammatory monocyte-macrophage responses in vitro, in resolving skin blisters in vivo, and after cardiopulmonary bypass surgery," *Circulation Research*, vol. 94, no. 1, pp. 119–126, 2004.

[25] C. A. Schaer, F. Vallelian, A. Imhof, G. Schoedon, and D. J. Schaer, "CD163-expressing monocytes constitute an endotoxin-sensitive Hb clearance compartment within the vascular system," *Journal of Leukocyte Biology*, vol. 82, no. 1, pp. 106–110, 2007.

[26] M. Langlois, J. Delanghe, and M. De Buyzere, "Relation between serum IgA concentration and haptoglobin type," *Clinical Chemistry*, vol. 42, no. 10, pp. 1722–1723, 1996.

[27] I. A. Tabbara, "Hemolytic anemias: diagnosis and management," *Medical Clinics of North America*, vol. 76, no. 3, pp. 649–668, 1992.

[28] C. D. Reiter, X. Wang, J. E. Tanus-Santos et al., "Cell-free hemoglobin limits nitric oxide bioavailability in sickle-cell disease," *Nature Medicine*, vol. 8, no. 12, pp. 1383–1389, 2002.

[29] R. T. Eberhardt, L. McMahon, S. J. Duffy et al., "Sickle cell anemia is associated with reduced nitric oxide bioactivity in peripheral conduit and resistance vessels," *American Journal of Hematology*, vol. 74, no. 2, pp. 104–111, 2003.

[30] K. A. Nath, V. Shah, J. J. Haggard et al., "Mechanisms of vascular instability in a transgenic mouse model of sickle cell disease," *American Journal of Physiology*, vol. 279, no. 6, pp. R1949–R1955, 2000.

[31] W. Y. Wong, D. Elliott-Mills, and D. Powars, "Renal failure in sickle cell anemia," *Hematology/Oncology Clinics of North America*, vol. 10, no. 6, pp. 1321–1331, 1996.

[32] J. D. Studt, J. A. Kremer Hovinga, G. Antoine et al., "Fatal congenital thrombotic thrombocytopenic purpura with apparent ADAMTS13 inhibitor: in vitro inhibition of ADAMTS13 activity by hemoglobin," *Blood*, vol. 105, no. 2, pp. 542–544, 2005.

[33] M. W. Radomski, R. M. J. Palmer, and S. Moncada, "Endogenous nitric oxide inhibits human platelet adhesion to vascular endothelium," *Lancet*, vol. 2, no. 8567, pp. 1057–1058, 1987.

[34] Y. Kayanoki, S. Kawata, E. Yamasaki et al., "Reduced nitric oxide production by L-arginine deficiency in lysinuric protein intolerance exacerbates intravascular coagulation," *Metabolism*, vol. 48, no. 9, pp. 1136–1140, 1999.

[35] J. Shao, T. Miyata, K. Yamada et al., "Protective role of nitric oxide in a model of thrombotic microangiopathy in rats," *Journal of the American Society of Nephrology*, vol. 12, no. 10, pp. 2088–2097, 2001.

[36] J. J. B. Schnog, J. A. Hovinga, S. Krieg et al., "ADAMTS13 activity in sickle cell disease," *American Journal of Hematology*, vol. 81, no. 7, pp. 492–498, 2006.

[37] S. Krishnan, J. Siegel, G. Pullen, M. Hevelow, C. Dampier, and M. Stuart, "Increased von Willebrand factor antigen and high molecular weight multimers in sickle cell disease associated with nocturnal hypoxemia," *Thrombosis Research*, vol. 122, no. 4, pp. 455–458, 2008.

[38] A. C. Makis, E. C. Hatzimichael, and K. L. Bourantas, "The role of cytokines in sickle cell disease," *Annals of Hematology*, vol. 79, no. 8, pp. 407–413, 2000.

[39] T. M. Wick, J. L. Moake, M. M. Udden, and L. V. McIntire, "Unusually large von Willebrand factor multimers preferentially promote young sickle and nonsickle erythrocyte adhesion to endothelial cells," *American Journal of Hematology*, vol. 42, no. 3, pp. 284–292, 1993.

[40] M. Furlan and B. Lämmle, "Aetiology and pathogenesis of thrombotic thrombocytopenic purpura and haemolytic uraemic syndrome: the role of von Willebrand factor-cleaving protease," *Best Practice and Research: Clinical Haematology*, vol. 14, no. 2, pp. 437–454, 2001.

[41] D. D. Wagner, "Cell biology of von Willebrand factor," *Annual Review of Cell Biology*, vol. 6, pp. 217–246, 1990.

[42] R. Pendu, V. Terraube, O. D. Christophe et al., "P-selectin glycoprotein ligand 1 and $\beta$2-integrins cooperate in the adhesion of leukocytes to von Willebrand factor," *Blood*, vol. 108, no. 12, pp. 3746–3752, 2006.

[43] M. Furlan, R. Rubles, M. Solenthaler, M. Wassmer, P. Sandoz, and B. Lämmle, "Deficient activity of von Willebrand factor-cleaving protease in chronic relapsing thrombotic thrombocytopenic purpura," *Blood*, vol. 89, no. 9, pp. 3097–3103, 1997.

[44] H. M. Tsai and E. C. Y. Lian, "Antibodies to von Willebrand factor-cleaving protease in acute thrombotic thrombocytopenic purpura," *New England Journal of Medicine*, vol. 339, no. 22, pp. 1585–1594, 1998.

[45] G. Remuzzi, M. Galbusera, M. Noris et al., "Von Willebrand factor cleaving protease (ADAMTS13) is deficient in recurrent and familial thrombotic thrombocytopenic purpura and hemolytic uremic syndrome," *Blood*, vol. 100, no. 3, pp. 778–785, 2002.

[46] Z. Zhou and P. Guchhait, "Extracellular Hemoglobin regulation of von Willebrand factor activity," *US Hematology*. In press.

[47] Q. Zhang, Y. F. Zhou, C. Z. Zhang, X. Zhang, C. Lu, and T. A. Springer, "Structural specializations of A2, a force-sensing domain in the ultralarge vascular protein von Willebrand factor," *Proceedings of the National Academy of Sciences of the United States of America*, vol. 106, no. 23, pp. 9226–9231, 2009.

[48] X. Zhang, K. Halvorsen, C. Z. Zhang, W. P. Wong, and T. A. Springer, "Mechanoenzymatic cleavage of the ultralarge vascular protein von willebrand factor," *Science*, vol. 324, no. 5932, pp. 1330–1334, 2009.

# 22

# Management of Sickle Cell Disease: A Review for Physician Education in Nigeria (Sub-Saharan Africa)

**Ademola Samson Adewoyin**

*Department of Haematology and Blood Transfusion, University of Benin Teaching Hospital, PMB 1111, Benin City, Edo State, Nigeria*

Correspondence should be addressed to Ademola Samson Adewoyin; drademola@yahoo.com

Academic Editor: Maria Stella Figueiredo

Sickle cell disease (SCD) predominates in sub-Saharan Africa, East Mediterranean areas, Middle East, and India. Nigeria, being the most populous black nation in the world, bears its greatest burden in sub-Saharan Africa. The last few decades have witnessed remarkable scientific progress in the understanding of the complex pathophysiology of the disease. Improved clinical insights have heralded development and establishment of disease modifying interventions such as chronic blood transfusions, hydroxyurea therapy, and haemopoietic stem cell transplantation. Coupled with parallel improvements in general supportive, symptomatic, and preventive measures, current evidence reveals remarkable appreciation in quality of life among affected individuals in developed nations. Currently, in Nigeria and other West African states, treatment and control of SCD are largely suboptimal. Improved knowledge regarding SCD phenotypes and its comprehensive care among Nigerian physicians will enhance quality of care for affected persons. This paper therefore provides a review on the aetiopathogenesis, clinical manifestations, and management of SCD in Nigeria, with a focus on its local patterns and peculiarities. Established treatment guidelines as appropriate in the Nigerian setting are proffered, as well as recommendations for improving care of affected persons.

## 1. Introduction

Sickle cell disease (SCD) is one of the most common genetic diseases worldwide and its highest prevalence occurs in Middle East, Mediterranean regions, Southeast Asia, and sub-Saharan Africa especially Nigeria [1, 2].

SCD is a chronic haemolytic disorder that is marked by tendency of haemoglobin molecules within red cells to polymerise and deform the red cell into a sickle (or crescent) shape resulting in characteristic vasoocclusive events and accelerated haemolysis. It is inherited in an autosomal recessive fashion either in the homozygous state or double heterozygous state. When inherited in the homozygous state, it is termed sickle cell anaemia (SCA). Other known SCD genotypes include haemoglobin SC disease, sickle beta plus thalassaemia, and sickle beta zero thalassemia (which has similar severity with sickle cell anaemia), haemoglobin SD Punjab disease, haemoglobin SO Arab disease, and others.

In Nigeria, SCD forms a small part of the clinical practice of most general duty doctors, as there is gross absence of dedicated sickle cell centres. Thus, it may be difficult to keep abreast of current knowledge and practices in the treatment of SCD. The purpose of this paper therefore is to provide a comprehensive and concise review of SCD and its management for physician education in Nigeria. Particular attention is given to its local epidemiology, clinical phenotypes and complications, current treatment guidelines, practice challenges, and recommendations for improved care. Relevant literatures and local references including clinical studies, reviews, and texts were gathered, summarized, and presented in this paper.

## 2. Epidemiology

About 5–7% of the global population carries an abnormal haemoglobin gene [3, 4]. The most predominant form of haemoglobinopathy worldwide is sickle cell disease. The greatest burden of the disease lies in sub-Saharan Africa and Asia [5].

The prevalence of sickle cell trait ranges between 10 and 45% in various parts of sub-Saharan Africa [6–8]. In Nigeria, carrier prevalence is about 20 to 30% [9, 10]. SCD affects about 2 to 3% of the Nigerian population of more than 160 million [9]. Recent estimate from a large retrospective study by Nwogoh et al. in Benin City, South-South Nigeria revealed an SCD prevalence of 2.39% and a carrier rate of about 23% [11].

## 3. Brief History and Genetic Origin of SCD

In 1874, Dr. Horton, a Sierra Leonian medical Doctor, reportedly gave the first description of clinical symptoms and signs which is now referred to as sickle cell disease [12]. Herrick, a Chicago physician, also gave a formal description of the disease in 1910 when he observed abnormal sickle shaped red cells in the blood of a dental student from West Indies who had anaemia [13]. In 1927, Hahn and Gillespie observed that sickling of red cells was associated with conditions of low oxygen tension. In 1949, Linus Pauling and colleagues demonstrated that haemoglobin in these patients was different from normal subjects using protein electrophoresis [14]. However, Venon Ingram and J. A. Hunt in 1956 sequenced the sickle haemoglobin molecule and showed that the abnormality was due to valine substitution for glutamate on the 6th position of the sickle beta-haemoglobin gene. Marotta and coworkers in 1977 showed that the corresponding change in codon 6 of the beta-globin gene was GAG to GTG [14]. Since then, further insights have been gained into understanding the origin, complex pathophysiology, and treatment of the disease through molecular biology techniques.

Africa and Asia are considered as the birthplace of the sickle cell mutation. Sickle cell disease is believed to be a consequence of natural mutation of the beta-globin gene (HBB) affecting the gametes and transferred to subsequent generations. Using restriction fragment length polymorphism analysis, four main African haplotypes and one Asian haplotype of the beta-globin chain genes have been characterized and are believed to originate differently in these regions. The main African haplotypes include Senegal, Benin, Bantu (central-African republic), and Cameroon haplotype [15–18]. The Bantu haplotype is associated with the most severe disease phenotype while the Asian (also called Arab-Indian) haplotype is associated with a mild phenotype [19].

SCD is found in other parts of the world including USA and Europe due to migration and interracial marriages [5, 20]. The high prevalence of SCD in sub-Saharan Africa has been attributed to survival advantage conferred by the sickle cell trait against *Plasmodium falciparum*. Resistance of individuals with sickle cell trait to *Plasmodium falciparum* creates a selective pressure that has maintained the sickle cell gene within human populations in malaria endemic regions like sub-Saharan Africa. This phenomenon is termed balanced polymorphism [21, 22].

## 4. Aetiopathogenesis of Sickle Cell Disease

SCD is a qualitative haemoglobinopathy resulting from a structural change in the sequence of amino acids on the beta globin chain of the haemoglobin molecule due to a point mutation. The sickling mutation causes a single base change from adenine to thymine on the 17th nucleotide of the beta globin chain gene (HBB). This invariably translates into substitution of valine for glutamate on the 6th amino acid of the beta globin chain. The abnormal biochemistry of this mutant haemoglobin induces polymerization of Hb S molecules within the red cells, so called sickling. On the sickle haemoglobin, the glutamate protein molecule, which is hydrophilic, polar, and negatively charged, is replaced by a less polar, hydrophobic, neutral amino acid, valine. Under deoxy conditions, the abnormal valine residue causes intraerythrocytic hydrophobic interaction of sickle haemoglobin tetramers, leading to their precipitation and polymer formation, so called gelation [23]. Eventually, all cytosolic haemoglobin molecules precipitate into seven (one inner and six outer) double strands with cross-links which are called tactoids. Upon reoxygenation, unsickling occurs and the red cell assumes its normal shape. However, repeated sickling and unsickling of the red cell damages the red cell membrane, due to herniation of sickle haemoglobin polymers through the cytoskeleton, thus rendering the red cell permanently sickled. These appear as irreversibly sickled cells (ISCs) on peripheral blood cytology.

The kinetics of red cell sickling is highly heterogenous. Several variables are known to affect the rate and degree of sickling of the red cells. Intracellular dehydration of sickle red cells increases mean cell haemoglobin concentration (MCHC) [14]. Higher MCHC favours sickling. As such, very high Hb S level of about 80 to 90% seen in the homozygous disease is associated with a worse disease while the presence of alpha thalassemia (one or two gene deletions) ameliorates the disease. Another variable is the presence of other interacting nonsickle haemoglobin. Of note is fetal haemoglobin (Hb F). Higher proportion of Hb F is associated with mild disease. When present, high levels of Hb F are uniformly dispersed within the red cell and it retards the sickling process. Thus, coinheritance of sickle haemoglobin with hereditary persistence of fetal haemoglobin (HPFH) is associated with mild disease [24]. Similarly, this advantage is positively utilized through clinical use of fetal haemoglobin inducing drug such as hydroxyurea. Vascular beds that have intrinsically sluggish venous outflow such as bone marrow, spleen, or inflamed tissues are at higher risk of infarctive events due to prolonged microvascular transit time [25]. Whenever and wherever microvascular transit time becomes longer than sickling delay time, sickling and vascular occlusion become imminent. Intracellular pH is another important variable. With acidosis, the haemoglobin molecules give off their oxygen more readily and sickling occurs more readily.

Repeated sickling of the red cell induces cellular injury which has been shown to activate membrane ion channels such as the Gardos pathway (calcium gated potassium channels) and KCL cotransporter [25]. There are influx of calcium ions and efflux of potassium and water, hence intracellular dehydration. High intracellular calcium levels provoke activity of proteolytic enzymes such as phospholipases and proteases causing the digestion of membrane phospholipids and proteins, respectively. Subsequently, there is perturbation of the membrane lipids with exteriorization of lipids such as phosphatidyl serine and ethanolamine which are normally located in the inner leaflets of the membrane lipid bilayer [26].

The diverse clinical heterogeneity of SCD is related to two main pathogenetic processes: chronic haemolysis and high viscosity/vascular occlusion. Infarctive events in SCD result from erythrostasis caused by rigid sickled cells in various vascular beds especially organs with sluggish blood flow such as the spleen and the bone marrow. Capillaries are about 2-3 microns in diameter. Sickle cells due to loss of flexibility are unable to transit the microvasculature, hence vessel occlusion. Aside from these mechanistic processes, sickle cells are also shown to exhibit increased adhesiveness to vascular endothelium, leucocytes, platelets, and themselves [27–29]. Sickle reticulocytes are even more adhesive to the endothelium than sickle discocytes [30]. Molecular interactions between the red cells and the vascular endothelium include CD36 and thrombospondin, VLA4 and VCAM-1, respectively [30, 31]. Fibronectin and von Willebrand factor are also involved in these interactions. Currently, it is known that increased adhesiveness of different cellular surfaces with formation of heterocellular aggregates is believed to propagate the phenomenon of vascular occlusion, especially in the postcapillary venules [26]. Also note that destruction of red cell membrane causes exposure of membrane proteins, thereby inciting autoantibody formation. These antibodies such as IgG anti-band 3 antibodies are believed to promote erythrophagocytosis [25].

Episodic microvascular occlusion in sickle cell disease even in steady state results in ischaemic-reperfusion injury which sets the stage for an increased inflammatory tone, thus significant elevations in total leucocyte counts, platelet counts, and positive serum acute phase reactants. Even in steady state, SCD is a chronic inflammatory condition; the attendant inflammation induced oxidative stress further contributes to progressive tissue damage [32, 33]. The leucocytes in SCD also express higher levels of L-selectins and also have stimulated adhesiveness. Increased adhesiveness coupled with phosphatidyl serine exposure on the red cell surface makes SCD a procoagulant and a hypercoagulable state [34].

Erythrocyte lifespan in SCD averages about 16–20 days in contrast to about 100–120 days in normal state [35, 36]. Haemolysis in sickle cell disease is both extravascular and intravascular. Abnormal shape of the ISCs creates an abnormal rheology, associated with heightened clearance by the reticuloendothelial system. Because of their increased fragility and reduced deformability, some red cells undergo intravascular haemolysis. High plasma haemoglobin level is associated with low haptoglobin levels and high levels of lactate dehydrogenase (LDH), arginase-1, and AST [37]. Plasma haemoglobin is an avid scavenger of nitric oxide (NO). High plasma haemoglobin levels resulting from chronic haemolysis reduce NO bioavailability. Normally, NO relaxes the endothelium and maintains vascular tone (vasodilator) [37]. Low circulating levels of NO propagate vasospasm which is observed even in large vessels in SCD. Contributing to this is dysfunction of endothelial nitric oxide synthetase [37]. This is the underlying basis of vasculopathic complications such as

cerebrovascular diseases, priapism, pulmonary hypertension, and chronic leg ulcers. Arginase 1 is normally involved in formation of urea in protein excretion. Accelerated haemolysis of red cells leads to higher levels of arginase 1. As such, more ornithine is produced, further depleting plasma arginine levels. Excess ornithine is channeled to alternate pathways which produce excess prolenes and polyamines. These byproducts promote endothelial smooth muscle proliferations, further narrowing the vascular chamber [38]. Chronic haemolysis results in excess breakdown of haemoglobin molecules and high levels of bilirubin, which is associated with formation of bilirubin pigment stones in the gall bladder (cholelithiasis).

Some authorities have attempted to categorize SCD patients into two clinical subphenotypes based on the overriding pathogenic process [25, 39]. Clinically, there is some degree of overlap between the two groups. Some patients experience more of viscosity/vasoocclusive complications and tend to have higher baseline haematocrit levels. Others experience more of vasculopathic complications due to more intense haemolysis associated with a lower baseline haematocrit [14, 39].

## 5. Clinical Phenotypes and Complications in Sickle Cell Disease

There is marked intraindividual and interindividual variability in SCD. Clinical heterogeneity of the disease has been explained by both genetic and environmental factors. Known genetic factors contributing to variations in clinical severity of the disease include the pattern of sickle cell inheritance, nature of b-globin haplotype, Hb F level, and FCP loci [15]. Other modulators of the disease include presence of alpha thalassemia and other probable genetic influences as well as environmental factors such as access to optimal health care, ambient living conditions, and availability of finance [15].

*Physical Effects of Sickle Cell Disease.* Body habitus in SCD ranges from a normal build to a tall, lanky physique depending on the clinical severity. Other physical changes include prognathism, arachnodactyly, and increased AP chest diameter (barrel chest) [40, 41]. In childhood, sickle cell patients may be shorter or smaller than normal. Puberty is often delayed but considerable growth takes place in late adolescence such that adults with sickle cell anaemia are at least as tall as normal [14]. However, adults that have suffered vertebral infarction and collapse may be shorter than normal. Many of these physical changes are due to the chronic hypoxaemia associated with severe anaemia. Severe haemolysis in infancy causes marrow hyperplasia of the skull and facial bones, resulting in frontal bossing, prognathism, or malocclusion [42]. The abnormal facies results from extension of the marrow into the cortical bone causing widening of the diploe spaces and thinning of the bone cortex. The chronic haemolytic process is associated with pallor, jaundice, splenomegaly in early childhood.

### 5.1. Acute Sickle Syndromes/Complications

*5.1.1. Bone Pain Crisis (BPC).* BPC is the most consistent and characteristic feature of SCD [43]. The pain results from activation of nociceptive afferent nerve endings in the ischemic bones. Commonly affected bones include the long bones such as femur and humerus, vertebrae, pelvis, ribs, and sternum [24]. Multiple sites may be involved. An early manifestation of bone infarction is the hand and foot syndrome. This is characterized by dactylitis involving the small bones of the hand or foot, marked by diffuse swelling over the involved area. It often resolves spontaneously within one to two weeks and is rare after 2-3 years of life. Frequency of bone pain crisis is higher in patients with homozygous sickle cell disease, low Hb F, and higher baseline haemoglobin. It is said to be more common in young adults but its frequency tends to wane at older ages. Pain episodes vary in intensity and tend to resolve within a few days. In about 57% of cases, no precipitating factor is identified [44]. However, known precipitants include exposure to cold, dehydration, intercurrent infections such as malaria, physical exertion, tobacco smoke, alcohol use, hard drugs, high altitude, hypoxic conditions, physical pain, pregnancy, hot weather, emotional stress, or onset of menses [32, 45]. Suggested treatment guideline for uncomplicated BPC is presented as follows.

*Treatment Guidelines for Bone Pain Crisis*

(i) Principles of treatment include adequate analgesia, hydration, warmth, prophylactic or therapeutic antibiotics if pyrexial after necessary culture samples are taken, as well as oxygenation if hypoxic (Sp $O_2$ < 90%) [45–48].

(ii) Oral hydration must be adequate with at least 1.5 L/m$^2$ of water based fluid per day in children and 60–70 mL/kg in adults. If parenteral, not more than 1.5 times maintenance is given in order to prevent volume overload considering baseline anaemia in most patients [49, 50].

(iii) Patients and parents should be encouraged to keep a stock of simple analgesics at home in event of a painful episode. However, mild to moderate pain that does not succumb to home-based oral analgesia and hydration within 2 days requires hospitalization.

(iv) Analgesia should be commenced within 15 to 30 minutes of presentation in the emergency room or day hospital. Effective analgesia should be achieved within 1 hour. There should be an ongoing assessment of analgesic efficacy every 30 minutes until pain is controlled, thereafter every 2 hours [49, 50].

(v) Treatment should be individualized. The choice of analgesia depends on the severity of the pain and the patient's prior analgesic needs/history.

(vi) Nonopioids such as simple paracetamol and NSAIDS (nonsteroidal anti-inflammatory drugs) may be used in mild VOC. Weak opioids such as tramadol and DF118 (dihydrocodeine) are used for moderate pain while severe pain requires stronger opioids/narcotics such as morphine [45, 46].

(vii) Adjuvants for pain control help in achieving better analgesia. They may include mild sedatives such as promethazine or diazepam. Combination of paracetamol or NSAIDS with opiates gives better analgesia because of their synergistic actions. Oversedation should be avoided. Laxatives should be prescribed for prevention and treatment of constipation, a side effect of opioid use.

(viii) More than five to seven days of sequential NSAID use should be avoided to reduce the risk of peptic ulceration and GIT haemorrhage. Also, NSAIDS are potentially nephrotoxic and are better avoided in established renal disease.

(ix) Severe VOC requires parenteral opioid analgesia and hydration in a hospital setting. The dose of the analgesia should be titrated with the severity of the pain until adequate control is achieved in a fixed dose schedule (FDS), interspersed with short-acting agents for breakthrough pains.

(x) Prophylactic incentive spirometry is recommended for prevention of acute chest syndrome especially in BPC involving the chest wall. In the absence of a spirometer, 10 deep breaths every 2 hours while awake between 8 a.m. and 10 p.m. are an alternative.

(xi) If pain persists, patient controlled analgesia (PCA) should be considered where available. PCA is sparsely available in Nigeria, except in very few private facilities. PCA reduces the risk of pain undertreatment.

(xii) Short-acting opioids in clinical use include tramadol, morphine, hydrocodeine, hydromorphine, fentanyl, oxymorphone, and oxycodeine. Longer acting opioids include methadone and slow release preparations of tramadol, morphine, and oxycodeine. Access to a wide range of opioids may not always be readily available in Nigeria; however, the available ones should be used.

(xiii) In difficult cases, where pain is unremitting after 48 hours of well conducted analgesia, exchange blood transfusion (EBT) may be offered [51].

(xiv) Hospitalization for severe BPC occurring on 3 or more occasions per year is an indication for initiation of hydroxyurea therapy or chronic transfusion therapy in patients that are intolerant of hydroxyurea.

(xv) Pain in SCD is majorly nociceptive in origin. However, it may also have a neuropathic component marked by tingling/burning sensation or numbness. In such cases, drugs such as pregabalin or carbamazepine will be useful [46].

(xvi) Pain control in SCD is essentially pharmacologic. However, nonpharmacologic measures such as physical therapy with heat or ice packs, relaxation, distraction, music, menthol rub, meditation, and transcutaneous electrical nerve stimulation (TENS) are also helpful [46].

Treatment of acute sickle cell pain in a dedicated day hospital is associated with better outcome due to prompt triage and familiarity with analgesic needs of individual patients, hence reduced risk of pain undertreatment. Invariably, there is reduction in overall patient admission rates and better outcomes compared to emergency room settings [52–54]. However, most institutions in Nigeria lack daycare settings for management of sickle cell crisis.

Furthermore, it is important to note that BPC may be complicated by a concurrent hyperhaemolytic crisis with resultant acute severe anaemia or may even progress to acute chest syndrome or multiorgan failure syndrome (MOFS). MOFS is defined as sudden onset, severe organ dysfunction simultaneously involving at least two major organ systems (such as the liver, lung, and kidney) in the setting of an acute sickle cell crisis. MOFS is partly explained by significant vasoocclusive events in vital organs with major functional compromise and organ failure [55]. This life-threatening complication requires immediate intensive care and a multispecialist attention including the intensivists, nephrologist, hepatologist, respiratory physicians, and others.

### 5.1.2. Acute Abdominal Pain.

Acute abdominal pain in SCD may be due to sequestration crisis, vasoocclusion of mesenteric vessels, gall bladder/biliary tract disorders, or other non-SCD specific causes. In a Nigerian study by Akingbola et al., the aetiology of acute abdominal pain in a population of adult Nigerian SCD patients presenting in a tertiary facility were found to include SCD related complications such as abdominal VOC and acute cholecystitis, as well as other infective causes such as cystitis, gastroenteritis, appendicitis, and bowel obstruction [56]. About 38% of the cases were due to abdominal infarction/crisis [56]. In Ile-Ife, Akinola et al. observed abdominal pain due to VOC in 26% of sickle cell anaemia patients [57]. Microvascular occlusion may involve the mesenteric bed causing ischaemic abdominal pain. Abdominal pain of presumed vasoocclusive origin is termed abdominal crisis. Girdle syndrome, otherwise called mesenteric syndrome, is a rare complication owing to extensive collateral blood supplies to the mesentery and bowel wall [58]. Girdle syndrome or mesenteric syndrome is said to be present when there is an established paralytic ileus, which may be associated with vomiting, silent distended abdomen, dilated bowel loops, and air-fluid levels on abdominal radiography. Typically, a patient with girdle syndrome presents with generalized abdominal pain and rarely in shock if there is massive bowel gangrene (third space losses). Other abdominal findings may include localized or rebound tenderness, board-like rigidity, and lack of movement on respiration. Abdominal radiography and ultrasound scan are helpful as well as investigations to rule out differentials such as pancreatitis, acute appendicitis, cholecystitis, biliary colic, splenic abscess, ischaemic colitis, and other forms of acute abdomen. Intravenous hydration, analgesia, and antibiotics are indicated. For an established ileus, NPO (nothing by mouth) should be commenced, as well as nasogastric aspiration, if there is vomiting. Urgent surgical opinion should be sought. Exchange blood transfusion may be necessary in mesenteric (girdle) syndrome. Biliary/gall bladder anomalies commonly observed in SCD include cholelithiasis and biliary sludge [59]. Recent studies among Nigerian patients observed an age-related prevalence of about 5 to 10% for cholelithiasis [60, 61].

### 5.1.3. Visceral Sequestration Crisis.

Infants and children less than 7 years are at greatest risk of sequestration crisis especially splenic sequestration. Children above this age group and adults are at less risk of splenic sequestration because the spleen tends to become fibrotic with repeated infarctions and cannot enlarge [24]. However, in haemoglobin SC disease, older children and adults can experience sequestration crisis. If not corrected rapidly, acute sequestration results in hypovolaemia, severe anaemia, and possibly death. A typical patient is irritable with rapidly enlarging spleen or liver and pain in the upper abdomen. Features of acute anaemia include worsening pallor, generalized weakness, and tachycardia. Early presentation in the hospital and close monitoring are important. Blood transfusion is necessary if haemoglobin level falls 2 g/dL below steady state haemoglobin levels or evidence of cardiac decompensation. A major sequestration crisis is defined by haemoglobin level below 6 g/dL. There is risk for recurrence; therefore parents and caregivers must be taught how to examine the child's spleen regularly and report any abnormal finding to the physician immediately. Splenectomy is recommended after the second episode in children above two years of age. For children below 2 years of age, chronic blood transfusion should be offered [62]. Majority of SCD sequestration crisis involves the spleen. Though less common, the liver and lymph nodes may also be sites of sequestration in SCD.

### 5.1.4. Aplastic Crisis.

Aplastic crisis usually occurs in those less than 16 years of age. It is commonly caused by parvovirus B19 infection which causes transient selective suppression of erythroid progenitors. In Nigeria, prevalence of parvovirus B19 infection is shown to be similar among sickle cell patients and the general population [63]. In normal subjects, parvovirus B19 infection is asymptomatic. However, in patients with chronic haemolytic anaemia such as SCD, parvoviral infection is potentially devastating. Reticulocytopenia often lasts about 7 to 10 days, followed by spontaneous remission with reticulocytosis. Aplastic crisis may follow a recent upper respiratory tract infection and the patient may have flu-like symptoms such as headache, mild fever, and lethargy. Other findings include pallor and worsening anaemia. The condition is self-limiting. Treatment is to give red cell transfusion support until erythroid activity resumes.

### 5.1.5. Worsening (Acute) Anaemia in SCD.

Baseline haemoglobin level in sickle cell disease ranges between 6 and 9 g/dL [64]. A study among adult SCD patients in Lagos by Akinbami et al. shows mean steady state haemoglobin levels of $7.92 \pm 1.49$ g/dL [65]. Average haemoglobin concentration of an SCD patient over a minimum of 4 weeks is considered steady state (or stable) haemoglobin level in the absence of any form of crisis in the preceding three months. Anaemia in

SCD is usually well compensated. Occasionally, some patients have high steady state haematocrit level above 10 g/dL and they tend to present with more vasoocclusive complications. This has been termed high haematocrit syndrome [26]. Therapeutic phlebotomy when haemoglobin level is higher than 12 g/dL may benefit such patients [59]. However, in most other patients, significant decline of more than 2 g/dL below steady state level has functional consequences. Untreated severe anaemia is symptomatic and may precipitate heart failure. Causes of worsening anaemia in sickle cell disease may include hyperhaemolysis from any cause, aplastic crisis, megaloblastic crisis, iron deficiency, haemorrhage, renal failure, sequestration crisis, and extreme bone marrow necrosis. Treatment requires both definitive and supportive care. If patient shows signs of cardiac decompensation, blood transfusion should be given. The cause of worsening anaemia should be sought and treated accordingly.

*5.1.6. Cerebrovascular Disease (CVD).* CVD is a significant cause of morbidity and mortality in sickle cell disease [56]. CVD or stroke refers to a sudden onset focal or global neurologic deficit of vascular origin lasting more than 24 hours. It may be ischaemic or haemorrhagic. TIA or stroke occurs in 25% of patients with sickle cell disease. Overt stroke occurs in 10 to 15% of homozygous patients under the age of 10 years [66–68]. The prevalence of overt stroke among SCA children in Port Harcourt, Nigeria, is reported as 4.3% [69]. In Abuja, Nigeria, Oniyangi et al. reported a stroke prevalence of 5.2% among SCD children seen in a tertiary center [70]. The risk of CVD is higher in those with low baseline haemoglobin, low fetal haemoglobin, high white blood cell count, and high systolic blood pressure. CVD is rare in infants. Incidence of CVD is higher in Hb SS disease compared with SC disease, S/b+thalassemia, and S/b zero thalassemia [36, 59].

Infarctive CVD is commonest and occurs in patients aged less than 20 years and older than 30 years (peak incidence: 10–15 years) [71]. Infarction is often associated with stenosis or occlusion of affected vessels most commonly the distal internal carotid, proximal middle cerebral, and anterior cerebral arteries. The patient may present with antecedent history of TIA or seizures, which eventually progresses to an overt stroke, characterized by hemiparesis, speech, or visual impairment, or even coma if immediate therapy is not instituted. Suggested guideline on acute and long-term treatment of an ischaemic stroke in SCD is provided as follows.

*Treatment Guidelines for Sickle Cell Ischaemic Stroke*

   (i) After initial evaluation of patient's airway, breathing, and circulation (ABC of resuscitation), further stabilization should be pursued through prevention and control of hypoxaemia, hypotension, hyperthermia, and glycaemic imbalance, which would worsen the cerebral insult.

   (ii) Presence of seizures should be controlled with appropriate anticonvulsants. Prophylactic antiseizure therapy is not necessary.

   (iii) Urgent noncontrast CT/MRI is required to distinguish haemorrhage and infarction. This important distinction has to be made early, as this will impact subsequent therapeutic decisions.

   (iv) In the early stage of brain ischaemia (<3 hours), cranial CT may be negative or show only subtle inconclusive signs. Magnetic resonance imaging (MRI) provides better details but should be deferred until treatment has been initiated.

   (v) Early institution of exchange transfusion is crucial to improving treatment outcome. EBT should be targeted at reducing sickle Hb level below 30%. Simple transfusions may be offered in the interim while EBT is being planned. Simple transfusions at 10–15 mL per kg red cells reduce sickle haemoglobin levels to about 60%.

   (vi) Adequate hydration not more than 1.5 times the maintenance should be instituted with isotonic fluids preferably 0.9% normal saline.

   (vii) In untransfused SCD patients, stroke recurrence rate is 67%, with 70% of recurrent strokes occurring in the first 3 years after the initial stroke [72]. As such, EBT should be followed up with hypertransfusion therapy to maintain sickle Hb level below 30% at a haemoglobin concentration of about 10 to 11 g/dL.

   (viii) Chronic blood transfusion (CBT) has been shown to be beneficial in primary and secondary prevention of CVD [70, 73–75]. However, clear definitions on when and how CBT should be stopped is yet to be made. Often times, transfusions continue till late adolescence or early adulthood.

   (ix) Hydroxyurea therapy reduces cerebral blood flow. Though less effective, hydroxyurea may be considered an alternative to chronic transfusion therapy, where transfusion is not feasible [67, 68].

   (x) Thrombolysis with recombinant tissue plasminogen activator (rTPA) within the first 3 hours of ischaemic CVD in adult patients should be considered after careful patient evaluation [76]. TPA is not recommended in children. However, the current prospect of TPA use among Nigerian patients is remote due to challenges of its availability, cost, delayed diagnosis, and clinical experience with its use.

   (xi) Antiplatelet agent, aspirin 325 mg, is recommended if TPA is not used and should be avoided for the first 24 hours if TPA is used [77].

   (xii) Adult SCD patients should be evaluated and treated for modifiable risk factors such as dyslipidaemia.

   (xiii) Acute stroke should be treated in a dedicated stroke unit with input of both neurologist and haematologist.

Haemorrhagic stroke tends to occur between 20 and 29 years of age and is associated with low steady state haemoglobin levels and high steady state leucocyte counts [71]. Hemorrhage often results from rupture of vessels within the circle of Willis. Clinical presentation is similar to ischaemic CVD. However, patients with haemorrhagic CVDs are more likely to present with coma. In haemorrhagic CVD, patient may present with severe headache, vomiting, and other features suggesting raised intracranial pressure. Haemorrhagic CVD is rare but more fatal. Cerebral oedema is worse in haemorrhagic stroke. Prompt confirmation of diagnosis through imaging studies is required. Treatment of cerebral oedema with hypertonic solution such as mannitol is desirable. Antiplatelet and anticoagulants are contraindicated in haemorrhagic stroke. Though its exact role in haemorrhagic CVD is not clear, EBT is recommended especially for patients billed to undergo magnetic resonance angiography [76]. Surgical interventions by vascular surgeons may include ligation of accessible aneurysms and surgical vascular bypass procedure for moyamoya syndrome. Nimodipine, a calcium channel blocker, improves outcome in adults with subarachnoid haemorrhage by counteracting delayed arterial vasospasm [76, 78].

Risk evaluation for an overt ischaemic stroke and the need for early preventive intervention are performed by assessment of cerebral blood flow velocity using transcranial Doppler (TCD) ultrasound. Cerebral blood flow in excess of 2 meters per second portends a high risk for CVD. Typically, TCD ultrasound assessment is commenced by age of 2 years. TCD between 1.7 and 2 should be reassessed in 3-4 months. If stable, assessment should be annual until 16 years of age [59]. Cerebral blood flow in excess of 2 meters/second is an indication for commencement of hypertransfusion therapy and this is shown to reduce stroke occurrence by about 90% [66]. MRI scan every 5 years may also be used in periodic evaluation of the brain for silent infarctions where resources are available [79].

Subclinical cerebral infarcts (SCI) in sickle cell disease patients occur in 27% and 37% of patients before their 6th and 14th birthdays, respectively [80]. Silent stroke is defined by an abnormal MRI in the absence of history and physical signs of an overt CVD. Risk factors for SCI include male gender, low steady state haemoglobin levels, higher baseline systolic blood pressure, and previous seizures [80]. Subclinical strokes are associated with neuropsychiatric dysfunction in apparently healthy SCD patients [79, 81] and are a risk factor for overt stroke [82]. In confirmed silent brain infarctions with neurocognitive delay and behavioural disturbances, chronic transfusion therapy is indicated.

*5.1.7. Acute Chest Syndrome (ACS).* ACS is a leading cause of mortality in sickle cell disease even among Nigerian patients, accounting for about 25% of all deaths [83–85]. Risk factors for acute chest syndrome includes older age, low fetal haemoglobin level, high haematocrit level, homozygous SS disease, chest VOC, smoking, general anaesthesia and surgery, asthma, and possibly opioid use [86]. ACS is defined by new pulmonary infiltrates (on chest radiography) in at least one complete lung segment, fever, and at least one respiratory symptom (pleuritic chest pain, cough, dyspnoea, and tachypnoea) [86]. ACS may follow a painful crisis especially in adults. ACS may also complicate the immediate

postoperative state. As such, there is need to maintain proper protocols for preventing or treating ACS during BPC and after surgery.

The underlying pathophysiology of ACS includes vasoocclusion of pulmonary vessels and microbial involvement. Implicated microbes include bacteria such as Pneumococcus, *Haemophilus influenza*, respiratory viruses, and atypical organisms such as *Mycoplasma*, Chlamydia, or *Legionella*. Respiratory viruses are more likely in children while bacterial causes are more frequent in adults [24]. Furthermore, hypoxia induced by ACS can trigger widespread sickling and vasoocclusion, with possibility of multiorgan failure and death. Fat laden pulmonary macrophages in the airways are observed in about half of the cases, suggesting possible contributions from bone marrow fat embolisation [83]. Bone pain crisis involving the chest cage can also trigger ACS as a result of pain induced hypoventilation, which encourages sickling in the pulmonary bed and microbial growth. Similarly, oversedation with opioids may predispose to ACS.

During BPC or in the immediate postoperative period, care should be taken to prevent ACS. In such patients, prophylactic incentive spirometry is helpful [87]. In the absence of a spirometer, 10 deep breaths every 2 hours of the day is an alternative. Treatment of an established ACS also includes incentive spirometry/chest physiotherapy, parenteral broad-spectrum antibiotics, effective pain relief, and supplemental oxygen therapy (2–4 liters per minute). Opioid is the mainstay of pain control in SCD. Its liberal use is encouraged in order to prevent pain undertreatment, prolonged treatment, and hypoventilation. However, care should be taken to avoid oversedation. Recommended antibiotic combinations include quinolones, 2nd or 3rd generation cephalosporin alongside macrolides (for atypical bacteria). Antibiotic choice should be further directed by local susceptibility profile if available.

Bronchodilator therapy is also required as most patients may have a bronchoreactive component. EBT is indicated in worsening lung consolidation or persistent hypoxia, any neurological deficit (confusion, motor deficit, epilepsy), intractable pain or opioid intolerance, haemodynamic instability, nosocomial infections, acute worsening of anaemia or cardiovascular insufficiency, and acute enlargement of spleen or liver [59]. Mechanical ventilation is required in rapidly progressive cases. Inhaled nitric oxide and steroid may be helpful in life-threatening cases. Evidence suggests that recurrent episodes of ACS can be prevented by hydroxyurea [88]. Also chronic transfusion therapy is beneficial in secondary prevention of ACS and is indicated in patients with two or more episodes annually, who are unresponsive to hydroxyurea [89].

*5.1.8. Priapism.* Priapism is another acute complication of sickle cell disease. It is defined as persistent, purposeless, painful penile erection that is unassociated with sexual pleasure. Generally, reports of lifetime prevalence of priapism in sickle cell disease range from 2 to 35% [90]. Its prevalence is found to be as high as 44.9% among Nigerian male SCD patients [91]. Peak incidence occurs in 2nd and 3rd decade (median age: 18.5 years) [24, 91]. SCD priapism is a "low-flow" type. The penile ischaemia results from outflow obstruction (poor venous drainage) caused by sickled cells. Usually, it affects the corpora cavernosa alone while the spongiosum is spared. A typical genital examination reveals a hard penis with soft glans; tricorporeal involvement is rare. The priapism may also be defined as stuttering, minor, or major (prolonged) depending on the duration of the attack and its frequency. Stuttering priapism typically last about 30 minutes to 2 hours, tends to become recurrent (occurs several times a week), and may herald episodes of prolonged priapism. Minor attacks occur infrequently or isolated. Major or severe attacks last longer than 3 to 4 hours and should be treated as a urological emergency. Severe (major) and recurrent priapism (penile ischaemia) is associated with irreversible organ damage, fibrosis, and impotence.

The goal of treatment is to preserve erectile function and prevent recurrences. As such, there is need for early presentation in the hospital if home remedies are unsuccessful within 2 hours of onset. At the onset, patients should be counseled to drink extra fluid, use home-based simple or compound analgesia, and attempt to void. Other self-help strategies such as warm baths and gentle exercises like jogging may be helpful. Oral dose of pseudoephedrine or terbutaline may be given. If the priapism persists more than 2 hours, hospital care is required. This includes intravenous hydration and opioid analgesia. If the priapism persists more than 3 hours, aspiration and irrigation of the corpora with dilute phenylephrine, epinephrine, or etilefrine is indicated. Frequently, aspiration of blood from the cavernosal bodies is performed with a 23-gauge sterile needle, followed by irrigation with a 1 : 1,000,000 dilution of epinephrine in saline, after adequate counseling, conscious sedation, and local anaesthesia [92]. If detumescence is achieved lasting more than one hour, patient may be discharged home on oral analgesic, pseudoephedrine, and clinic follow-up. Penile aspiration and irrigation may be repeated up to 3 or 4 episodes if detumescence is not achieved early.

Simple early self-intracavernosal injection (SICI) of etilefrine and other adrenergic agonists such as metaraminol may achieve detumescence within one hour of onset, hence removing the need for hospital-based surgical aspiration and irrigation [93–95]. Sympathomimetics (adrenergic agonists) may be associated with untoward effects such as blood pressure changes and are yet to be licensed for SICI. EBT is indicated in recalcitrant cases. Surgical shunt procedures such as proximal shunt of quackel or distal shunt of winter may be tried, if conservative measures remain unsuccessful. However, surgical penile shunts may also be unsuccessful and may induce impotence [96]. Often, priapism will resolve with one or a combination of medical interventions.

In preventing priapism, male sickle cell patients ought to be adequately informed and counseled about priapism from adolescence. Patients with frequent episodes (≥2 per month, ≥4 per year) should receive priapism prophylaxis with oral pseudoephedrine 30 mg daily if they are less than 10 years of age and 60 mg per day if they are older than 10 years. Etilefrine and diethylstilbestrol (DES) may be used prophylactically although evidence for its usefulness is limited [97, 98]. DES use has been limited by its feminizing effects, though a short course of 5 mg daily may be used to abort a stuttering episode [99]. Similarly use of injectable leuprolide, a GnRH antagonist, which works through endogenous suppression of androgen production, is associated with longstanding hypogonadism and rebound priapism after discontinuation [97]. Use of hydroxyurea may also be beneficial [97]. There is recent evidence that use of phosphodiesterase (PDE) 5 inhibitor such as sildenafil is useful in preventing recurrent episodes of priapism [100–102]. Though not always successful, penile prosthesis may be remedial in those with established erectile difficulties persisting more than 12 months [103].

*5.1.9. Ocular Disease.* Central retinal artery occlusion by sickled red cell sludge is an ocular emergency. It manifests as sudden change in vision. It is treated like stroke. Treatment requires EBT, hyperoxygenation, and reduction of intraocular pressure with carbonic anhydrase inhibitors [24]. Prognosis is however poor.

*5.1.10. Osteomyelitis.* Osteomyelitis is one of the commonest skeletal complications of SCD [104, 105]. About 29% of Nigerian SCD patients experience this complication in their lifetime [106]. It often originates from bacteremia, as also observed in septic arthritis. Diagnosis may be quite difficult due to its similar presentation to acute bone infarction. Diagnosis requires a high index of suspicion. Serial blood cultures, as well as culture of local bone aspirates, may be required [59]. The commonest cause of osteomyelitis in SCD population is *salmonella* spp, followed by *staphylococcus* species [24, 107, 108]. Treatment requires involvement of the orthopedic surgeon and clinical microbiologist. Broad spectrum antibiotic based on the common local isolates and their susceptibility profile should be commenced after culture samples have been taken.

### 5.2. Chronic Morbidities in Sickle Cell Disease

*5.2.1. Delayed Growth and Development.* Children with sickle cell disease have normal body weight at birth. However, by one year of life, there might be obvious weight lag when compared with normal infants. This weight deficit persists till adulthood and typically imparts a thin (asthenic) build [14]. Obesity may be seen in some cases [24]. Pubertal growth spurt may be delayed 1-2 years compared to their peers. Growth deficits in children with SCD may be due to multiple factors including severe anaemia, long-term effects of repeated vasoocclusion, endocrine failure, low dietary intake, and low socioeconomic status [109]. However, delay in skeletal maturation allows for bone growth such that final adult height is reached. Menarche may also be delayed for 1-2 years in females [24].

*5.2.2. Chronic Pain Syndromes.* There are two forms of chronic pain in SCD: chronic pain due to obvious tissue damage such as AVN or leg ulcers, and intractable chronic pain with no obvious cause. Suboptimal treatment of recurrent severe acute painful crisis may progress to an intractable chronic pain syndrome. There is need for prompt and adequate treatment of acute pain episodes. Opioids coupled with nonopioids and adjuvant remain the mainstay of analgesia in SCD [45].

### 5.2.3. Immunological and Infectious Complication.
SCD patients have a subnormal immunity, which partly accounts for their increased susceptibility to infections [32]. Immunologic dysfunction in SCD is attributable to autosplenectomy with the resultant defective cellular and humoral immunity [110]. About 30% loss of splenic function occurs by first year of life and 90% by sixth year of life [111]. Normal splenic synthesis of immunoglobulins, properdin, and tuftsin is impaired, leading to increased susceptibility to infections. They are particularly susceptible to encapsulated organisms such as pneumococcus especially in children aged less than 5 years, hence the rationale behind pneumococcal vaccination and penicillin prophylaxis from four months of life till age five in western societies. Previous infections with *pneumococcus* confer lifelong prophylaxis. Studies reveal that, without preventive actions, invasive pneumococcal infection is 30 to 600 times more likely to occur in SCD children compared to normal persons [112]. *Haemophilus influenza* is the next most common organism and affects children older than 5 years. In Africa, *Salmonella, Klebsiella, Escherichia coli,* and *staphylococcus* seem to be more common than *pneumococcus* [113, 114]. As such, routine prophylaxis against *pneumococcus* is not an established practice in Nigeria [115]. However, there is recent compelling evidence from other parts of Africa that *pneumococcus* contributes significantly to infections in SCD [116–118]. Since infection has been documented as the commonest cause of death among SCD patients in Nigeria, the role of pneumococcus in SCD related infections and mortalities needs to be clarified through further research. There is a need for vaccination and chemoprophylaxis against common infections [83]. Current national immunization schedule in Nigeria routinely includes vaccinations against polio, tuberculosis, Diphtheria, tetanus, pertussis, hepatitis B, *Haemophilus influenza* infections, measles, and Yellow fever. Before one year of life, the infant should have completed the vaccination schedule and is entitled to subsequent booster doses [119]. However, for persons affected with sickle cell disease, additional compulsory vaccinations should be administered to cover for *Streptococcus pneumonia, Influenza virus,* and *Neisseria meningococcus, human papillomavirus (HPV)*. Children less than two years of age should have four doses of the 7 valent pneumococcal vaccine between 2 and 15 months of life. The 23 valent pneumococcal vaccine should be administered at age of 2 years and older and should be repeated every 3 to 5 years till 10 years of age and every 5 years for those older than 10 years. Influenza vaccines should be administered during cold seasons beginning at 6 months of life. HIB vaccine should be commenced at 2 months of life. Meningococcal vaccination is recommended for patient at 5 years and older and is repeated every two years. HPV vaccine is administered to females under 26 years.

Also contributing to increased risk of infection in sickle cell disease is repeated tissue infarctions, which are potential foci for pathogens. Similarly, iron overload in patients that have had several transfusions favors growth of iron dependent bacteria such as *Yersinia enterocolitica*. Furthermore, micronutrient deficiency especially zinc deficiency is associated with lymphopenia and decreased immunity [120]. About 60–70% of SCD patients are zinc deficient. In Nigeria, a case-control study showed the serum zinc level to be significantly lower among SCD children compared with healthy controls [121]. Other studies have also shown significant deficiencies of other micronutrients such as magnesium and selenium [122, 123].

### 5.2.4. Sickle Cell Chronic Lung Disease.
Sickle cell chronic lung disease (SCCLD) is an age related morbidity. It affects at least a third of adult SCD patients [59]. Patterns of the lung involvement among Nigerian patients include restrictive lung disease, obstructive lung disease, chronic hypoxaemia, and pulmonary hypertension (PHT) [59, 124–126]. A Study in Nigeria reported a prevalence of 18.9% for SCCLD among adult SCD patients [127]. Chronic complications occur more frequently in those with history of acute chest syndrome. In about 20% of patients, echocardiography shows elevated pulmonary artery systolic blood pressure >35 mmHg. Incidence of PHT is higher in patients with high haemolytic rates and high LDH. PHT is associated with 10-fold increase in the relative risk of death and it confers poor prognosis [128]. Primary PHT is not the only cause of elevated TRV (tricuspid regurgitation jet velocity) in SCD patients. Patients with elevated TRV have increased risk of mortality in the next 3 years [59]. Treatment includes hydroxyurea therapy, chronic transfusion, vasodilator use, anticoagulation, and oxygen therapy.

### 5.2.5. Hepatobiliary Complications.
Chronic liver damage in sickle cell disease is caused by intrahepatic trapping of sickle cells, transfusion transmitted hepatotropic infections, and transfusion siderosis [59, 129]. Evidence suggests that post-transfusion hepatitis and other transfusion transmissible infections are still a significant problem in Nigeria [130, 131]. In Ibadan, Nigeria, Fashola and Otegbayo observed a post-transfusion viral hepatitis prevalence rate of 12.5% in 2002 [130]. In rare instances, vasoocclusion in the liver with cholestasis may precipitate acute liver failure. Pigment gallstones are found in about two-thirds of sickle cell patients, especially those with sickle cell anaemia [129]. Symptomatic gallstones require cholecystectomy. Cholecystitis is treated with antibiotics. Treatment of asymptomatic cholelithiasis may require watchful waiting. Gall stones associated with common bile duct stones require endoscopic retrograde cholangiopancreatography (ERCP). The risk of hepatic damage is reduced by ensuring viral safety of all transfused blood components and prompt institution of iron chelation therapy if iron overload is present. In hepatic failure, liver transplantation is a veritable option.

*5.2.6. Other Abdominal Complications.* Incidence of peptic ulcer disease (PUD) is higher in SCD patients. PUD occurs in about 35% of SCD patients with epigastric pain [58]. In Ile-Ife, Nigeria, Akinola et al. observed PUD among 28% and 50% of Hb SS and Hb SC disease patients presenting with abdominal pains, respectively. Interestingly, duodenal ulcers are not associated with high acid outputs; rather, ulcers are secondary to decreased mucosal resistance, possibly due to bowel ischaemia and NSAID abuse.

*5.2.7. Renal Complications.* The hypoxic, acidotic, and hypertonic state of the renal medulla favors vasoocclusion and destruction of the vasa recta. By the first year of life, SCD infants may develop hyposthenuria manifesting as nocturia or enuresis [24]. Local studies have shown that the prevalence of nocturnal enuresis is higher among children with homozygous sickle cell disease [132]. This further makes them susceptible to dehydration, especially in hot climate. In addition, distal type IV tubulopathy in SCD promotes acidosis, further predisposing to vasoocclusive events. Papillary necrosis (usually of the left kidney) presents with haematuria. Other possible causes of haematuria include infections, stones, and tumor. Recommended guidelines for treatment and prevention of sickle cell nephropathy (SCN) are presented as follows.

*Recommended Guidelines for Management of Sickle Cell Nephropathy*

(i) SCN is an age-related morbidity. Among Nigerian patients, its prevalence and severity increases with advancing age, longer survival, and homozygous SS disease [133, 134].

(ii) Relevant clinical history and examination findings such as facial puffiness, loin pain, painless haematuria, leg and abdominal swelling, frothy urine, worsening anaemia, and hypertension, which may suggest renal disease, should be elicited at regular intervals during visits.

(iii) At least once annually during maintenance visits, SCD patients should be assessed for their renal status. Recommended laboratory assays include urinalysis (on every visit), serum electrolytes, urea and creatinine (semiannually), creatinine clearance/estimated glomerular filtration rate (eGFR), and tests for microalbuminuria (albumin creatinine ratio, ACR; urinary protein to creatinine ratio, uPCR). A normal creatinine level does not exclude renal disease in SCD due to supranormal kidneys precipitated by hyperfiltration and increased secretion of creatinine and uric acid. Emphasis and therapeutic decisions should be placed on significant adverse changes in the renal markers rather than single absolute values.

(iv) Consultations and comanagement with experienced nephrologist is recommended in the following setting: patients with uPCR >50 mg/mmol (442 mg/g), persistent microscopic haematuria, declining renal function (>10% fall in eGFR per annum), or eGFR <60 mL/min/1.73 m$^2$. Further evaluations including renal biopsy are necessitated in settings of sudden onset heavy proteinuria with or without nephrotic syndrome [135, 136].

(v) Treatment of haematuria includes bed rest, hydration, and blood transfusion if indicated in events of a significant blood loss. Most times, haematuria is caused by papillary necrosis. However, the possibility of a renal medullary cell carcinoma must be excluded in these patients.

(vi) Progression of SCN to ESRD is often heralded by worsening proteinuria, anaemia, and hypertension. This may be delayed with adequate control of hypertension and proteinuria. Introduction of angiotensin converting enzyme inhibitors (ACEIs) or angiotensin receptor blockers (ARBs) reduces proteinuria [136]. For blood pressure control, diuretics are better avoided.

(vii) Similarly, early commencement of hydroxyurea helps to delay progression to ESRD except hydroxyurea is contraindicated for other reasons.

(viii) NSAIDS for pain control are better avoided in patients with established SCN, in order to prevent worse organ damage. NSAIDS cause significant decline in renal blood flow and glomerular filtration.

(ix) Urinary tract infection in these patients should be treated aggressively. Patients with ESRD should be on regular EBT especially if renal transplant is being planned. End stage renal disease is managed with repeated dialysis, erythropoietin therapy, and/or renal transplant.

*5.2.8. Ocular Disease.* Incidence of ocular disease is higher in Hb SC disease, Hb SB+thal compared to Hb SS [59, 137]. Repeated vasoocclusion in the vascular beds of the eye especially the retina causes progressive ophthalmopathy, which manifests as comma-shaped conjunctival vessels, iris atrophy, retinal pigmentary changes, and retinal hemorrhages. Neovascularization leads to sea-fanning, so called proliferative retinopathy. Eventually, vitreous haemorrhage and retinal detachment may occur. For prevention, annual eye examination is recommended for all SCD patients from the 2nd decade of life [59]. Treatment options for proliferative retinopathy include laser photocoagulation and vitrectomy.

*5.2.9. Sickle Cell Leg Ulcer.* Leg ulcers are frequent in adults SCD patients especially males with SS phenotype and patients with low steady state haemoglobin levels [138, 139]. In a report from Benin City, Nigeria, Bazuaye et al. observed a prevalence rate of 9.6 and 22.4% for current ulcers and previous ulcers, respectively [139]. Ulcers commonly arise near the medial or lateral malleolus and may be single or multiple. The aetiology is often multifactorial and they include vasoocclusion of skin microvasculature, made worse by trauma, infection, warm climate, and iron overload [24]. Commonly isolated microbes include *pseudomonas aeruginosa*, *staphylococcus aureus*, and *streptococcus* species. Chronic SCD ulcers are painful and resistant to healing. Treatment of these ulcers requires multidisciplinary approach involving the haematologist, plastic surgeon, specialist nurses, and orthopaedic surgeon [24]. Generally, treatment includes pain relief (including local pain control before wound dressing), elevation of the leg, debridement (to remove necrotic tissue), elastic dressing/support bandage, and zinc sulphate therapy (600 mg/day). Some patients may benefit from chronic blood transfusion and skin grafting.

*5.2.10. Musculoskeletal Complications.* Known musculoskeletal complications in SCD include medullary hyperplasia, dystrophic intramedullary calcification, H-vertebra, osteolysis, osteopenia, septic arthritis, dactylitis, ulcers, pathologic fracture, and osteomyelitis. H-vertebra or Cod-fish vertebra is due to infarction of the vertebral body, giving a fish-mouth appearance on radiography. In a study by Balogun et al., musculoskeletal complications occurred in 31.4% of adult Nigerian SCD patients [140]. Avascular osteonecrosis of the femoral and humeral head is particularly associated with reduced quality of life. AVN develops in about 50% of patients who survive to above 35 years of age and about 60% of patients who survive to 60 years of age [141]. Another recent study revealed that AVN occurred in about 13 per 1000 Nigerian SCD patients [142]. Exact mechanism for development of AVN is yet to be clearly described. Even patients with high fetal haemoglobin levels may not be totally protected from developing AVN. However, high steady state platelet count has been correlated with AVN in Nigerian SCD patients [142]. Other clinical and laboratory correlations of AVN include high haematocrit, coexistence of alpha thalassemia, and frequent VOC [143–145].

In older patients, humeral head necrosis is more common than femoral head necrosis, although femoral head necrosis is associated with more devastating pain due to weight bearing [146]. Treatment of musculoskeletal complications of SCD requires comanagement with an orthopedic surgeon with special interest in SCD. Persisting pain in a joint or at least a stage 3 arthropathy is indication for referral to an orthopedic specialist [146]. X-ray features of AVN may not be obvious until repair processes have changed the density of the bone. MRI is the investigation of choice in SCD patients with persisting hip or shoulder pain. Every patient with confirmed AVN should be staged with MRI. Initial conservative treatment should include counseling/patient education, analgesia, partial weight bearing on crutches, and physiotherapy. Option of joint replacement/arthroplasty is available for patients with severe joint destruction.

*5.2.11. Cardiovascular System Changes.* Sickle cell disease is associated with cardiac abnormalities including dilated cardiomyopathy, ventricular hypertrophy, cardiac iron overload, dysrhythmias, pulmonary hypertension, myocardial infarction, and sudden death [147, 148]. Chronic anaemia in SCD potentiates ventricular hypertrophy and dilatation which may progress to left ventricular diastolic dysfunction and exercise intolerance [147]. Pulmonary arterial hypertension is defined by end systolic pressure in the right ventricle greater

than 25 mmHg (normal is less than 15 mmHg). In a cohort of Nigerian SCD patients, 2 (3.6%) out of 56 met the criteria for pulmonary hypertension [125]. Tricuspid regurgitation jet velocity of >2.5 m/sec is associated with a high risk of pulmonary hypertension and is an independent risk factor for death [128].

*5.2.12. Transfusion Related Morbidities.* Blood transfusion is a key therapeutic modality in SCD. In a cohort of Nigerian SCD children, the prevalence of blood transfusion is as high as 57% [149]. Benefits of transfusion in sickle cell disease include correction of the baseline anaemia, dilution of sickle haemoglobin levels, and suppression of endogenous sickle red cell production, as well as reduction in chronic haemolysis and circulating sickle cell levels [150–152]. Transfusion modalities in SCD include simple transfusions, exchange blood transfusion, or chronic blood transfusion (hypertransfusion). Simple transfusion refers to top up correction of anaemia. Indications for chronic blood transfusion include prevention of first stroke, prevention of repeat stroke, TCD USS >2 m/sec, delayed growth and development in children, frequent ACS, severe disease, severe SCD lacking HLA match, sickle chronic lung disease, pregnant women with bad obstetric history and frequent bone pains, and sickle cell leg ulcers [150, 151]. Indications for exchange blood transfusion include moderate to severe ACS, refractory painful VOC, stroke, central retinal artery thrombosis, and acute refractory priapism [36]. The choice of blood component for transfusion in SCD should be a sickle negative, recently donated (less than 7 days old), leucodepleted, and phenotypically matched for at least Rh and Kell antigens, racial and minority matched red cell concentrate. Cytomegalovirus (CMV) negative component should be used for transfusion in all CMV negative children, as they may be candidates for bone marrow transplantation. Target haemoglobin level should not exceed 10-11 g/dL in SCD as there are concerns for hyperviscosity and vasoocclusion [26, 153].

Transfusion of blood and blood components is not without risks. In particular, delayed haemolytic transfusion reaction and alloimmunisation are among the immunologic complications of blood transfusion associated with sickle cell disease. Due to their tendency for repeated transfusion from chronic prophylactic transfusion or otherwise, the risk of iron overload in body tissues with irreversible organ damages ensues, hence the need for close monitoring and prompt iron chelation when indicated. Reports on alloimmunisation rate among Nigerian SCD patients are lacking and may be related to the lack of routine alloantibody screening and extended red cell phenotyping in most blood banks in Nigeria.

Among nonimmunologic complications of transfusion therapy in SCD in Nigeria, transmission of viruses and iron overload is of note [89, 131]. Recent evidence suggests that transmission of viruses is still a major challenge to transfusion safety in Nigeria [131]. This calls for a better national transfusion service. SCD patients, particularly those on hypertransfusion therapy, are at particular risk for iron overload, with resultant damage to vital organs [89]. Iron status should be monitored in SCD patients, particularly those who have received a cumulative transfusion dose of more than 20 to 30 units. Chelation therapy should be instituted promptly if serum ferritin levels exceed 1000 ug/L [154].

*5.2.13. Psychosocial Issues/Psychiatric Complications.* Psychosocial complications of SCD include poor self-image, negative thoughts and feelings about the condition, stigmatization, depression, cognitive impairments, fears, anxieties, hatred for parents and others, dropping out of school, and tendency for substance abuse [24, 155]. These complications are associated with the chronic nature, recurrent pain, reduced health related quality of life, and unpredictable course of the disease. Some degree of psychologic trauma is also rendered to parents and health caregivers. A recent report by Anie et al. revealed that about half of Nigerian SCD patients had depressive feelings [156]. Adequate psychological support should be provided for patients by physicians, other health care staff, parents, and support groups. Those requiring more definite intervention should be comanaged with clinical psychologists and psychiatrists.

A study in Jamaica revealed that 29% of SS patients had a psychiatric disorder, compared to 25% in the control population [157]. Association of psychiatric morbidity included leaving school early, difficulties in social adjustment, impaired cognition, and previous psychiatric difficulties [157]. Asthenic body builds and abnormal facies may be associated with poor self-image. Such patients should be identified early and treated. Other complications such as undereducation and underemployment may require the services of medical social worker and occupational therapy unit.

## 6. Special Care Situations

*6.1. Sickle Cell Disease and Pregnancy.* Typically, pregnancy in female SCD patients is attended by anaemia which may be worsened by pregnancy related plasma volume expansion and folate deficiency. VOC is more common in 3rd trimester [158]. Increased incidence of preeclampsia, maternal mortality, and perinatal complications such as abortions, stillbirths, low birth weight, and neonatal deaths are associated with SCD pregnancy [158–160]. As such, pregnant SCD patients require special care by specialists including experienced obstetrician, haematologist, midwives, and anaesthesiologist. Preferably, oral contraception should be recommended for sexually active SCD females and pregnancy should be planned. Folate supplementation should be ensured. A local study has shown that preconceptual care and early antenatal booking produce better outcome and less obstetric complications in SCD pregnancies [161]. Hypertransfusion is indicated in cases of bad obstetric history and severe sickle cell disease in pregnancy. SCD and pregnancy are procoagulant states. Coupled with obstetric surgeries, the risk of VTE is significantly increased and appropriate anticoagulation may also be necessary in their care-plan [45].

*6.2. Perioperative Care in Sickle Cell Disease.* Perioperative complications of surgery in SCD patients include hypoxia, dehydration, bone pain crisis, significant anaemia, and acute chest syndrome [162]. Anaesthesia may be associated with hypoxia and dehydration [163]. Good anaesthetic expertise and experience is indicated when undertaking surgical procedure in SCD patients [163]. Early surgical complications such as pain and haemorrhage should be well controlled. Optimal analgesia and tact surgical skills are indicated. Other strategies to improve perioperative outcomes in SCD include conservative preoperative blood transfusion therapy, epidural analgesia, and adequate postoperative pain control with opiate and nonopiate analgesia [164, 165]. Aggressive or exchange transfusion therapy has not been associated with better surgical outcomes [162, 164].

*6.3. Sickle Cell Disease and Radiology.* Infusion of radiologic contrast media may precipitate VOC. Hypertonic nature of contrast media triggers marked intracellular dehydration and marked increment in red cell MCHC, thus precipitating sickling. This complication may be averted by preprocedure red cell exchange to achieve target sickle haemoglobin level of 50%. Traditional iodinated contrast media (due to its high osmolality) are relatively contraindicated in SCD. Isotonic contrasts are safer to use in SCD [166].

## 7. Laboratory Diagnosis of Sickle Cell Disease

The science behind laboratory diagnosis of sickle cell disorder entails phenotypic testing for the presence the sickle haemoglobin and genetic analysis. Physicochemical properties of the sickle haemoglobin such as decreased solubility and sickling under deoxy conditions, its pattern of mobility in an electric field, and rate of elution from solution unto adsorbents are applied in its laboratory detection. Phenotypic tests may be used as screening tests or diagnostic tests. Screening tests chosen for the purpose of mass screening should be highly sensitive and cheap to run. Examples of screening tests include sickling test, solubility test, and alkaline haemoglobin electrophoresis. On the other hand, high specific, diagnostic tests include isoelectric focusing, citrate agar electrophoresis, and high performance liquid chromatography [167, 168]. Quantification of haemoglobin variants and globin chain studies are used in evaluation of compound heterozygous disease states such as sickle thalassemia syndrome [167, 169]. Hb A2 levels in excess of 3.5% are suggestive of haemoglobin S-beta thalassemia [168]. Other ancillary laboratory investigations useful in detection and monitoring of the disease include FBC, reticulocyte count, and peripheral blood film. Reticulocyte count usually range from 5 to 15% in sickle cell disease. On peripheral blood film examination, findings may include irreversible sickled red cells, polychromasia, occasional nucleated red cells, and schistocytes, as well as Howell-Jolly bodies [24, 111]. Target cells are seen in sickle haemoglobinopathies. In sickle cell thalassemia syndromes, target cells are seen alongside microcytes and moderate-severe hypochromia. Red cell indices may suggest macrocytosis due to increased reticulocytosis or compliance with hydroxyurea therapy. However, oval macrocytosis with hypersegmented neutrophils may suggest folic acid deficiency. Biochemical changes include high LDH, low haptoglobin, high total and indirect bilirubin, and high AST [35]. Genetic studies such as PCR are used for prenatal and preimplantation diagnosis [170].

## 8. Prognosis and Life Expectancy

Severe SCD is associated with poor outcomes, if no intervention is rendered. Known modulators of clinical severity include fetal haemoglobin levels, beta globin haplotype, amd coinheritance of alpha-thalassemia, as well as geographical and other unknown genetic factors [15, 16]. In a study by Emmanuelchide et al., a higher leucocyte count was associated with more SCD complications in a Nigerian SCD population [171]. Another recent Nigerian study in a cohort of 115 children with SCD showed the presence of dactylitis at first presentation and higher total WBC, neutrophil count, platelet count, and serum bilirubin levels to be significantly higher among those with severe disease, while a higher fetal haemoglobin level was associated with a milder disease [172]. Other notable poor prognostic factors include low haemoglobin F production, Hb less than 7 g/dL, Hb greater than 7 g/dL, high VOC rate, pulmonary HTN, and nocturnal hypoxaemia (more strokes) [59].

From a large cooperative study in USA in 1994, the median survival for SCA was reported as 42 and 48 years in men and women, respectively. For haemoglobin SC disease, it was reported as 60 years and 68 years for men and women, respectively [84]. In USA, 95% of children with SCD survive till adulthood [173]. In Jamaica, survival estimates for persons with SCA were reported as 53 years and 58.5 years for men and women, respectively [174].

Life expectancy in SCD is substantially reduced especially in those with severe disease. In a 10-year retrospective study reported in 2009 from Ilorin, Nigeria, by Chijioke and Kolo, the mean age of sickle cell anaemia patients was found to be 23 years compared to 40 years in the control population, suggesting reduced life expectancy [175]. Findings from that study also revealed that age correlated negatively with survival [175]. As recently reported by Ogun et al., the leading causes of mortality in Nigerian SCD patients include infections, acute chest syndrome, anaemia, acute sequestration crisis, and stroke. According to the study, the mean age at death was 21.3 years. Though some patients now attain fifth decade, most mortality occurs in their second and third decades of life [83].

## 9. Sickle Cell Disease Control and Current Challenges in Nigeria

Control of SCD begins with public education and definite strategies to prevent further transmission of the trait. Carrier detection and genetic counseling have been proven to be successful in curbing the spread of other haemoglobinopathies like thalassaemia [176]. Carrier detection should be offered at designated centres after proper genetic counselling through antenatal and newborn screening, couple/premarital screening, and other forms of population screening. Genetic counselling by trained personnel helps individuals at risk to take informed decisions about their reproductive life choices. The option of prenatal diagnosis and selective abortion in Nigeria is controversial and relatively unavailable. Local studies show that a significant proportion of Nigerians are averse to selective abortion, even if legally permitted [177–179]. Early detection and diagnosis of sickle cell disease is crucial to reducing mortality and mortality associated with sickle cell disease, as affected persons are offered early supportive and preventive treatments. Despite the huge burden of SCD, currently, there is lack of national or regional SCD newborn screening programme in Nigeria, as at the time of this publication. Specialized centers dedicated to care of SCD patients with requisite multidisciplinary teams and other facilities are grossly absent. Ideally, SCD infants diagnosed prenatally or through newborn screening should be routed to comprehensive SCD centers for optimal treatment [180]. Conversely, Nigerian SCD is still associated with delayed diagnosis [181].

Continuous training of healthcare professionals involved in care of SCD patients is also desirable. Further efforts should be directed at education of the patients and their parents or caregivers. The health caregivers should also constantly undergo professional refresher and update courses in order to optimize their knowledge and skills in care of SCD. Recent surveys still suggest a dearth of public health knowledge on sickle cell disease in Nigeria [182]. Despite Nigeria being the most populous black nation on earth with the highest burden of sickle cell disease, till now, there are no coordinated nationwide efforts aimed at controlling the disease. Current evidence suggests that the care available for patients with SCD in Nigeria is still suboptimal [183]. Secondary control measures such as chronic transfusion therapy and use of hydroxyurea are faced with peculiar challenges in developing nations such as Nigeria [89]. Such challenges include unavailability of blood and blood components, the need for patients and relatives to regularly source for blood and blood donors, cost of iron chelation, risk of transfusion transmissible infections, and overall cost of chronic blood transfusion [73, 89]. A recent study estimated the mean annual cost of hypertransfusion in Ibadan among paediatric SCD patient to be 3,276 US Dollars (SD = 1,168) [73]. Also, treatment of iron overload with metal chelators, which is a potentially inevitable complication of chronic transfusion, increases cost.

Furthermore, HSCT, which is the only potentially curative disease modifying intervention in sickle cell disease, is currently available in Nigeria and has been reported [171]. However, its practice is bewildered by ample challenges including poor government commitment, weak political will, poor infrastructure, unaffordability by the average eligible Nigerian SCD patient, lack of local bone marrow registries, absence of specialized molecular diagnostic laboratories, and epileptic electric power supply [184, 185].

## 10. Comprehensive Care in Sickle Cell Disease and Recommendations in Nigeria

Comprehensive care incorporates provision of holistic healthcare services including state-of-the-art diagnosis, standard therapies, preventive care, rehabilitative therapy, and other ancillary services, by a team of specialists in a given location, with maximum accessibility for all patients. Comprehensive sickle cell centers are grossly lacking in Nigeria. Holistic care has been shown to provide better outcomes in sickle cell disease evidenced by significant reduction in mortality, hospitalizations, and blood transfusion rates among Nigerian patients [186]. As well, WHO recommends that in areas where hemoglobin disorders are common, special dedicated centers with a high degree of autonomy are required in appropriate numbers and locations, with a high degree of autonomy [187]. Treatment of SCD requires a multispecialist team including professionals such as hematologist, pediatrician, orthopedic surgeons, plastic surgeons, ophthalmologists, nephrologist, specialist nurses, clinical psychologists, and social workers.

Provision of comprehensive health centers is crucial to improving SCD disease outcomes in Nigeria. At such facilities, treatment should be tailored to individual patient's needs. At diagnosis, proper education regarding the nature of the disease, possible complications, and its prevention and treatment should be offered to the patient and parents. Regular health maintenance visits should be scheduled and patients should be counseled on the need for adherence [188]. Compliance on the part of the patient depends on having adequate information on the disease and confidence in the health professionals. Similarly, timely and regular medical education should be provided to health care professionals involved in management of SCD in order to improve their expertise and skills. Also, establishment of support groups among patients is encouraged.

Comprehensive care centers must possess facilities for outpatient care, day-case admissions (day hospital services), and hospitalizations on a 24-hour basis [52]. Patients should have direct access (including phone contact) to such centers and their physicians. For acute complications and emergencies, a quick triage is carried out and prompt therapy is instituted. Standard protocols should be provided for management of specific complications, as well as general health maintenance. Scheduled review and strict adherence to protocols are advised.

Patients and parents should be counseled on avoidance of known precipitants of sickle cell crisis. Keeping a diary of pain episodes is helpful in identifying and avoiding triggers for pain crisis. Infections especially malaria have been reported as a major precipitant of sickle cell crisis among Nigerian patients. As such, vector control and chemoprophylaxis for malaria is recommended in all patients [189]. All forms of undue physical exertion or exhaustion should be discouraged. Mothers should be regularly reminded about routine national vaccination schedule as well as vaccination against organisms to which SCD children and adults are particularly susceptible, especially encapsulated organisms.

Adequate and regular hydration is important. At least 60–70 mL/kg of oral fluids or at least $1.5 L/m^2$ every 24 hours is recommended [45, 187]. Hydration helps with haemodilution, which reduces the propensity for sickling and vasoocclusion. Regular hydration also prevents dehydration which they are prone to due to impaired concentrating ability of the kidneys. Exercise caution with fluid administration especially in those with renal disease or severe anaemia. Excessive fluids may precipitate pulmonary oedema and death.

Moreover, physicians should administer, monitor, and encourage patient's compliance with routine medications at follow-up visits. Routine medications include prophylactic antimalarial [190] and folic acid. Others may include antioxidants, aspirin, and prophylactic antibiotic (oral penicillin from 2-3 months of life until at least age 5 in areas where pneumococcal infection is prevalent). Malaria has been described as one of the major precipitants of VOC for patients in Malaria endemic regions including Nigeria, hence the rationale behind continuous life-long chemoprophylaxis [190–192]. However, according to a local study, no significant benefit or advantage was associated with routine chemoprophylaxis for malaria in SCD patients as both patients and controls had equal rates of asymptomatic parasitaemia and similar frequency of malarial attacks [193]. In Nigeria, the actual benefits of malaria chemoprophylaxis in SCD need to be clarified through further research.

Early institution of broad spectrum antibiotics is recommended in febrile SCD patients [187]. Antibiotic use should be guided by local bacteriological profile and should be commenced after necessary bacterial cultures are taken. A switch to appropriate antibiotic is based on sensitivity pattern of the offending isolate especially if the fever is persistent (unresponsive to the former antibiotic).

## 11. Disease Modifying Therapies

*11.1. Hydroxyurea Therapy.* Currently, hydroxyurea (HU) is the only approved disease modifying drug in SCD used for selected patients above 24 months of age [194]. HU is a cytotoxic agent that has been mainly used in treatment of CML and other myeloproliferative disorders. Its usefulness in SCD is related to its ability to induce increased levels of fetal haemoglobin production in sickle cells thus mitigating tendencies for red cell sickling. The exact mechanism is not fully understood, but, as a ribonucleotide reductase inhibitor, it prevents formation of deoxyribonucleotides, causing S-phase arrest of all replicating cells, thereby inducing stress erythropoiesis, which favors increased production of fetal haemoglobin [24]. HU is also known to increase steady state haemoglobin levels and reduce leucocyte and platelet counts. Also, as a rheological agent, HU improves cell hydration, limits interaction of the sickle cells with the vascular endothelium, and acts as a nitric oxide donor [195]. HU is of benefit to patients with moderate to severe sickle cell disease. Indications for HU therapy include recurrent VOC (3 or more severe episodes requiring admission in the last 12 months), recurrent ACS (2 or more episodes in a lifetime), severe symptomatic anaemia, and recurrent priapism, alternative to transfusion to prevent new or recurrent stroke especially where transfusion is not feasible [194]. Usually, HU therapy is commenced at 10–15 mg/kg once daily. Baseline investigations prior to commencement of hydroxyurea should include FBC, reticulocyte count, %Hb F, electrolyte urea and creatinine level, liver function test, uric acid, and LDH levels. Full blood counts are monitored weekly for the first 4 weeks, fortnightly for the next 8 weeks, and thereafter monthly if the counts remain stable [14, 194]. Its dose is increased by 2.5 to 5 mg/kg/day every 12 weeks (range of 4 weeks to 6 months) if absolute neutrophil count (ANC) >2000, Haemoglobin concentration >4.5 g/dL, and platelet count >80,000/$\mu$L [14, 195]. As marrow suppression occurs, HU is withheld to allow for marrow recovery and then restarted at a dose of 2.5 mg/kg less than dose causing myelosuppression. This is known as the maximum tolerable dose [88, 195]. However, the ceiling dose for HU therapy is 35 mg/kg [151]. Minimum time interval for evaluation of therapeutic efficacy is 6 to 9 months [165]. Hb F levels should be monitored. HbF level in excess of 20% significantly ameliorates the disease. Complications of HU include myelotoxicity, mouth ulceration, macrocytosis and megaloblastoid changes, nausea, skin toxicity rashes, and hyperpigmentation [88, 194].

*11.2. Haemopoietic Stem Cell Transplantation (HSCT).* Suggested eligibility criteria for HSCT in SCD include the following [196, 197]: (A) age <17 years; (B) at least one of the following complications: brain infarct/ischaemia (MRI), secondary cognitive impairment with cerebral vasculopathy, severe and recurrent ACS, ≥3 VOC per annum requiring hospitalization (>3 Hospitalisations for severe VOC in consecutive 3 to 4 years), moderate glomerular dysfunction, multiple epiphyseal aseptic necrosis, and grade I/II sickle chronic lung disease; (C) availability of HLA matched sibling donor. Exclusion criteria include donor with major haemoglobinopathy and one or more of the following: Karnofsky performance <70%, Portal fibrosis (moderate or severe), renal failure (GFR <30%), major intellectual impairment, stage III or IV chronic sickle lung disease, cardiomyopathy, or HIV infection. Older adults are considered less favorable candidates for HSCT due to the higher risk for severe organ toxicities and greater susceptibility to severe graft versus host disease [198]. HSCT should be performed in centers experienced in transplant for sickle cell disease.

*11.3. Future Therapies.* Aside from Hydroxyurea, other promising drugs that have been shown to modulate Hb F production but are still under investigation/trials include decitabine, 5-azacytidine, and short chain fatty acids such as butyrates [199, 200]. Other novel therapies are also being investigated. Their therapeutic efficacy is designed based on their targets against specific pathophysiological processes in SCD such as the abnormal membrane cation transport systems, increased/stimulated red cell-endothelial adhesiveness, endothelial activation and vasospasm, cellular dehydration, prooxidant state, and hypercoagulability in SCD. Gardos channel blockers such as clotrimazole and its analog, Senicapoc (ICA 17043), have been shown to reduce red cell dehydration and abate haemolytic rate and are well tolerated in SCD patients [201, 202]. Administration of magnesium salts is also observed to reduce red cell dehydration by inhibiting the KCL cotransporter. It is reported that infusion of magnesium sulfate reduced the length of hospital stay in patients with VOC [203]. However, this is not yet an established practice. Similarly, antiadhesive agents such as anti-P-selectin and heparin, as well as agents such as warfarin and aspirin for normalization of hypercoagulable state and Flocor for reduction of whole blood viscosity, and specific monoclonal antibodies for inhibition of red cell-endothelial adhesion are also being considered [199]. Inhalational nitric oxide and its precursor, L-arginine, are shown to be beneficial in acute vasoocclusive crisis and other ischaemic complications by increasing NO bioavailability [200, 203].

Theoretically, gene therapy offers a great hope of cure. However, effective vector for safe transfer and stable, erythroid specific expression of normal beta globin gene are still under investigation [204, 205].

## 12. Conclusion

Sickle cell disease is a major public health disease worldwide. There is still a high burden of the disease in Nigeria. There is still a significantly high rate of SCD complications and mortality among Nigerian patients. Current evidence suggests that available care is suboptimal. Largely speaking, prevention, control, and treatment of SCD in Nigeria are still in infancy. Yester efforts albeit present measures appear meager in the face of the enormous disease burden. There is need for a better coordinated effort towards control of SCD by the government at all levels and other concerned stakeholders. Appropriate interventional programmes backed by an effective national policy should be instituted. In addition, physicians involved in the care of SCD patients should be conversant with current knowledge and standard practices in the treatment of sickle cell disease in order to improve treatment outcomes.

## Conflict of Interests

The author declares that there is no conflict of interests regarding the publication of this paper.

## References

[1] B. Modell, Ed., *Guidelines for the Control of Haemoglobin Disorders*, WHO, Sardinia, Italy, 1989.

[2] G. R. Serjeant, "Sickle-cell disease," *The Lancet*, vol. 350, no. 9079, pp. 725–730, 1997.

[3] B. Modell and M. Darlison, "Global epidemiology of haemoglobin disorders and derived service indicators," *Bulletin of the World Health Organization*, vol. 86, no. 6, pp. 480–487, 2008.

[4] World Health Organisation 2008, "Management of haemoglobin disorders," in *Proceedings of the Report of Joint WHO-TIF Meeting*, Nicosia, Cyprus, November 2007.

[5] F. B. Piel, A. P. Patil, R. E. Howes et al., "Global epidemiology of Sickle haemoglobin in neonates: a contemporary geostatistical model-based map and population estimates," *The Lancet*, vol. 381, no. 9861, pp. 142–151, 2013.

[6] WHO Regional office for Africa, Sickle cell disease prevention and control, 2013, http://www.afro.who.int/en/nigeria/nigeria-publications/1775-sickle cell disease.html.

[7] G. R. Serjeant and B. E. Serjeant, "The epidemiology of sickle cell disorder: a challenge for Africa," *Archives of Ibadan Medicine*, vol. 2, no. 2, pp. 46–52, 2001.

[8] A. L. Okwi, W. Byarugaba, C. M. Ndugwa, A. Parkes, M. Ocaido, and J. K. Tumwine, "An up-date on the prevalence of sickle cell trait in Eastern and Western Uganda," *BMC Blood Disorders*, vol. 10, article 5, 2010.

[9] A. F. Fleming, J. Storey, L. Molineaux, E. A. Iroko, and E. D. Attai, "Abnormal haemoglobins in the Sudan savanna of Nigeria. I. Prevalence of haemoglobins and relationships between sickle cell trait, malaria and survival," *Annals of Tropical Medicine and Parasitology*, vol. 73, no. 2, pp. 161–172, 1979.

[10] P. N. Uzoegwu and A. E. Onwurah, "Prevalence of haemoglobinopathy and malaria diseases in the population of old Aguata Division, Anambra State, Nigeria," *Biokemistri*, vol. 15, no. 2, pp. 57–66, 2003.

[11] B. Nwogoh, A. S. Adewoyin, O. E. Iheanacho, and G. N. Bazuaye, "Prevalence of haemoglobin variants in Benin City, Nigeria," *Annals of Biomedical Sciences*, vol. 11, no. 2, pp. 60–64, 2012.

[12] J. A. B. Horton, *The Diseases of Tropical Climates and Their Treatment*, Churchill, London, UK, 1874.

[13] J. B. Herrick, "Peculiar elongated and sickle-shaped red blood corpuscles in a case of severe anemia," *Archives of Internal Medicine*, vol. 6, no. 5, pp. 517–521, 1910.

[14] E. Beutler, "Disorders of haemoglobin structure: sickle cell anaemia and related abnormalities," in *Williams Haematology*, M. A. Lichtman and W. J. Williams, Eds., vol. 47, pp. 667–700, McGraw-Hill, New York, NY, USA, 2006.

[15] G. R. Serjeant, "The natural history of sickle cell disease," *Cold Spring Harbor Perspectives in Medicine*, vol. 3, no. 10, Article ID a011783, 2013.

[16] J. Pagnier, J. G. Mears, O. Dunda-Belkhodja et al., "Evidence for the multicentric origin of the sickle cell hemoglobin gene in Africa," *Proceedings of the National Academy of Sciences of the United States of America*, vol. 81, no. 6 I, pp. 1771–1773, 1984.

[17] A. E. Kulozik, J. S. Wainscoat, G. R. Serjeant et al., "Geographical survey of $\beta$(S)-globin gene haplotypes: evidence for an independent Asian origin of the sickle-cell mutation," *American Journal of Human Genetics*, vol. 39, no. 2, pp. 239–244, 1986.

[18] C. Lapoumeroulie, O. Dunda, R. Ducrocq et al., "A novel sickle gene of yet another origin in Africa: the Cameroon type," *Human Genetics*, vol. 89, no. 3, pp. 333–337, 1992.

[19] M. H. Steinberg, "Predicting clinical severity in sickle cell anaemia," *British Journal of Haematology*, vol. 129, no. 4, pp. 465–481, 2005.

[20] B. Modell, M. Darlison, H. Birgens et al., "Epidemiology of haemoglobin disorders in Europe: an overview," *Scandinavian Journal of Clinical and Laboratory Investigation*, vol. 67, no. 1, pp. 39–69, 2007.

[21] D. Desai and H. Dhanani, "Sickle cell disease: history and origin," *The Internet Journal of Hematology*, vol. 1, no. 2, 2003.

[22] A. C. Allison, "Protection afforded by sickle-cell trait against subtertian malareal infection," *British Medical Journal*, vol. 1, no. 4857, pp. 290–294, 1954.

[23] C. Madigan and P. Malik, "Pathophysiology and therapy for haemoglobinopathies; Part I: sickle cell disease," *Expert Reviews in Molecular Medicine*, vol. 8, no. 9, pp. 1–23, 2006.

[24] A. Lal and E. P. Vinchinsky, "Sickle cell disease," in *Postgraduate Haematology*, A. V. Hoffbrand, D. Catovsky, E. G. D. Tuddenham, and A. R. Green, Eds., vol. 7, pp. 109–125, Blackwell Publishing, 6th edition, 2011.

[25] M.-H. Odièvre, E. Verger, A. C. Silva-Pinto, and J. Elion, "Pathophysiological insights in sickle cell disease," *Indian Journal of Medical Research*, vol. 134, no. 10, pp. 532–537, 2011.

[26] W. F. Rosse, M. Narla, L. D. Petz, and M. H. Steinberg, "New views of sickle cell disease pathophysiology and treatment," *Haematatogy*, vol. 2000, no. 1, pp. 2–17, 2000.

[27] M. H. Steinberg, "Management of sickle cell disease," *The New England Journal of Medicine*, vol. 340, no. 13, pp. 1021–1030, 1999.

[28] P. S. Frenette, "Sickle cell vasoocclusion: heterotypic, multicellular aggregations driven by leukocyte adhesion," *Microcirculation*, vol. 11, no. 2, pp. 167–177, 2004.

[29] J. E. Brittain and L. V. Parise, "The $\alpha 4\beta 1$ integrin in sickle cell disease," *Transfusion Clinique et Biologique*, vol. 15, no. 1-2, pp. 19–22, 2008.

[30] J. E. Brittain, J. Han, K. I. Ataga, E. P. Orringer, and L. V. Parise, "Mechanism of CD47-induced $\alpha 4\beta 1$ integrin activation and adhesion in sickle reticulocytes," *The Journal of Biological Chemistry*, vol. 279, no. 41, pp. 42393–42402, 2004.

[31] J. E. Elion, M. Brun, M. H. Odièvre, C. L. Lapouméroulie, and R. Krishnamoorthy, "Vaso-occlusion in sickle cell anemia: role of interactions between blood cells and endothelium," *Hematology Journal*, vol. 5, no. 3, pp. S195–S198, 2004.

[32] S. G. Ahmed, "The role of infection in the pathogenesis of vaso-occlusive crisis in patients with sickle cell disease," *Mediterranean Journal of Hematology and Infectious Diseases*, vol. 3, no. 1, Article ID e2011028, 2011.

[33] F. Fasola, K. Adedapo, J. Anetor, and M. Kuti, "Total antioxidants status and some hematological values in sickle cell disease patients in steady state," *Journal of the National Medical Association*, vol. 99, no. 8, pp. 891–894, 2007.

[34] M. Westerman, A. Pizzey, J. Hirschman et al., "Microvesicles in haemoglobinopathies offer insights into mechanisms of hypercoagulability, haemolysis and the effects of therapy," *British Journal of Haematology*, vol. 142, no. 1, pp. 126–135, 2008.

[35] S. D. Roseff, "Sickle cell disease: a review," *Immunohematology*, vol. 25, no. 2, pp. 67–74, 2009.

[36] M. M. Hsieh, J. F. Tisdale, and G. P. Rodgers, "Haemolytic anaemia: thalassemias and sickle cell disorders," in *The Bethesda Handbook of Clinical Haematology*, G. P. Rodgers and N. S. Young, Eds., vol. 4, pp. 37–56, Lippincott Williams & Wilkins, Philadelphia, Pa, USA, 3rd edition, 2013.

[37] P. S. Frenette and G. F. Atweh, "Sickle cell disease: old discoveries, new concepts, and future promise," *The Journal of Clinical Investigation*, vol. 117, no. 4, pp. 850–858, 2007.

[38] R. P. Hebbel, R. Osarogiagbon, and D. Kaul, "The endothelial biology of sickle cell disease: inflammation and a chronic vasculopathy," *Microcirculation*, vol. 11, no. 2, pp. 129–151, 2004.

[39] G. J. Kato, M. T. Gladwin, and M. H. Steinberg, "Deconstructing sickle cell disease: reappraisal of the role of hemolysis in the development of clinical subphenotypes," *Blood Reviews*, vol. 21, no. 1, pp. 37–47, 2007.

[40] T. M. Walker, D. T. Dunn, and G. R. Serjeant, "The metacarpal index in homozygous sickle-cell disease," *British Journal of Radiology*, vol. 61, no. 724, pp. 280–281, 1988.

[41] N. C. G. Stevens, R. J. Hayes, and G. R. Serjeant, "Body shape in young children with homozygous sickle cell disease," *Pediatrics*, vol. 71, no. 4, pp. 610–614, 1983.

[42] F. A. Oredugba and K. O. Savage, "Anthropometric finding in Nigerian children with sickle cell disease," *Pediatric Dentistry*, vol. 24, no. 4, pp. 321–325, 2002.

[43] O. S. Platt, B. D. Thorington, D. J. Brambilla et al., "Pain in sickle cell disease: rates and risk factors," *The New England Journal of Medicine*, vol. 325, no. 1, pp. 11–16, 1991.

[44] V. Vijay, J. D. Cavenagh, and P. Yate, "The anaesthetist's role in acute sickle cell crisis," *British Journal of Anaesthesia*, vol. 80, no. 6, pp. 820–828, 1998.

[45] S. Delicou and K. Maragkos, "Pain management in patients with Sickle cell disease—a review," *European Medical Journal*, vol. 1, pp. 30–36, 2013.

[46] S. K. Ballas, "Current issues in sickle cell pain and its management," *ASH Education Book*, vol. 2007, no. 1, pp. 97–105, 2007.

[47] S. H. Yale, N. Nagib, and T. Guthrie, "Approach to the vaso-occlusive crisis in adults with sickle cell disease," *American Family Physician*, vol. 61, no. 5, pp. 1349–1356, 2000.

[48] I. Okpala and A. Tawil, "Management of pain in sickle-cell disease," *Journal of the Royal Society of Medicine*, vol. 95, no. 9, pp. 456–458, 2002.

[49] L. R. Solomon, "Pain management in adults with sickle cell disease in a medical center emergency department," *Journal of the National Medical Association*, vol. 102, no. 11, pp. 1025–1032, 2010.

[50] D. C. Rees, A. D. Olujohungbe, N. E. Parker, A. D. Stephens, P. Telfer, and J. Wright, "Guidelines for the management of the acute painful crisis in sickle cell disease," *British Journal of Haematology*, vol. 120, no. 5, pp. 744–752, 2003.

[51] S. C. Davies and M. Brozovic, "The presentation, management and prophylaxis of sickle cell disease," *Blood Reviews*, vol. 3, no. 1, pp. 29–44, 1989.

[52] A. H. Adewoye, V. Nolan, L. McMahon, Q. Ma, and M. H. Steinberg, "Effectiveness of a dedicated day hospital for management of acute sickle cell pain," *Haematologica*, vol. 92, no. 6, article 854, 2007.

[53] L. J. Benjamin, G. I. Swinson, and R. L. Nagel, "Sickle cell anemia day hospital: an approach for the management of uncomplicated painful crises," *Blood*, vol. 95, no. 4, pp. 1130–1137, 2000.

[54] M. A. Ware, I. Hambleton, I. Ochaya, and G. Serjeant, "Day-care management of sickle cell painful crisis in Jamaica: a model applicable elsewhere?" *British Journal of Haematology*, vol. 104, no. 1, pp. 93–96, 1999.

[55] K. L. Hassell, J. R. Eckman, and P. A. Lane, "Acute multiorgan failure syndrome: a potentially catastrophic complication of severe sickle cell pain episodes," *The American Journal of Medicine*, vol. 96, no. 2, pp. 155–162, 1994.

[56] T. S. Akingbola, B. Kolude, E. C. Aneni et al., "Abdominal pain in adult sickle cell disease patients: a Nigerian experience," *Annals of Ibadan Postgraduate Medicine*, vol. 9, no. 2, pp. 100–104, 2011.

[57] N. O. Akinola, R. A. Bolarinwa, and A. F. Faponle, "The import of abdominal pain in adults with sickle cell disorder," *West African Journal of Medicine*, vol. 28, no. 2, pp. 83–86, 2009.

[58] E. C. Ebert, M. Nagar, and K. D. Hagspiel, "Gastrointestinal and hepatic complications of sickle cell disease," *Clinical Gastroenterology and Hepatology*, vol. 8, no. 6, pp. 483–489, 2010.

[59] F. Galacteros and M. de Montalembert, "Sickle cell disease: a short guide to management," in *ESH Handbook on Disorders of Erythropoiesis, Erythrocytes and Iron Metabolism*, C. Beaumont, P. Beris, Y. Beuzard, and C. Brugnara, Eds., vol. 13, pp. 276–309, 2009.

[60] M. E. Odunvbun and A. A. Adeyekun, "Ultrasonic assessment of the prevalence of gall stones in sickle cell disease children seen at the University of Benin Teaching Hospital, Benin City, Nigeria," *Nigerian Journal of Paediatrics*, vol. 41, no. 4, pp. 370–374, 2014.

[61] C. A. Agholor, A. O. Akhigbe, and O. M. Atalabi, "The prevalence of cholelithiasis in Nigerians with sickle cell disease as diagnosed by ultrasound," *British Journal of Medicine and Medical Research*, vol. 4, no. 15, pp. 2866–2873, 2014.

[62] National Heart and Lung and Blood Institute, *The Management of Sickle Cell Disease*, NIH Publication 02-2117, National Institutes of Health, 2002.

[63] M. C. Iheanacho, A. S. Akanmu, and B. Nwogoh, "Seroprevalence of human parvovirus B19 antibody in paediatric sickle cell disease patients seen at the Lagos University Teaching Hospital," *Annals of Biomedical Sciences*, vol. 13, no. 1, pp. 123–129, 2014.

[64] "Genetic disorders of haemoglobin," in *Essential Haematology*, A. V. Hoffbrand, P. A. H. Moss, and J. E. Pettit, Eds., vol. 6, pp. 72–93, Blackwell Publishing, Southampton, UK, 5th edition, 2006.

[65] A. Akinbami, A. Dosunmu, A. Adediran et al., "Steady state hemoglobin concentration and packed cell volume in homozygous sickle cell disease patients in Lagos, Nigeria," *Caspian Journal of Internal Medicine*, vol. 3, no. 2, pp. 405–409, 2012.

[66] R. J. Adams, V. C. Mckie, L. H. Su et al., "Prevention of a first stroke by transfusions in children with sickle cell anemia and abnormal results on transcranial Doppler ultrasonography," *The New England Journal of Medicine*, vol. 339, pp. 5–11, 1998.

[67] O. S. Platt, "Preventing stroke in sickle cell anemia," *The New England Journal of Medicine*, vol. 353, no. 26, pp. 2743–2745, 2005.

[68] R. E. Ware, S. A. Zimmerman, and W. H. Schultz, "Hydroxyurea as an alternative to blood transfusions for the prevention of recurrent stroke in children with sickle cell disease," *Blood*, vol. 94, no. 9, pp. 3022–3026, 1999.

[69] I. O. George and A. I. Frank-Biggs, "Stroke in Nigerian children with sickle cell anaemia," *Journal of Public Health and Epidemiology*, vol. 3, no. 9, pp. 407–409, 2011.

[70] O. Oniyangi, P. Ahmed, O. T. Otuneye et al., "Strokes in children with sickle cell disease at the National Hospital, Abuja, Nigeria," *Nigerian Journal of Paediatrics*, vol. 40, no. 2, pp. 158–164, 2013.

[71] A. Ferster, P. Tahriri, C. Vermylen et al., "Five years of experience with hydroxyurea in children and young adults with sickle cell disease," *Blood*, vol. 97, no. 11, pp. 3628–3632, 2001.

[72] D. Powars, B. Wilson, C. Imbus, C. Pegelow, and J. Allen, "The natural history of stroke in sickle cell disease," *The American Journal of Medicine*, vol. 65, no. 3, pp. 461–471, 1978.

[73] I. A. Lagunju, B. J. Brown, and O. O. Sodeinde, "Chronic blood transfusion for primary and secondary stroke prevention in Nigerian children with sickle cell disease: a 5-year appraisal," *Pediatric Blood and Cancer*, vol. 60, no. 12, pp. 1940–1945, 2013.

[74] S. T. Miller, E. Wright, M. Abboud et al., "Impact of chronic transfusion on incidence of pain and acute chest syndrome during the Stroke Prevention Trial (STOP) in sickle-cell anemia," *The Journal of Pediatrics*, vol. 139, no. 6, pp. 785–789, 2001.

[75] T. L. McCavit, L. Xuan, S. Zhang, G. Flores, and C. T. Quinn, "National trends in incidence rates of hospitalization for stroke in children with sickle cell disease," *Pediatric Blood & Cancer*, vol. 60, no. 5, pp. 823–827, 2013.

[76] J. J. Strouse, S. Lanzkron, and V. Urrutia, "The epidemiology, evaluation and treatment of stroke in adults with sickle cell disease," *Expert Review of Hematology*, vol. 4, no. 6, pp. 597–606, 2011.

[77] W. C. Wang, "The pathophysiology, prevention, and treatment of stroke in sickle cell disease," *Current Opinion in Hematology*, vol. 14, no. 3, pp. 191–197, 2007.

[78] M. R. Mayberg, H. H. Batjer, R. Dacey et al., "Guidelines for the management of aneurysmal subarachnoid hemorrhage," *Stroke*, vol. 25, no. 11, pp. 231–232, 1994.

[79] O. S. Platt, "Prevention and management of stroke in sickle cell anemia," *Hematology*, pp. 54–57, 2006.

[80] M. R. DeBaun, F. D. Armstrong, R. C. McKinstry, R. E. Ware, E. Vichinsky, and F. J. Kirkham, "Silent cerebral infarcts: a review on a prevalent and progressive cause of neurologic injury in sickle cell anemia," *Blood*, vol. 119, no. 20, pp. 4587–4596, 2012.

[81] M. R. DeBaun, J. Schatz, M. J. Siegel et al., "Cognitive screening examinations for silent cerebral infarcts in sickle cell disease," *Neurology*, vol. 50, no. 6, pp. 1678–1682, 1998.

[82] S. T. Miller, E. A. Macklin, C. H. Pegelow et al., "Silent infarction as a risk factor for overt stroke in children with sickle cell anemia: a report from the cooperative study of sickle cell disease," *Journal of Pediatrics*, vol. 139, no. 3, pp. 385–390, 2001.

[83] G. O. Ogun, H. Ebili, and T. R. Kotila, "Autopsy findings and pattern of mortality in Nigerian sickle cell disease patients," *The Pan African Medical Journal*, vol. 18, article 30, 2014.

[84] O. S. Platt, D. J. Brambilla, W. F. Rosse et al., "Mortality in sickle cell disease. Life expectancy and risk factors for early death," *The New England Journal of Medicine*, vol. 330, no. 23, pp. 1639–1644, 1994.

[85] A. Gray, E. N. Anionwu, S. C. Davies, and M. Brozovic, "Patterns of mortality in sickle cell disease in the United Kingdom," *Journal of Clinical Pathology*, vol. 44, no. 6, pp. 459–463, 1991.

[86] R. N. Paul, O. L. Castro, A. Aggarwal, and P. A. Oneal, "Acute chest syndrome: sickle cell disease," *European Journal of Haematology*, vol. 87, no. 3, pp. 191–207, 2011.

[87] P. S. Bellet, K. A. Kalinyak, R. Shukla, M. J. Gelfand, and D. L. Rucknagel, "Incentive spirometry to prevent acute pulmonary complications in sickle cell diseases," *The New England Journal of Medicine*, vol. 333, no. 11, pp. 699–703, 1995.

[88] S. Charache, M. L. Terrin, R. D. Moore et al., "Effect of hydroxyurea on the frequency of painful crises in Sickle cell anemia," *The New England Journal of Medicine*, vol. 332, no. 20, pp. 1317–1322, 1995.

[89] A. S. Adewoyin and J. C. Obieche, "Hypertransfusion therapy in sickle cell disease in Nigeria," *Advances in Hematology*, vol. 2014, Article ID 923593, 8 pages, 2014.

[90] G. M. Crane and N. E. Bennett, "Priapism in sickle cell anemia: emerging mechanistic understanding and better preventative strategies," *Anemia*, vol. 2011, Article ID 297364, 6 pages, 2011.

[91] B. Nwogoh, A. Adewoyin, G. N. Bazuaye, and I. A. Nwannadi, "Prevalence of priapism among male sickle cell disease patients at the University of Benin Teaching Hospital, Benin City," *Nigerian Medical Practitioner*, vol. 65, no. 1-2, pp. 3–7, 2014.

[92] E. M. Isoa, "Current trends in the management of sickle cell disease: an overview," *Benin Journal of Postgraduate Medicine*, vol. 11, no. 1, pp. 50–64, 2009.

[93] R. Virag, D. Bachir, K. Lee, and F. Galacteros, "Preventive treatment of priapism in sickle cell disease with oral and self-administered intracavernous injection of etilefrine," *Urology*, vol. 47, no. 5, pp. 777–781, 1996.

[94] M. McDonald and R. A. Santucci, "Successful management of stuttering priapism using home self-injections of the alpha-agonist metaraminol," *International Braz J Urol*, vol. 30, no. 2, pp. 121–122, 2004.

[95] C. Teloken, E. P. Ribeiro, M. Chammas Jr., P. E. Teloken, and C. A. V. Souto, "Intracavernosal etilefrine self-injection therapy for recurrent priapism: one decade of follow-up," *Urology*, vol. 65, no. 5, p. 1002, 2005.

[96] J. Cherian, A. R. Rao, A. Thwaini, F. Kapasi, I. S. Shergill, and R. Samman, "Medical and surgical management of priapism," *Postgraduate Medical Journal*, vol. 82, no. 964, pp. 89–94, 2006.

[97] G. J. Kato, "Priapism in sickle-cell disease: a hematologist's perspective," *The Journal of Sexual Medicine*, vol. 9, no. 1, pp. 70–78, 2012.

[98] A. D. Gbadoé, Y. Atakouma, K. Kusiaku, and J. K. Assimadi, "Management of sickle cell priapism with etilefrine," *Archives of Disease in Childhood*, vol. 85, no. 1, pp. 52–53, 2001.

[99] G. R. Serjeant, K. De Ceulaer, and G. H. Maude, "Stilboestrol and stuttering priapism in homozygous sickle-cell disease," *The Lancet*, vol. 2, no. 8467, pp. 1274–1276, 1985.

[100] A. L. Burnett, U. A. Anele, I. N. Trueheart, J. J. Strouss, and J. F. Casella, "Randomised Clinical Trial of sildenafil for preventing recurrent ischaemic priapism in Sickle cell disease," *American Journal of Medicine*, vol. 127, no. 7, pp. 664–668, 2014.

[101] A. Lane and R. Deveras, "Potential risks of chronic sildenafil use for priapism in sickle cell disease," *The Journal of Sexual Medicine*, vol. 8, no. 11, pp. 3193–3195, 2011.

[102] P. M. Pierorazio, T. J. Bivalacqua, and A. L. Burnett, "Daily phosphodiesterase type 5 inhibitor therapy as rescue for recurrent ischemic priapism after failed androgen ablation," *Journal of Andrology*, vol. 32, no. 4, pp. 371–374, 2011.

[103] L. Douglas, H. Fletcher, and G. R. Serjeant, "Penile prostheses in the management of impotence in sickle cell disease," *British Journal of Urology*, vol. 65, no. 5, pp. 533–535, 1990.

[104] A. Mallouh and Y. Talab, "Bone and joint infection in patients with sickle cell disease," *Journal of Pediatric Orthopaedics*, vol. 5, no. 2, pp. 158–162, 1985.

[105] A. Almeida and I. Roberts, "Bone involvement in sickle cell disease," *British Journal of Haematology*, vol. 129, no. 4, pp. 482–490, 2005.

[106] W. W. Ebong, "Acute osteomyelitis in Nigerians with sickle cell disease," *Annals of the Rheumatic Diseases*, vol. 45, no. 11, pp. 911–915, 1986.

[107] M. Sadat-Ali, "The status of acute osteomyelitis in sickle cell disease. A 15 year review," *International Surgery*, vol. 83, no. 1, pp. 84–87, 1998.

[108] M. W. Burnett, J. W. Bass, and B. A. Cook, "Etiology of osteomyelitis complicating sickle cell disease," *Pediatrics*, vol. 101, no. 2, pp. 296–297, 1998.

[109] E. M. Barden, D. A. Kawchak, K. Ohene-Frempong, V. A. Stallings, and B. S. Zemel, "Body composition in children with sickle cell disease," *The American Journal of Clinical Nutrition*, vol. 76, no. 1, pp. 218–225, 2002.

[110] C. Booth, B. Inusa, and S. K. Obaro, "Infection in sickle cell disease: a review," *International Journal of Infectious Diseases*, vol. 14, no. 1, pp. e2–e12, 2010.

[111] F. Rahim, "The sickle cell disease," Haematology Updates, 2010.

[112] N. B. Halasa, S. M. Shankar, T. R. Talbot et al., "Incidence of invasive pneumococcal disease among individuals with sickle cell disease before and after the introduction of the pneumococcal conjugate vaccine," *Clinical Infectious Diseases*, vol. 44, no. 11, pp. 1428–1433, 2007.

[113] O. Akinyanju and A. O. Johnson, "Acute illness in Nigerian children with sickle cell anaemia," *Annals of Tropical Paediatrics*, vol. 7, no. 3, pp. 181–186, 1987.

[114] H. O. Okuonghae, M. U. Nwankwo, and E. C. Offor, "Pattern of bacteraemia in febrile children with sickle cell anaemia," *Annals of Tropical Paediatrics*, vol. 13, no. 1, pp. 55–64, 1993.

[115] S. Obaro, "Pneumococcal infections and sickle cell disease in Africa: does absence of evidence imply evidence of absence?" *Archives of Disease in Childhood*, vol. 94, no. 9, pp. 713–716, 2009.

[116] J. A. Berkley, B. S. Lowe, I. Mwangi et al., "Bacteremia among children admitted to a rural hospital in Kenya," *The New England Journal of Medicine*, vol. 352, no. 1, pp. 39–47, 2005.

[117] A. Roca, B. Sigaúque, L. Quintó et al., "Invasive pneumococcal disease in children >5 years of age in rural Mozambique," *Tropical Medicine and International Health*, vol. 11, no. 9, pp. 1422–1431, 2006.

[118] T. N. Williams, S. Uyoga, A. Macharia et al., "Bacteraemia in Kenyan children with sickle-cell anaemia: a retrospective cohort and case-control study," *The Lancet*, vol. 374, no. 9698, pp. 1364–1370, 2009.

[119] National Immunization Policy Nigeria, "National primary health care development agency 2013," 2014.

[120] P. J. Fraker, L. E. King, T. Laakko, and T. L. Vollmer, "The dynamic link between the integrity of the immune system and zinc status," *Journal of Nutrition*, vol. 130, supplement 5, pp. S1399–S1406, 2000.

[121] E. O. Temiye, E. S. Duke, M. A. Owolabi, and J. K. Renner, "Relationship between painful crisis and serum zinc level in children with sickle cell anaemia," *Anemia*, vol. 2011, Article ID 698586, 7 pages, 2011.

[122] B. O. Idonije, O. I. Iribhogbe, and G. R. A. Okogun, "Serum trace element levels in sickle cell disease patients in an urban city in Nigeria," *Nature and Science*, vol. 9, no. 3, pp. 67–71, 2011.

[123] O. G. Arinola, J. A. Olaniyi, and M. O. Akiibinu, "Evaluation of antioxidant levels and trace element status in Nigerian sickle cell disease patients with Plasmodium parasitaemia," *Pakistan Journal of Nutrition*, vol. 7, no. 6, pp. 766–769, 2008.

[124] E. S. Klings, D. F. Wyszynski, V. G. Nolan, and M. H. Steinberg, "Abnormal pulmonary function in adults with sickle cell anemia," *American Journal of Respiratory and Critical Care Medicine*, vol. 173, no. 11, pp. 1264–1269, 2006.

[125] A. O. Dosunmu, T. M. Balogun, O. O. Adeyeye et al., "Prevalence of pulmonary hypertension in sickle cell anaemia patients of a tertiary hospital in Nigeria," *Nigerian Medical Journal*, vol. 55, no. 2, pp. 161–165, 2014.

[126] A. O. Dosunmu, R. A. Akinola, J. A. Onakoya et al., "Pattern of chronic lung lesions in adults with sickle cell disease in Lagos, Nigeria," *Caspian Journal of Internal Medicine*, vol. 4, no. 4, pp. 754–758, 2013.

[127] A. E. Fawibe, "Sickle cell chronic pulmonary disease among Africans: the need for increased recognition and treatment," *African Journal of Respiratory Medicine*, pp. 13–16, 2008.

[128] M. T. Gladwin, V. Sachdev, M. L. Jison et al., "Pulmonary hypertension as a risk factor for death in patients with sickle cell disease," *The New England Journal of Medicine*, vol. 350, no. 9, pp. 886–895, 2004.

[129] H. Issa and A. H. Al-Salem, "Hepatobiliary manifestations of sickle cell anemia," *Gastroenterology Research*, vol. 3, no. 1, pp. 1–8, 2010.

[130] F. A. Fashola and I. A. Otegbayo, "Post transfusion viral hepatitis in sickle cell anaemia: retrospective—prospective analysis," *Nigerian Journal of Clinical Practice*, vol. 5, no. 1, pp. 16–19, 2002.

[131] E. U. Ejeliogu, S. N. Okolo, S. D. Pam, E. S. Okpe, C. C. John, and M. O. Ochoga, "Is human immunodeficiency virus still transmissible through blood transfusion in children with sickle cell anaemia in Jos, Nigeria?" *The British Journal of Medicine and Medical Research*, vol. 4, no. 21, pp. 3912–3923, 2014.

[132] G. O. Ogunrinde, R. O. Zubair, S. M. Mado, S. Musa, and L. W. Umar, "Prevalence of nocturnal enuresis in children with homozygous sickle cell disease in zaria," *Nigerian Journal of Paediatrics*, vol. 34, pp. 31–35, 2007.

[133] A. Abdu, M. Emokpae, P. Uadia, and A. Kuliya-Gwarzo, "Proteinuria among adult sickle cell anemia patients in Nigeria," *Annals of African Medicine*, vol. 10, no. 1, pp. 34–37, 2011.

[134] J. C. Aneke, A. O. Adegoke, A. A. Oyekunle et al., "Degrees of kidney disease in Nigerian adults with sickle-cell disease," *Medical Principles and Practice*, vol. 23, no. 3, pp. 271–274, 2014.

[135] C. C. Sharpe and S. L. Thein, "How I treat renal complications in sickle cell disease," *Blood*, vol. 123, no. 24, pp. 3720–3726, 2014.

[136] K. I. Ataga and E. P. Orringer, "Renal abnormalities in sickle cell disease," *American Journal of Hematology*, vol. 63, pp. 205–211, 2000.

[137] P. I. Condon and G. R. Serjeant, "Ocular findings in homozygous sickle cell anemia in Jamaica," *The American Journal of Ophthalmology*, vol. 73, no. 4, pp. 533–543, 1972.

[138] M. Koshy, R. Entsuah, A. Koranda et al., "Leg ulcers in patients with sickle cell disease," *Blood*, vol. 74, no. 4, pp. 1403–1408, 1989.

[139] G. N. Bazuaye, A. I. Nwannadi, and E. E. Olayemi, "Leg Ulcers in Adult sickle cell disease patients in Benin City, Nigeria," *Gomal Journal of Medical Sciences*, vol. 8, no. 2, pp. 190–194, 2010.

[140] R. A. Balogun, D. C. Obalum, S. O. Giwa, T. O. Adekoya-Cole, C. N. Ogo, and G. O. Enweluzo, "Spectrum of musculo-skeletal disorders in sickle cell disease in Lagos, Nigeria," *Journal of Orthopaedic Surgery and Research*, vol. 5, article 2, 2010.

[141] P. Hernigou, A. Habibi, D. Bachir, and F. Galacteros, "The natural history of asymptomatic osteonecrosis of the femoral head in adults with sickle cell disease," *Journal of Bone and Joint Surgery—Series A*, vol. 88, no. 12, pp. 2565–2572, 2006.

[142] A. J. Madu, A. K. Madu, G. K. Umar, K. Ibekwe, A. Duru, and A. O. Ugwu, "Avascular necrosis in sickle cell (homozygous S) patients: predictive clinical and laboratory indices," *Nigerian Journal of Clinical Practice*, vol. 17, no. 1, pp. 86–89, 2014.

[143] H. Hawker, H. Neilson, R. J. Hayes, and G. R. Serjeant, "Haematological factors associated with avascular necrosis of the femoral head in homozygous sickle cell disease," *British Journal of Haematology*, vol. 50, no. 1, pp. 29–34, 1982.

[144] M. Mukisi-Mukaza, A. Elbaz, Y. Samuel-Leborgne et al., "Prevalence, clinical features, and risk factors of osteonecrosis of the femoral head among adults with sickle cell disease," *Orthopedics*, vol. 23, no. 4, pp. 357–363, 2000.

[145] A. D. Adekile, R. Gupta, F. Yacoub, T. Sinan, M. Al-Bloushi, and M. Z. Haider, "Avascular necrosis of the hip in children with sickle cell disease and high Hb F: magnetic resonance imaging findings and influence of $\alpha$-thalassemia trait," *Acta Haematologica*, vol. 105, no. 1, pp. 27–31, 2001.

[146] "Sickle cell disease in childhood. Standards and guidelines for clinical care," UK Forum on Haemoglobin Disorders, 2010.

[147] M. T. Gladwin and V. Sachdev, "Cardiovascular abnormalities in sickle cell disease," *Journal of the American College of Cardiology*, vol. 59, no. 13, pp. 1123–1133, 2012.

[148] N. I. Oguanobi, E. C. Ejim, B. C. Anisiuba et al., "Clinical and electrocardiographic evaluation of sickle-cell anaemia patients with pulmonary hypertension," *ISRN Hematology*, vol. 2012, Article ID 768718, 6 pages, 2012.

[149] B. Otaigbe, "Prevalence of blood transfusion in sickle cell anaemia patients in South-South Nigeria: a two-year experience," *International Journal of Biological and Medical Research*, vol. 1, no. 1, pp. 13–18, 2013.

[150] H. H. Al-Saeed and A. H. Al-Salem, "Principles of blood transfusion in sickle cell anemia," *Saudi Medical Journal*, vol. 23, no. 12, pp. 1443–1448, 2002.

[151] Z. Y. Aliyu, A. R. Tumblin, and G. J. Kato, "Current therapy of sickle cell disease," *Haematologica*, vol. 91, no. 1, pp. 7–11, 2006.

[152] N. Win, "Blood transfusion therapy for Haemoglobinopathies," in *Practical Management of Haemoglobinopathies*, I. E. Okpala, Ed., pp. 99–106, Blackwell Publishing, 2004.

[153] C. D. Josephson, L. L. Su, K. L. Hillyer, and C. D. Hillyer, "Transfusion in the patient with sickle cell disease: a critical review of the literature and transfusion guidelines," *Transfusion Medicine Reviews*, vol. 21, no. 2, pp. 118–133, 2007.

[154] E. P. Vinchinsky, "Transfusion therapy in sickle cell disease," 2014, http://sickle.bwh.harvard.edu/transfusion.html.

[155] J. L. Levenson, "Psychiatric issues in adults with sickle cell disease," *Primary Psychiatry*, vol. 15, no. 5, pp. 45–49, 2008.

[156] K. A. Anie, F. E. Egunjobi, and O. O. Akinyanju, "Psychosocial impact of sickle cell disorder: perspectives from a Nigerian setting," *Globalization and Health*, vol. 6, article 2, 2010.

[157] C. Hilton, M. Osborn, S. Knight, A. Singhal, and G. Serjeant, "Psychiatric complications of homozygous sickle cell disease among young adults in the Jamaican cohort study," *The British Journal of Psychiatry*, vol. 170, pp. 69–76, 1997.

[158] V. J. Rappaport, M. Velazquez, and K. Williams, "Hemoglobinopathies in pregnancy," *Obstetrics and Gynecology Clinics of North America*, vol. 31, no. 2, pp. 287–317, 2004.

[159] R. P. Naik and S. Lanzkron, "Baby on board: what you need to know about pregnancy in the hemoglobinopathies," *Hematology*, vol. 2012, pp. 208–214, 2012.

[160] B. B. Afolabi, N. C. Iwuala, I. C. Iwuala, and O. K. Ogedengbe, "Morbidity and mortality in sickle cell pregnancies in Lagos, Nigeria: a case control study," *Journal of Obstetrics & Gynaecology*, vol. 29, no. 2, pp. 104–106, 2009.

[161] A. Omole-Ohonsi, O. A. Ashimi, and T. A. Aiyedun, "Preconception care and sickle cell anemia in pregnancy," *Journal of Basic and Clinical Reproductive Sciences*, vol. 1, no. 1, pp. 12–18, 2012.

[162] Z. M. Al-Samak, M. M. Al-Falaki, and A. A. Pasha, "Assessment of perioperative transfusion therapy and complications in sickle cell disease patients undergoing surgery," *Middle East Journal of Anesthesiology*, vol. 19, no. 5, pp. 983–995, 2008.

[163] W. A. Marchant and I. Walker, "Anaesthetic management of the child with sickle cell disease," *Paediatric Anaesthesia*, vol. 13, no. 6, pp. 473–489, 2003.

[164] E. P. Vichinsky, C. M. Haberkern, L. Neumayr et al., "A comparison of conservative and aggressive transfusion regimens in the perioperative management of sickle cell disease," *The New England Journal of Medicine*, vol. 333, no. 4, pp. 206–213, 1995.

[165] H. M. Dix, "New advances in the treatment of sickle cell disease: focus on perioperative significance," *Journal of the American Association of Nurse Anesthetists*, vol. 69, no. 4, pp. 281–286, 2001.

[166] P. Losco, G. Nash, P. Stone, and J. Ventre, "Comparison of the effects of radiographic contrast media on dehydration and filterability of red blood cells from donors homozygous for hemoglobin A or hemoglobin S," *American Journal of Hematology*, vol. 68, no. 3, pp. 149–158, 2001.

[167] T. R. Kotila, "Guidelines for the diagnosis of the haemoglobinopathies in Nigeria," *Annals of Ibadan Postgraduate Medicine*, vol. 8, no. 1, pp. 25–29, 2011.

[168] Y. Daniel, "Haemoglobinopathy diagnostic tests: blood counts, sickle solubility test, haemoglobin electrophoresis and high-performance liquid chromatography," in *Practical Management of Haemoglobinopathies*, I. E. Okpala, Ed., pp. 10–19, Blackwell Publishing, 2004.

[169] B. J. Bain, "Haemoglobinopathy diagnosis: algorithms, lessons and pitfalls," *Blood Reviews*, vol. 25, no. 5, pp. 205–213, 2011.

[170] G. M. Clarke and T. N. Higgins, "Laboratory investigation of hemoglobinopathies and thalassemias: review and update," *Clinical Chemistry*, vol. 46, no. 8, part 2, pp. 1284–1290, 2000.

[171] O. Emmanuelchide, O. Charle, and O. Uchenna, "Hematological parameters in association with outcomes in sickle cell anemia patients," *Indian Journal of Medical Sciences*, vol. 65, no. 9, pp. 393–398, 2011.

[172] S. A. Adegoke and B. P. Kuti, "Evaluation of clinical severity of sickle cell anaemia in Nigerian children," *Journal of Applied Hematology*, vol. 4, no. 2, pp. 58–64, 2013.

[173] C. T. Quinn, Z. R. Rogers, and G. R. Buchanan, "Survival of children with sickle cell disease," *Blood*, vol. 103, no. 11, pp. 4023–4027, 2004.

[174] K. J. J. Wierenga, I. R. Hambleton, and N. A. Lewis, "Survival estimates for patients with homozygous sickle-cell disease in Jamaica: a clinic-based population study," *The Lancet*, vol. 357, no. 9257, pp. 680–683, 2001.

[175] A. Chijioke and P. M. Kolo, "The longevity and clinical pattern of adult sickle cell anaemia in Ilorin," *European Journal of Scientific Research*, vol. 32, no. 4, pp. 528–532, 2009.

[176] M. Angastiniotis, S. Kyriakidou, and M. Hadjiminas, "How thalassaemia was controlled in Cyprus.," *World Health Forum*, vol. 7, no. 3, pp. 291–297, 1986.

[177] M. A. Durosinmi, A. I. Odebiyi, I. A. Adediran, N. O. Akinola, D. E. Adegorioye, and M. A. Okunade, "Acceptability of prenatal diagnosis of sickle cell anaemia (SCA) by female patients and parents of SCA patients in Nigeria," *Social Science and Medicine*, vol. 41, no. 3, pp. 433–436, 1995.

[178] A. S. Adeyemi and D. A. Adekanle, "Knowledge and attitude of female health workers towards prenatal diagnosis of sickle cell disease," *Nigerian Journal of Medicine*, vol. 16, no. 3, pp. 268–270, 2007.

[179] M. B. Kagu, U. A. Abjah, and S. G. Ahmed, "Awareness and acceptability of prenatal diagnosis of sickle cell anaemia among health professionals and students in North Eastern Nigeria," *Nigerian Journal of Medicine*, vol. 13, no. 1, pp. 48–51, 2004.

[180] World Health Organisation, *Guidelines for the Control of Haemoglobin Disorders*, WHO, Sardinia, Italy, 1994.

[181] S. O. Akodu, I. N. Diaku-Akinwumi, and O. F. Njokanma, "Age at diagnosis of sickle cell anaemia in lagos, Nigeria," *Mediterranean Journal of Hematology and Infectious Diseases*, vol. 5, no. 1, Article ID e2013001, 2013.

[182] F. A. Olatona, K. A. Odeyemi, A. T. Onajole, and M. C. Asuzu, "Effects of health education on knowledge and attitude of youth corps members to sickle cell disease and its screening in Lagos State," *Journal of Community Medicine & Health Education*, vol. 2, article 163, 2012.

[183] N. Galadanci, B. J. Wudil, T. M. Balogun et al., "Current sickle cell disease management practices in Nigeria," *International Health*, vol. 6, no. 1, pp. 23–28, 2014.

[184] A. A. Oyekunle, "Haemopoietic stem cell transplantation: prospects and challenges in Nigeria," *Annals of Ibadan Postgraduate Medicine*, vol. 4, no. 1, pp. 17–27, 2006.

[185] N. Bazuaye, B. Nwogoh, D. Ikponmwen et al., "First successful allogeneic hematopoietic stem cell transplantation for a sickle cell disease patient in a low resource country (Nigeria): a case report," *Annals of Transplantation*, vol. 19, no. 1, pp. 210–213, 2014.

[186] O. O. Akinyanju, A. I. Otaigbe, and M. O. O. Ibidapo, "Outcome of holistic care in Nigerian patients with sickle cell anaemia," *Clinical and Laboratory Haematology*, vol. 27, no. 3, pp. 195–199, 2005.

[187] I. E. Okpala, "Sickle cell crisis," in *Practical Management of Haemoglobinopathies*, I. E. Okpala, Ed., pp. 63–71, Blackwell Publishing, 2004.

[188] I. Okpala, V. Thomas, N. Westerdale et al., "The comprehensive care of sickle cell disease," *European Journal of Haematology*, vol. 68, no. 3, pp. 157–162, 2002.

[189] J. Makani, S. F. Ofori-Acquah, O. Nnodu, A. Wonkam, and K. Ohene-Frempong, "Sickle cell disease: new opportunities and challenges in Africa," *The Scientific World Journal*, vol. 2013, Article ID 193252, 16 pages, 2013.

[190] O. Oniyangi and A. A. A. Omari, "Malaria chemoprophylaxis in sickle cell disease," *The Cochrane Library*, vol. 1, pp. 1–18, 2009.

[191] E. O. Ibe, A. C. J. Ezeoke, I. Emeodi et al., "Electrolyte profile and prevalent causes of sickle cell crisis in Enugu, Nigeria," *African Journal of Biochemistry Research*, vol. 3, no. 11, pp. 370–374, 2009.

[192] R. A. Bolarinwa, N. O. Akinola, O. A. Aboderin, and M. A. Durosinmi, "The role of malaria in vaso-occlusive crisis of adult patients with sickle cell disease," *Journal of Medicine and Medical Sciences*, vol. 1, pp. 407–411, 2010.

[193] R. Kotila, A. Okesola, and O. Makanjuola, "Asymptomatic malaria parasitaemia in sickle-cell disease patients: how effective is chemoprophylaxis?" *Journal of Vector Borne Diseases*, vol. 44, no. 1, pp. 52–55, 2007.

[194] R. E. Ware, "How I use hydroxyurea to treat young patients with sickle cell anemia," *Blood*, vol. 115, no. 26, pp. 5300–5311, 2010.

[195] S. C. Davies and A. Gilmore, "The role of hydroxyurea in the management of sickle cell disease," *Blood Reviews*, vol. 17, no. 2, pp. 99–109, 2003.

[196] S. C. Davies and I. A. G. Roberts, "Bone marrow transplant for sickle cell disease—an update," *Archives of Disease in Childhood*, vol. 75, no. 1, pp. 3–6, 1996.

[197] I. Roberts, "Current status of allogeneic transplantation for haemoglobinopathies," *British Journal of Haematology*, vol. 98, no. 1, pp. 1–7, 1997.

[198] S. Shenoy, "Hematopoietic stem cell transplantation for sickle cell disease: current practice and emerging trends," *Hematology*, vol. 2011, pp. 273–279, 2011.

[199] L. De Franceschi, "Pathophysiology of sickle cell disease and new drugs for the treatment," *Mediterranean Journal of Hematology and Infectious Diseases*, vol. 1, no. 1, 2009.

[200] L. De Franceschi and R. Corrocher, "Established and experimental treatments for sickle cell disease," *Haematologica*, vol. 89, no. 3, pp. 348–356, 2004.

[201] K. I. Ataga and J. Stocker, "Senicapoc (ICA17043): a potential therapy for the prevention and treatment of hemolysis-associated complications in sickle cell anemia," *Expert Opinion on Investigational Drugs*, vol. 18, no. 2, pp. 231–239, 2009.

[202] K. I. Ataga, W. R. Smith, L. M. De Castro et al., "Efficacy and safety of the Gardos channel blocker, senicapoc (ICA-17043), in patients with sickle cell anemia," *Blood*, vol. 111, no. 8, pp. 3991–3997, 2008.

[203] I. E. Okpala, "New therapies for sickle cell disease," *Hematology/Oncology Clinics of North America*, vol. 19, no. 5, pp. 975–987, 2005.

[204] M. J. Stuart and R. L. Nagel, "Sickle-cell disease," *The Lancet*, vol. 364, no. 9442, pp. 1343–1360, 2004.

[205] M. C. Walters, "Stem cell therapy for sickle cell disease: transplantation and gene therapy," *Hematology*, vol. 2005, no. 1, pp. 66–73, 2005.

# 23

# Factors Associated with Growth Retardation in Children Suffering from Sickle Cell Anemia: First Report from Central Africa

**Aimé Lukusa Kazadi,[1] René Makuala Ngiyulu,[1] Jean Lambert Gini-Ehungu,[1] Jean Marie Mbuyi-Muamba,[2] and Michel Ntetani Aloni[1]**

[1]*Division of Paediatric Haemato-Oncology and Nephrology, Department of Paediatrics, University Hospital of Kinshasa, Faculty of Medicine, University of Kinshasa, Kinshasa, Democratic Republic of the Congo*
[2]*Department of Internal Medicine, Faculty of Medicine, University of Kinshasa, Kinshasa, Democratic Republic of the Congo*

Correspondence should be addressed to Aimé Lukusa Kazadi; aimekaz@yahoo.fr

Academic Editor: Aurelio Maggio

*Background.* The aim of this study was to investigate and determine the risk factors associated with poor growth among SCA children. *Methods.* A cross-sectional study was conducted in Kinshasa, the capital's country. The nutritional status was assessed using the Z scores of the anthropometric indices. *Results.* We gathered data on the 256 patients, 138 females (53.9%), who entered the study. The mean age at presentation was 8.4 ± 4.9 years of age. Underweight, stunting, and wasting were found, respectively, in 47.7%, 10.5%, and 50.3% of SCA children. A history of hand-foot syndrome, more than 3 blood transfusions, being less than 12 months of age when receiving the first transfusion, more than two severe sickle crises per year, a medical history of severe infections, and the presence of hepatomegaly were associated with poor growth. When comparing sickle cell patients under 12 years of age ($n = 159$) to a group of 296 age-matched children with normal Hb-AA, a significantly higher proportion of subjects with stunting and underweight were found among SCA. *Conclusion.* Nutritional status encountered in Congolese sickle cell children has been described for the first time in this study. A high prevalence of poor growth in SCA children was found in our study.

## 1. Introduction

Sickle cell anaemia (SCA) is the commonest genetic diseases in sub-Saharan Africa [1]. In the Democratic Republic of Congo (DRC), the HBB*S allele prevalence in neonates ranges from 0.96% to 1.4%. According to 2010 estimation, the DRC contributed to the global burden of SCA with 39,800 [CI: 32,600–48,800] neonates each year [2].

SCA is an inflammatory disease characterized by chronic haemolysis, vasoocclusive crises, severe infection, and organ damage [1]. It is known that the sickle cell neonates have a normal weight at birth [3, 4]. However, the disease with its attendant increased energy requirements has a negative effect on growth with a slow prepubertal growth and a delayed velocity compared with normal children [5]. Many factors as endocrine and/or metabolic dysfunction, haematological status, and nutritional status may play an important role in growth failure [5, 6].

Great progress has been made in the care of children with SCA in recent decades [7, 8]. Management of this haemoglobinopathy has been changing and is excellent as we have patients with advanced age in developed countries [8, 9]. However, in developing countries such as the DRC, these cures are compromised by financial, human and laboratories resources deficiencies, inconsistent drug supplies, and delayed time of diagnosis [10, 11].

The determinants of low growth are not well understood and are probably due to phenotypic polymorphism due to haplotype, genetics factors, foetal haemoglobin level, specific nutrient deficiencies, and environmental factors [12–14].

Most studies are performed in sickle cell patients living in variable conditions that may affect growth and contribute to the difficulty to understand the mechanisms of growth in this population [15].

In the Democratic Republic of Congo (DRC), there is still very little information on nutritional status of children with SCA, because most provinces of this country lack paediatricians and vital hospital statistics scarcely contain sur information [16]. Additionally, 80% of the population lives in extreme poverty and more than 70% are estimated to suffer from malnutrition. Furthermore, the severity of the disease added to the poverty living conditions may influence the sickle cell children's growth curve [17]. Despite the high incidence and prevalence of SCA and the risk of failure to thrive in these patients, there was a paucity of studies from Central Africa, highlighting a large knowledge gap for low-resource settings.

It is necessary for health planning to have the main characteristics of children with SCA living in the DRC. This information will give the whole view of patients and may serve to rule out public health and in-hospital politics in our midst.

Thus, the aim of this study was to determine the prevalence and secondly to investigate the risk factors associated with failure to thrive among SCA children living in Kinshasa, the DRC. Our findings were compared to the results of previous studies reported in the literature.

## 2. Methods

This cross-sectional study was conducted in three paediatric health facilities in Kinshasa, namely, Centre de santé Saint Sacrement de Binza (West), the Sickle Cell Center of Yolo (Centre), and Centre de Santé Saint Marc (East). These health facilities provide most of the paediatric sickle cell follow-up in Kinshasa, DRC. These hospitals also provide most of the nonprivate paediatrics beds in Kinshasa for sickle cell patients.

Patients were consecutively selected in the outpatient clinic of the three health institutions. For the growth comparison, each sickle cell child under twelve years of age was matched with one or two control AA children for age, sex, and place of residence.

The following clinical and laboratory information were collected and analyzed: (i) demographic characteristics, (ii) anthropometric parameters, (iii) age at the first pain crisis and at the first blood transfusion, (iv) number of severe sickle cell crises per year, (v) blood transfusion, and (vi) haematologic parameters.

## 3. Data Collection Procedure and Analysis

Height and weight were measured using standardized techniques. Weighing scale was calibrated to zero before taking every measurement. The children were weighed with minimum clothing and without shoes.

Measurement of height was done in a lying position with wooden board for children under 2 years of age and measurement of height for children over 2 years of age was in a standing position in centimeters to the nearest 1 cm.

The nutritional status of the study population was assessed using the Z scores of the anthropometric indices: weight-for-height Z score (WHZ), height-for-age Z score (HAZ), and weight-for-age Z score (WAZ). These indicators were calculated according to the references of the National Centre for Health Statistics/WHO/CDC [18]. Abnormal status is defined as having an indicator Z score less than −2.0. WHZ determined the severity of wasting, HAZ the severity of stunting, and WAZ underweight.

At the end, the nutritional status of SCA patients was compared to healthy peers age-matched haemoglobin-AA group. Because sex steroid hormones effects on the growth pattern start on average at 12 [19], we only compare children under 12 years of age for this purpose, in both groups.

Blood samples were collected from all subjects. Sickle cell screening was performed using isoelectric focusing (IEF) technique with the Multiphor II apparatus (GE Healthcare, Little Chalfont, England). The separation of different haemoglobin (F, A, S, and other types of haemoglobin) was obtained after application on thin layer home-made agarose gel containing ampholytes pH 6–8 (ref. 2117–003; Pharmalyte pH 6.7–7.7; GE Healthcare).

## 4. Data Management

The information that was obtained was analyzed using Epi info version 6 (CDC). After data cleaning (control for quality and coherence), they were exported on SPSS 22.0 for further analysis. All data from discrete variables are represented as means ± standard deviation (SD). Frequency of various clinical and laboratory findings are expressed as percentages. The confidence interval at 95% was calculated. Pearson chi-square or Fisher's exact test was used to assess differences in categorical data between groups. The analysis of Student's $t$-test or Mann–Whitney test was used for comparisons of means. The relationship between growth in SCA children and study parameters was assessed using logistic regression models. Odds ratios were provided with their 95% confidence interval (95% CI) and were estimated for the factors that have a significant effect. A $p$ value $< 0.05$ was considered significant.

## 5. Results

5.1. Study Population and Baseline Characteristics. We gathered data on the 256 patients, 138 females (53.9%) and 118 males (46.1%), who entered the study. The mean age at presentation was 8.4 ± 4.9 years of age. Table 1 presents baseline characteristics of all patients.

5.2. Risk of Short Stature. Growth in height fell below the 5th percentile in 7.8% ($n = 20$) of sickle cell children. A history of hand-foot syndrome and the number of transfusions of more than 3 per patient were associated with an increased risk of short stature with OR, respectively, 4.3 and 4.8. However, the presence of hepatomegaly was also associated (OR 4.2) but with a nonsignificant CI 95%. All results are shown in Table 2.

TABLE 1: Characteristics of the study population.

| Parameters | Patients (n = 256) |
| --- | --- |
| Age, years | |
| Mean (SD) | 8.4 ± 4.9 |
| Age distribution, years | |
| <4 years, n (%) | (31.6) |
| 5–9 years, n (%) | (32.5) |
| 10–14 years, n (%) | (25) |
| ≥15 years, n (%) | (10.9) |
| Gender | |
| Male, n (%) | 118 (46.1) |
| Female, n (%) | 138 (53.9) |
| Anthropometrics parameters | |
| Mean weight (kg) (range) | 20.6 ± 9.8 (7–62) |
| Mean height (cm) (range) | 115 ± 24 (63–172) |
| Mean BMI, (range)* | 17.0 ± 1.8 (10.9–22.9) |
| Clinical findings | |
| Hepatomegaly, n (%) | 136 (53.1) |
| Splenomegaly, n (%) | 109 (41.7) |
| Sickle cell crises | |
| Haemolysis, n (%) | 136 (53.1) |
| Severe pain crisis, n (%) | 170 (66.4) |
| Hand-foot syndrome, n (%) | 85 (33.2) |
| Severe infection, n (%) | 45 (17.6) |
| splenic sequestration, n (%) | 19 (7.4) |
| Mean age at the first pain crisis (range), months | 18.2 ± 15.2 (2–108) |
| Mean age at the first transfusion (range), months | 29.2 ± 27.6 (2–132) |
| Number of severe pain crises/year, n (range) | 3.5 ± 2.9 (1–20) |
| Number of blood transfusions, n (range) | 4.1 ± 3.2 (0–30) |
| Laboratory features | |
| Mean Hb (g/dl) (range)* | 7.4 ± 1.5 (4.3–11) |
| Mean Ht (%) (range)* | 23.2 ± 4.5 (12.2–35) |
| Mean WBCs ($10^3$/mm³) (range)* | 14.5 = 5.4 (4.6–34.2) |
| Mean platelets ($10^3$/mm³) (range) | 315.5 ± 118.5 (114–582) |

*BMI, body mass index; Hb, hemoglobin; Ht, hematocrit; WBCs, white blood cells.

TABLE 2: Factors associated with a risk of stunting in the study population.

| Variables | OR | CI 95% | p |
| --- | --- | --- | --- |
| Underweight, WAZ | | | |
| *Hepatomegaly* | | | **<0.05** |
| Absence | **1** | | |
| Presence | **1.4** | **1–1.8** | |
| TAZ, risk of wasting | | | |
| *Number of sickle cell crises/year* | | | <0.01 |
| ≤2 | 1 | — | |
| >2 | 3.8 | 1.5–9.5 | |
| *Age at the first transfusion* | | | <0.01 |
| >12 months | 1 | — | |
| ≤12 months | 3.3 | 1.1–9.3 | |
| *Number of blood transfusions* | | | <0.05 |
| ≤3 | 1 | — | |
| >3 | 2.5 | 1.1–6 | |
| Risk of short stature | | | |
| *Hand-foot syndrome* | | | <0.01 |
| Absence | 1 | — | |
| Present | 4.3 | 1.3–13.7 | |
| *Number of blood transfusions* | | | <0.05 |
| ≤3 | 1 | — | |
| >3 | 4.8 | 1.1–21.5 | |
| *Hepatomegaly* | | | <0.05 |
| Absence | 1 | — | |
| Presence | 4.2 | 0.94–18.9 | |
| Wasting WHZ | | | |
| *Hand-foot syndrome* | | | <0.01 |
| Absence | 1 | — | |
| Present | 1.7 | 1.2–2.5 | |
| *Severe infections* | | | <0.05 |
| Absence | 1 | — | |
| Presence | 1.8 | 1.0–3.1 | |
| *Number of blood transfusions* | | | <0.05 |
| ≤3 | 1 | — | |
| >3 | 1.3 | 1.0–1.7 | |

5.3. *Underweight, WAZ.* In this series, underweight was found in 47.7% ($n$ = 122) of SCA children. The presence of hepatomegaly was weakly associated with an increased risk of wasting.

5.4. *Stunting TAZ.* In this series, stunting was found in 10.5% ($n$ = 27) of SCA children. Number of severe sickle cell crises of more than two per year, age at the first blood transfusion less than 12 months, and number of blood transfusions of more than three per patient were associated with an increased risk of stunting (Table 2).

5.5. *Wasting WHZ.* According the WHZ, wasting was found in 50.3% ($n$ = 129) of SCA children. A history of hand-foot syndrome is the main factor associated with an increased risk of wasting. Other factors such as history of severe infections and the number of transfusions of more than 3 per patient were weakly associated.

5.6. *Comparison with Normal Children (Hb-AA).* Among children under 12, a significantly higher proportion (34.9%) of subjects with stunting were children with Hb-SS, compared to 9.8% in children with Hb-AA. Additionally, more than a third (39.8%) of subjects with underweight were children

TABLE 3: Nutritional status according to Hb status in children under 12 years of age in the study population.

| Variables | Hb-SS, $n = 159$ | Hb-AA, $n = 296$ | $p$ |
|---|---|---|---|
| Stunting TAZ, $n$ (%) | 55 (34.6%) | 29 (9.8%) | <0.001 |
| Wasting WHZ, $n$ (%) | 23 (14.5%) | 37 (12.5%) | NS |
| Underweight WAZ, $n$ (%) | 63 (39.6%) | 36 (12.2%) | <0.001 |

with Hb-SS, compared to 12.2% in children with Hb-AA (Table 3).

In Hb-SS group, the prevalence of wasting (WHZ) tended to be higher than Hb-AA groups. However, there was no statistically significant difference between the two groups (Table 3).

## 6. Discussion

The aim of study is oriented to identify the factors associated with failure to thrive in a paediatric population. In Central Africa, a predominant region of Bantu haplotype, there is anecdotal information on growth in paediatric population suffering from SCA [20]. Our study is the first to investigate and determine the risk factors associated with failure to thrive among SCA children living in Kinshasa, the capital's country of the DRC.

Before going through discussing our results, it appears important to explain difficulties when using growth chart from different populations. Ideally, local charts would give better insight of the real situation and local realities. Unfortunately, to the better of our knowledge, available references for growth studies in our midst are the ones we used here from the National Centre for Health Statistics/WHO/CDC [18]. The advantage would be to have an international standard growth chart which allows comparison of children in different settings around the world.

Growth in height fell below the 5th percentile in 7.8% of sickle cell children. Similar observations on short stature were reported in other worldwide studies where the proportion varies from 5% to 54% [5, 21–24]. These wide variations are probably due to sample size, selection of reference growth data, and environmental and genetics factors which limited comparability between these studies.

A history of hand-foot syndrome, the number of transfusions of more than 3 per patient, and the presence of hepatomegaly were associated with an increased risk of short stature. These trends are in accordance with the results found in the literature [25].

In this series, underweight was found in 47.7% of SCA children. Similar observations were reported in other worldwide studies [24, 26–28]. The presence of hepatomegaly was weakly associated with an increased risk of wasting. This observation is probably due to the predominance of SCA without $\alpha\alpha$+thalassemia in Central Africa et the severity of this phenotype [29, 30]. In contrast to our findings, Al-Saqladi et al. found an association of low height-for-age Z score with increased age [22]. These differences between our study and the Yemen study presumably arise from differences in environmental and genetic factors that influence growth of sickle cell children

In this series, stunting was found in 10.5% ($n = 27$) of SCA children. These results are in consonance with previous studies where the prevalence varies from 16.4% to 43% [20, 24, 27, 31]. Number of severe sickle cell crises of more than two per year, age at the first blood transfusion less than 12 months, and number of blood transfusions of more than three per patient were associated with an increased risk of stunting. This may find explanation as these factors provide a trend of the severity of the disease. The severity of the clinical manifestations of the disease increases the energy expenditure and decreases the calorie intake [32]. The results found in this cohort confirm and extend the findings of several studies [20, 25, 33]. In contrast, Al-Saqladi et al. found an association of low height-for-age Z score with male gender in their series [22]. These differences between our study and the Yemen study presumably arise from differences in environmental and genetic factors that influence growth of sickle cell children.

According the WHZ, wasting was found in half of our of SCA children (50.3%). This prevalence is higher than the results reported by Henderson et al. in USA where 11% of sickle cell children were affected [31]. These differences may be due to selection of reference growth data and environmental and genetics factors. Only a history of hand-foot syndrome is strongly associated with an increased risk of wasting, while severe infections and the number of transfusions of more than 3 per patient were weakly associated. This is in accordance with those reported by other authors [24, 25]. In contrast, Al-Saqladi et al. in Yemen found an association of low weight-for-height Z score with increased age [22]. These differences between our study and the US study presumably arise from differences in environmental and genetic factors that influence growth of sickle cell children.

In this series, age, gender, increased volume of tonsil, age at the first transfusion, splenic sequestration, WBCs, and platelets levels were not associated with poor growth as described by other authors [31]. In contrast, these parameters were found to be associated with poor growth in previous worldwide studies [3, 20]. These differences between these studies presumably arise from differences in environmental and genetic factors that influence growth of sickle cell children.

From these findings, only little explanation may be advanced and speculated. Underweight and wasting are probably due to phenotypic polymorphism due to haplotype, genetics factors, fetal haemoglobin level, specific nutrient deficiencies, and environmental factors [12–14]. Indeed, the Bantu haplotype is predominant and the Congolese SCA patients displayed low levels of fetal haemoglobin (HbF) and F-cells that contribute to the severity of SCA [34]. To the best of our knowledge, it appears that factors associated with growth in SCA children are those that characterize more severe disease.

A significantly higher proportion of subjects with stunting were children with Hb-SS, compared to 9.8% in children with Hb-AA. The HAZ (stunting) scores were significantly more common among SCD children than controls, in previous worldwide studies [20, 35, 36]. In contrast, Barden et al. in Nigeria found no significant difference between normal and sickle cell children [36]. These differences between our study and the US study presumably arise from differences in environmental and genetic factors that influence growth of sickle cell children. Limitation from our study may arise in the fact that we did not assess nutritional intake of each patient as this was not the aim of the study. Mandese et al. showed that inadequate nutritional intake, weight, and Body Mass Index have significant impact on SCA severity indices such as number of hospital admissions per year, days of hospital admission per year, and mean haemoglobin F [32].

A significantly higher proportion (39.6%) of subjects being underweight were children with Hb-SS, compared to (12.2%) in children with Hb-AA. This observation is comparable with previous studies in African countries [35, 36]. In Hb-SS group, the prevalence of wasting (WH-Z score) tended to be higher than Hb-AA groups. However, there was no statistically significant difference between the two groups. This observation is also reported by previous studies in African and worldwide countries [35–38]. In USA, Malinauskas et al. found that WHZ did not differ from national reference data [25]. However, the sample size of the US study was limited to children under 6 years of age. This pattern is understandable because early event has by itself less impact on a chronic disease, and growth processes into phases which are influenced by different hormones [19].

The present study had some limitations due to its hospital-based cross-sectional design and a retrospective chart review. One additional limitation was biological measurements to perform during the study. Also, as Kinshasa accounts only for 15% of the DRC population, this study may not necessarily reflect the overview of the whole country. But this should be the general trend since our patients came from all different socioeconomic areas. Despite these limitations, these data provide insights into the relationship between poor growth and SCA in our midst.

## 7. Conclusion

Nutritional status encountered in Congolese sickle cell children has been described for the first time in this study. A high prevalence of poor growth in SCA children was found and was associated with more severe disease estimated by several clinical characteristics in our study. Stunting is more common compared to underweight in SCA children. These results reflect the chronicity of SCA. Additionally, Congolese SCA children are more underweight, wasted, and stunted than the Hb-AA children. The high prevalence of sickle cell anaemia in Sub-Saharan Africa underlines the need for screening of all SCA children to identify patients with the risk of developing poor growth and provide early management. Furthermore, our results strongly suggest that more research in our midst would provide valuable insights into the pathogenesis of poor growth.

## Competing Interests

The authors have no conflict of interests to disclose.

## Authors' Contributions

Aimé Lukusa Kazadi, Jean Marie Mbuyi-Muamba, Michel Ntetani Aloni, and Jean Lambert Gini-Ehungu conceived, designed, deployed, and directed the study at the Department of Paediatrics at Kinshasa University Hospital and wrote the manuscript. Aimé Lukusa Kazadi carried out recruitment and follow-up, sample collection, storage, and transport. Aimé Lukusa Kazadi and Michel Ntetani Aloni brought some precious corrections. Aimé Lukusa Kazadi, Jean Marie Mbuyi-Muamba, René Makuala Ngiyulu, and Michel Ntetani Aloni analyzed data. Michel Ntetani Aloni and Aimé Lukusa Kazadi edited the English and made corrections. All authors read and approved the final manuscript.

## Acknowledgments

The authors acknowledge all the physicians and nurses of the three health institutions of Kinshasa, DRC, for their assistance in collecting the data.

## References

[1] D. C. Rees, T. N. Williams, and M. T. Gladwin, "Sickle-cell disease," *The Lancet*, vol. 376, no. 9757, pp. 2018–2031, 2010.

[2] F. B. Piel, S. I. Hay, S. Gupta, D. J. Weatherall, and T. N. Williams, "Global burden of sickle cell anaemia in children under five, 2010–2050: modelling based on demographics, excess mortality, and interventions," *PLoS Medicine*, vol. 10, no. 7, Article ID e1001484, 2013.

[3] C. K. Phebus, M. F. Gloninger, and B. J. Maciak, "Growth patterns by age and sex in children with sickle cell disease," *The Journal of Pediatrics*, vol. 105, no. 1, pp. 28–33, 1984.

[4] O. S. Platt, W. Rosenstock, and M. A. Espeland, "Influence of sickle hemoglobinopathies on growth and development," *The New England Journal of Medicine*, vol. 311, no. 1, pp. 7–12, 1984.

[5] B. S. Zemel, D. A. Kawchak, K. Ohene-Frempong, J. I. Schall, and V. A. Stallings, "Effects of delayed pubertal development, nutritional status, and disease severity on longitudinal patterns of growth failure in children with sickle cell disease," *Pediatric Research*, vol. 61, no. 5, part 1, pp. 607–613, 2007.

[6] A. Singhal, J. Morris, P. Thomas, G. Dover, D. Higgs, and G. Serjeant, "Factors affecting prepubertal growth in homozygous sickle cell disease," *Archives of Disease in Childhood*, vol. 74, no. 6, pp. 502–506, 1996.

[7] L. Iughetti, E. Bigi, and D. Venturelli, "Novel insights in the management of sickle cell disease in childhood," *World Journal of Clinical Pediatrics*, vol. 5, no. 1, pp. 25–34, 2016.

[8] S. Chaturvedi and M. R. Debaun, "Evolution of sickle cell disease from a life-threatening disease of children to a chronic disease of adults: the last 40 years," *American Journal of Hematology*, vol. 91, no. 1, pp. 5–14, 2016.

[9] N. Matthie and C. Jenerette, "Sickle cell disease in adults: developing an appropriate care plan," *Clinical Journal of Oncology Nursing*, vol. 19, no. 5, pp. 562–568, 2015.

[10] T. N. Williams, "Sickle cell disease in Sub-Saharan Africa," *Hematology/Oncology Clinics of North America*, vol. 30, no. 2, pp. 343–358, 2016.

[11] M. N. Aloni and L. Nkee, "Challenge of managing sickle cell disease in a pediatric population living in kinshasa, democratic

republic of congo: a sickle cell center experience," *Hemoglobin*, vol. 38, no. 3, pp. 196–200, 2014.

[12] A. Habara and M. H. Steinberg, "Minireview: genetic basis of heterogeneity and severity in sickle cell disease," *Experimental Biology and Medicine*, vol. 241, no. 7, pp. 689–696, 2016.

[13] P. Bhatnagar, S. Purvis, E. Barron-Casella et al., "Genome-wide association study identifies genetic variants influencing F-cell levels in sickle-cell patients," *Journal of Human Genetics*, vol. 56, no. 4, pp. 316–323, 2011.

[14] W. R. Smith, P. Coyne, V. S. Smith, and B. Mercier, "Temperature changes, temperature extremes, and their relationship to emergency department visits and hospitalizations for sickle cell crisis," *Pain Management Nursing*, vol. 4, no. 3, pp. 106–111, 2003.

[15] A.-W. M. Al-Saqladi, R. Cipolotti, K. Fijnvandraat, and B. J. Brabin, "Growth and nutritional status of children with homozygous sickle cell disease," *Annals of Tropical Paediatrics*, vol. 28, no. 3, pp. 165–189, 2008.

[16] S. Wembonyama, S. Mpaka, and L. Tshilolo, "Medicine and health in the democratic republic of congo: from independence to the third republic," *Médecine Tropicale (Mars)*, vol. 67, no. 5, pp. 447–457, 2007.

[17] S. Tewari, V. Brousse, F. B. Piel, S. Menzel, and D. C. Rees, "Environmental determinants of severity in sickle cell disease," *Haematologica*, vol. 100, no. 9, pp. 1108–1116, 2015.

[18] WHO Multicentre Growth Reference Study Group, *WHO Child Growth Standards: Length/Height-for-Age, Weight-for-Age, Weight-for-Length, Weight-for-Height and Body Mass Index-for-Age: Methods and Development*, World Health Organization, Geneva, Switzerland, 2006.

[19] J. Karlberg, "A biologically-oriented mathematical model (ICP) for human growth," *Acta Paediatrica Scandinavica, Supplement*, vol. 78, no. 350, pp. 70–94, 1989.

[20] J. R. Mabiala-Babela, A. Massamba, J. B. Tsiba, J. G. A. Moulongo, S. Nzingoula, and P. Senga, "Body composition in Negro African children suffering from sickle cell disease. A mixed cross-sectional longitudinal study in Brazzaville, Congo," *Bulletin de la Societe de Pathologie Exotique*, vol. 98, no. 5, pp. 394–399, 2005.

[21] Z. D. Nogueira, N. Boa-Sorte, M. E. D. Q. Leite, M. M. Kiya, T. Amorim, and S. F. D. Fonseca, "Breastfeeding and the anthropometric profile of children with sickle cell anemia receiving follow-up in a newborn screening reference service," *Revista Paulista de Pediatria*, vol. 33, no. 2, pp. 154–159, 2015.

[22] A.-W. M. Al-Saqladi, H. A. Bin-Gadeen, and B. J. Brabin, "Growth in children and adolescents with sickle cell disease in Yemen," *Annals of Tropical Paediatrics*, vol. 30, no. 4, pp. 287–298, 2010.

[23] H. I. Hyacinth, O. A. Adekeye, and C. S. Yilgwan, "Malnutrition in sickle cell anemia: implications for infection, growth, and maturation," *Journal of Social, Behavioral and Health Sciences*, vol. 1, no. 1, pp. 1–7, 2013.

[24] M. J. Mitchell, G. J. O. Carpenter, L. E. Crosby, C. T. Bishop, J. Hines, and J. Noll, "Growth status in children and adolescents with sickle cell disease," *Pediatric hematology and oncology*, vol. 26, no. 4, pp. 202–215, 2009.

[25] B. M. Malinauskas, S. S. Gropper, D. A. Kawchak, B. S. Zemel, K. Ohene-Frempong, and V. A. Stallings, "Impact of acute illness on nutritional status of infants and young children with sickle cell disease," *Journal of the American Dietetic Association*, vol. 100, no. 3, pp. 330–334, 2000.

[26] O. Modebe and S. A. Ifenu, "Growth retardation in homozygous sickle cell disease: role of calorie intake and possible gender-related differences," *American Journal of Hematology*, vol. 44, no. 3, pp. 149–154, 1993.

[27] F. I. D. Konotey-Ahulu, *The Sickle Cell Disease Patient*, Tetteh-A'Domeno, Watford, UK, 1996.

[28] A. Chawla, P. G. Sprinz, J. Welch et al., "Weight status of children with sickle cell disease," *Pediatrics*, vol. 131, no. 4, pp. e1168–e1173, 2013.

[29] I. Lubega, C. M. Ndugwa, E. A. Mworozi, and J. K. Tumwine, "Alpha thalassemia among sickle cell anaemia patients in Kampala, Uganda," *African Health Sciences*, vol. 15, no. 2, pp. 682–689, 2015.

[30] R. Mouélé, O. Pambou, J. Feingold, and F. Galactéros, "$\alpha$-thalassemia in Bantu population from Congo-Brazzaville: its interaction with sickle cell anemia," *Human Heredity*, vol. 50, no. 2, pp. 118–125, 2000.

[31] R. A. Henderson, J. M. Saavedra, and G. J. Dover, "Prevalence of impaired growth in children with homozygous sickle cell anemia," *The American Journal of the Medical Sciences*, vol. 307, no. 6, pp. 405–407, 1994.

[32] V. Mandese, F. Marotti, L. Bedetti, E. Bigi, G. Palazzi, and L. Iughetti, "Effects of nutritional intake on disease severity in children with sickle cell disease," *Nutrition Journal*, vol. 15, no. 1, p. 46, 2016.

[33] M. Reid, "Nutrition and sickle cell disease," *Comptes Rendus Biologies*, vol. 336, no. 3, pp. 159–163, 2013.

[34] L. Tshilolo, V. Summa, C. Gregorj et al., "Foetal haemoglobin, erythrocytes containing foetal haemoglobin, and hematological features in Congolese patients with sickle cell anaemia," *Anemia*, vol. 2012, Article ID 105349, 7 pages, 2012.

[35] C. Osei-Yeboah, O. Rodrigues, and C. Enweronu-Laryea, "Nutritional status of children with sickle cell disease at Korle Bu Teaching Hospital, Accra, Ghana," *West African Journal of Medicine*, vol. 30, no. 4, pp. 262–267, 2011.

[36] E. M. Barden, D. A. Kawchak, K. Ohene-Frempong, V. A. Stallings, and B. S. Zemel, "Body composition in children with sickle cell disease," *American Journal of Clinical Nutrition*, vol. 76, no. 1, pp. 218–225, 2002.

[37] S. O. Akodu, I. N. Diaku-Akinwumi, O. A. Kehinde, and O. F. Njokanma, "Evaluation of arm span and sitting height as proxy for height in children with sickle cell anemia in Lagos, Nigeria," *Journal of the American College of Nutrition*, vol. 33, no. 6, pp. 437–441, 2014.

[38] B. A. Animasahun, E. O. Temiye, O. O. Ogunkunle, A. N. Izuora, and O. F. Njokanma, "The influence of socioeconomic status on the hemoglobin level and anthropometry of sickle cell anemia patients in steady state at the Lago; University Teaching Hospital," *Nigerian Journal of Clinical Practice*, vol. 14, no. 4, pp. 422–427, 2011.

# Permissions

# List of Contributors

**C. Kinsiama and J. A. Bazeboso**
Unité de Dépistage de la Drépanocytose, Centre Hospitalier Monkole, BP 817, Kinshasa XI, Democratic Republic of Congo

**L. Tshilolo**
Centre de Formation et d'Appui Sanitaire (CEFA), 10, Avenue Kemi, Mont Ngafula, Kinshasa, Democratic Republic of Congo
Unité de Dépistage de la Drépanocytose, Centre Hospitalier Monkole, BP 817, Kinshasa XI, Democratic Republic of Congo

**V. Summa, C. Gregorj and G. Avvisati**
Servizio di Ematologia, Università Campus Bio-Medico di Roma, 21, Via Alvaro del Portillo, 00128 Roma, Italy

**D. Labie**
INSERM, Institut Cochin, 4, rue du Faubourg Saint-Jacques, 75014 Paris, France

**Sunday J. Ameh and Florence D. Tarfa**
Department of Medicinal Chemistry and Quality Control, National Institute for Pharmaceutical Research and Development (NIPRD), PMB 21, Garki, Idu Industrial Area, Abuja, Nigeria

**Benjamin U. Ebeshi**
Department of Pharmaceutics & Medicinal Chemistry, Niger Delta University, Wilberforce Island, Amassoma, Nigeria

**S. O. Akodu, I. N. Diaku-Akinwumi, O. A. Kehinde and O. F. Njokanma**
Department of Paediatrics, Lagos State University Teaching Hospital, Ikeja 100001, Nigeria

**Erwin Weiss and John Stanley Gibson**
Department of Veterinary Medicine, University of Cambridge, Madingley Road, Cambridge CB3 0ES, UK

**David Charles Rees**
Department of Molecular Haematology, King's College School of Medicine, London SE5 9RS, UK

**Lori E. Crosby and Karen A. Kalinyak**
College of Medicine, University of Cincinnati, Cincinnati, OH 45221, USA
Behavioral Medicine and Clinical Psychology, Cincinnati Children's Hospital Medical Center, Cincinnati, OH 45229, USA

**Ilana Barach**
Department of Psychology, University of Cincinnati, Cincinnati, OH 45221, USA

**Meghan E. McGrady**
Behavioral Medicine and Clinical Psychology, Cincinnati Children's Hospital Medical Center, Cincinnati, OH 45229, USA
Department of Psychology, University of Cincinnati, Cincinnati, OH 45221, USA

**Adryan R. Eastin**
Behavioral Medicine and Clinical Psychology, Cincinnati Children's Hospital Medical Center, Cincinnati, OH 45229, USA

**Monica J. Mitchell**
Department of Psychology, University of Cincinnati, Cincinnati, OH 45221, USA
College of Medicine, University of Cincinnati, Cincinnati, OH 45221, USA
Behavioral Medicine and Clinical Psychology, Cincinnati Children's Hospital Medical Center, Cincinnati, OH 45229, USA

**Zeina A. Salman**
Center for Hereditary Blood Diseases, Basra Maternity and Children Hospital, Basra, Iraq

**Meaad K. Hassan**
Department of Pediatrics, College of Medicine, University of Basra, Basra, Iraq
Center for Hereditary Blood Diseases, Basra Maternity and Children Hospital, Basra, Iraq

**Edamisan Olusoji Temiye and James Kweku Renner**
Department of Paediatrics, College of Medicine, University of Lagos (CMUL), P.M.B 12003, Lagos, Nigeria

**Edem Samuel Duke**
Critical Rescue International (CRI), Plot 144, Oba Akran Road, Ikeja, Lagos, Nigeria

**Mbang Adeyemi Owolabi**
Department of Pharmaceutical Chemistry, Faculty of Pharmacy, College of Medicine, Idi-Araba, University of Lagos, P.M.B. 12003, Lagos, Nigeria

**Elisabeth H. Javazon**
Department of Biology, Morehouse College, 830 Westview Drive Southwest, Atlanta, GA 30314-3773, USA

**Mohamed Radhi**
Department of Pediatrics, UI Hospitals and Clinics, University of Iowa, 2633 Carver Pavilion, 200 Hawkins Drive, Iowa City, IA 52242, USA

**David R. Archer, Bagirath Gangadharan and Jennifer Perry**
Aflac Cancer and Blood Disorders Center, Emory University and Children's Healthcare of Atlanta, 2015 Uppergate Drive, Atlanta, GA 30322, USA

**Mário Angelo Claudino**
Laboratory of Multidisciplinary Research, São Francisco University (USF), 12916-900 Bragança Paulista, SP, Brazil

**Kleber Yotsumoto Fertrin**
Hematology and Hemotherapy Center, University of Campinas (UNICAMP), 13083-970 Campinas, SP, Brazil

**GenevieveM. Crane and Nelson E. Bennett Jr.**
Institute of Urology, Lahey Clinic, 41 Mall Road, Burlington, MA 01805, USA

**Solomon F. Ofori-Acquah and Ifeyinwa Osunkwo**
Department of Pediatrics, Division of Hematology/ Oncology, Emory University School of Medicine, 2015 Uppergate Dr. NE, Atlanta, GA 30322, USA

**Beatrice E. Gee and Iris D. Buchanan**
Department of Pediatrics, Morehouse School of Medicine, 720 Westview Drive, SW Atlanta, GA 30310-1495, USA

**Gary H. Gibbons and Jerry Manlove-Simmons**
Cardiovascular Research Institute, Morehouse School of Medicine, 720 Westview Drive, SW Atlanta, GA 30310-1495, USA

**Feyisayo Lawal**
Morehouse College, 830 Westview Dr SW, Atlanta, GA 30314, USA

**Alexander Quarshie**
Biostatistics Core, Morehouse School of Medicine, 720 Westview Drive, SW Atlanta, GA 30310-1495, USA

**Arshed A. Quyyumi**
Department of Medicine, Division of Cardiology, 1462 Clifton Road N.E. Suite 507, Atlanta, GA 30322, USA

**Kathryn Blake and John Lima**
Biomedical Research Department, Center for Clinical Pharmacogenomics and Translational Research, Nemours Children's Clinic, 807 Children's Way, Jacksonville, FL 32207, USA

**Samuel Olufemi Akodu, Olisamedua Fidelis Njokanma and Omolara Adeolu Kehinde**
Department of Paediatrics, Lagos State University Teaching Hospital, Ikeja, Lagos 100001, Nigeria

**Philip M. Keegan, Sindhuja Surapaneni and Manu O. Platt**
Wallace H. Coulter Department of Biomedical Engineering, Georgia Institute of Technology and Emory University, Atlanta, GA 30332, USA

**Samit Ghosh and Fang Tan**
Aflac Cancer and Blood Disorders Center, Division of Hematology/Oncology/BMT, Department of Pediatrics, Emory University School of Medicine, Atlanta, GA 30322, USA

**Solomon F. Ofori-Acquah**
Department of Pediatrics, Children's Healthcare of Atlanta, Atlanta, GA 30322, USA
Aflac Cancer and Blood Disorders Center, Division of Hematology/Oncology/BMT, Department of Pediatrics, Emory University School of Medicine, Atlanta, GA 30322, USA

**A. Hannemann and E. Weiss and J. S. Gibson**
Department of Veterinary Medicine, University of Cambridge, Madingley Road, Cambridge CB3 0ES, UK

**D. C. Rees**
Department of Molecular Haematology, King's College Hospital, London SE5 9RS, UK

**S. Dalibalta and J. C. Ellory**
Department of Physiology, Anatomy & Genetics, University of Oxford, Parks Road, Oxford OX1 3PT, UK

**M. A. Emokpae**
Department of Chemical Pathology, Aminu Kano Teaching Hospital, Kano 700001, Nigeria
Department of Medical Laboratory Science, School of Basic Medical Sciences, College of Medical Sciences, University of Benin, Benin City 300001, Nigeria

**P. O. Uadia**
Department of Biochemistry, University of Benin, Benin City 300001, Nigeria

**L. O. Ngolet, Innocent Kocko, Alexis Elira Dokekias and Georges Marius Moyen**
ClinicalHematologyUnit, Brazzaville Teaching Hospital, Auxence Ickonga Avenue, Brazzaville, Congo

**M. Moyen Engoba**
Pediatric Intensive Care Unit, Brazzaville Teaching Hospital, Brazzaville, Congo

**Jean-Vivien Mombouli**
National Laboratory of Public Health, Brazzaville Teaching Hospital, Brazzaville, Congo

**A. Ganguly, W. Boswell and H. Aniq**
Department of Radiology, Royal Liverpool University Hospital, Prescot Street, Liverpool L7 8XP, UK

**Rebecca J. Tanner and Christopher A. Harle**
Department of Health Services Research, Management and Policy, University of Florida, Gainesville, FL 32610, USA

**Arch G. Mainous III**
Department of Community Health and Family Medicine, University of Florida, Gainesville, FL 32610-0237, USA

**Richard Baker**
Department of Health Sciences, University of Leicester, 22-28 Princess RoadWest, Leicester LE1 6TP, UK

**Navkiran K. Shokar**
Department of Family and Community Medicine, Texas Tech University Health Science Center at El Paso, 9849 Kenworthy Street, El Paso, TX 79924, USA

**Mary M. Hulihan**
Division of Blood Disorders, CDC, National Center on Birth Defects and Developmental Disabilities, Mail-Stop E87, 1600 Clifton Road, Atlanta, GA 30333, USA

**Zhou Zhou, Molly Behymer and Prasenjit Guchhait**
Thrombosis Research Division, Cardiovascular Research Section, Department of Medicine, Baylor College of Medicine, One Baylor Plaza, N1319, Houston, TX 77030, USA

**Ademola Samson Adewoyin**
Department of Haematology and Blood Transfusion, University of Benin Teaching Hospital, PMB 1111, Benin City, Edo State, Nigeria

**Aimé Lukusa Kazadi, René Makuala Ngiyulu, Jean Lambert Gini-Ehungu and Michel Ntetani Aloni**
Division of Paediatric Haemato-Oncology and Nephrology, Department of Paediatrics, University Hospital of Kinshasa, Faculty of Medicine, University of Kinshasa, Kinshasa, Democratic Republic of the Congo

**Jean Marie Mbuyi-Muamba**
Department of Internal Medicine, Faculty of Medicine, University of Kinshasa, Kinshasa, Democratic Republic of the Congo

# Index